W9-CXC-228

Soft Neurological Signs

Soft Neurological Signs

Edited by

David E. Tupper, Ph.D.

Clinical Care Coordinator
Department of Neurobehavioral Rehabilitation Service
The Head Injury Center at Highgate
Troy, New York

G&S

Grune & Stratton, Inc.
Harcourt Brace Jovanovich, Publishers
Orlando New York San Diego London
San Francisco Tokyo Sydney Toronto

Library of Congress Cataloging-in-Publication Data

Soft neurological signs.

Includes bibliographies and index.
1. Pediatric neurology—Diagnosis. 2. Neurologic examination. 3. Neurologic manifestations of general diseases. I. Tupper, David E. [DNLM: 1. Child Behavior Disorders. 2. Neurologic Examination. 3. Neurologic Manifestations. WL 340 S679]
RJ488.S64 1987 616.89'075 86-27067
ISBN 0-8089-1841-9

Grune & Stratton, Inc.
Orlando, Florida 32887

Distributed in the United Kingdom by
Grune & Stratton, Ltd.
24/28 Oval Road, London NW 1

Library of Congress Catalog Number 86-27067
International Standard Book Number 0-8089-1841-9
Printed in the United States of America
86 87 88 89 10 9 8 7 6 5 4 3 2 1

To the memory of my mother,
Carol Ann Tupper (1933-1983)

D.E.T.

Contents

Preface

This book is an attempt to bring together some of the varied research, theory, and practice concerning neurobehavioral and EEG signs that have been considered as "soft" or "minor" indicators of neurological dysfunction. These signs have been variously interpreted as minimal, irregular, unreliable, or nonpersisting. One of the goals of the book is to help decipher the meaning of these signs for both clinical practice and future research and theory.

Each of the chapters covers a circumscribed aspect of the topic under the headings of assessment, past and present research, and the theoretical and practical importance of soft neurological signs. While the subject matter of the book typically invokes emphasis on research in developmental disabilities, authors are more practical in their discussion of soft signs and address directly specific etiologic, diagnostic, and prognostic issues relevant to the individual case. Descriptions and instructions for current soft sign examinations are also provided in the Appendices to make this a clinically useful volume. It is hoped that by pulling together the varied expertise on soft signs this book will provide a more stable base for clearer future understanding of these currently ambiguous signs.

The book is designed to be of interest to clinicians and researchers in the neurological sciences, particularly pediatric neurologists and child-clinical neuropsychologists, as well as to workers in the areas of developmental and learning disabilities such as school or educational psychologists. It should be useful both to those experienced in the assessment of soft signs as well as to those less experienced wishing to investigate or assess children manifesting difficulties suggestive of neurological dysfunction.

There are many people who need to be acknowledged here. Most of all, the contributors to this book who have spent a great deal of time preparing and working on their chapters. It is through their efforts that the book is even possible. I especially thank Drs. Hertzig and Peters for providing their soft sign evaluations for inclusion. Finally, I express my deep gratitude to my wife, Sharon, for helping me type my sections of the manuscirpt, and acknowledge my family, including Sharon, Jonathan, and my father, John Tupper, for providing support and encouragement throughout the book's preparation.

Contributors

Ruthmary Deuel, M.D., *Associate Professor, Departments of Pediatrics and Neurology, Washington University School of Medicine, St. Louis, Missouri*

Perry C. Goldstein, Ph.D., *Staff Psychologist, Department of Rehabilitation Psychology, Division of Neuropsychology Service, University of Miami/Jackson Memorial Medical Center, Miami, Florida*

Margaret E. Hertzig, M.D., *Associate Professor, Department of Psychiatry, Cornell University Medical Center, New York, New York*

John R. Hughes, M.D., Ph.D., *Professor of Neurology, Director of EEG, Director of Consultation Clinic for Epilepsy, Department of Neurology, Division of EEG, Epilepsy, University of Illinois College of Medicine at Chicago, Chicago, Illinois*

Paul L. Nichols, Ph.D., *Health Scientist Administrator, National Institute of Neurological and Communicative Disorders and Stroke, Bethesda, Maryland*

John E. Peters, *Director, Child Study Center, Division of Child Psychiatry, University of Arkansas for Medical Sciences, Little Rock, Arkansas*

Heinz F.R. Prechtl, M.B., D.Phil., *Professor and Chairman, Department of Developmental Neurology, University Hospital, Groningen, The Netherlands*

Jan C. Reeves, M.B., Ch.B., M.R.A.N.Z.C.P., *Department of Psychiatry and Behavioral Science, School of Medicine, University of Auckland, Auckland, New Zealand*

Ellen D. Rie, Ph.D., *Coordinator, The Parent-Child Program, Inc., Cleveland, Ohio*

Dora Jean Robinson, Ed.D., *Assistant Professor of Education, Department of Education/Special Education, Fontbonne College, St. Louis, Missouri*

Theodore Shapiro, M.D., *Professor and Director of Child and Adolescent Psychiatry, Department of Psychiatry, Cornell University Medical Center, New York, New York*

Eric Taylor, F.R.C.P., M.R.C.Psych., *Reader in Developmental Neuropsychiatry, Department of Child and Adolescent Psychiatry, Institute of Psychiatry, London University, London, England*

H. Gerry Taylor, Ph.D., *Associate Professor, Department of Psychology, McGill University; Director, Learning Center, McGill-Montreal Children's Hospital Learning Centre, Montreal, Quebec, Canada*

Bert C.L. Touwen, M.D., *Professor, Department of Developmental Neurology, University Hospital, Groningen, The Netherlands*

Abraham Towbin, M.D., *Medical Director, Mental Retardation Research Institute, Danvers, Massachusetts*

David E. Tupper, Ph.D., *Clinical Care Coordinator, Neurobehavioral Rehabilitation Service, The Head Injury Center at Highgate, Troy, New York*

John Werry, M.D., *Professor of Psychiatry, Department of Psychiatry and Behavioral Science, School of Medicine, University of Auckland, Auckland, New Zealand*

William Yule, Ph.D., *Reader in Applied Child Psychology, Department of Psychology, Institute of Psychiatry, London University, London, England*

David E. Tupper

1

The Issues With "Soft Signs"

Most everyone as they review this book will already recognize the myriad of issues that surround the concept and practice of soft neurological signs (and the related issues of understanding subtle neurological dysfunction). This is the case because often in the history of science and medicine there have been phenomena that have, at least on the surface, seemed rather intuitive. Sometimes, however, it has been found that these phenomena are intriguing not because they are clearly valid and useful scientifically or clinically, but because they defy our easy explanation and intuition and tell us something further about our own thinking and our approach to the problem we find so interesting. Such is the case with "soft signs."

It is probably too early to predict what the eventual outcome of our study of soft neurological signs will be, so the present volume is designed to provide for us only a current view of these intriguing signs and the phenomena to which they are supposedly related. This introductory chapter will briefly summarize, in the context of this volume, some of the major issues evident in our past search for the meaning of the so-called soft neurological signs. Generally, these issues (and the themes apparent in this book) concern the needs for clearer terminology, for better classificatory systems of signs, for better assessment devices with adequate psychometric properties for research and clinical practice, and for better understanding through appropriate research of the neurological and behavioral significance of these signs. These issues will be presented in turn.

SOFT NEUROLOGICAL SIGNS
ISBN 0-8089-1841-9

TERMINOLOGY ISSUES

The traditional definition of the neurological *sign* is that it is "any objective evidence or manifestation of an illness or disordered function of the body. Signs are more or less definitive and obvious ... in contrast to symptoms which are subjective" (*Taber's Cyclopedic Medical Dictionary*, 1973). Thus, with regard to neurobehavioral dysfunction, neurological signs identify in an objective manner an underlying disturbance that affects the individual's functioning. Though quantification of the neurological sign is useful, as long as the manifestation can be viewed objectively and clearly related to the underlying dysfunction, it represents a sign and not a symptom of neurological deficit. This logic is the basis for most items used in a traditional neurologic (Bickerstaff, 1973; DeJong, 1979), pediatric (Rutter, Graham, & Yule, 1970), or neuropsychologic (Boll, 1978) examination.

A sign thus defined can be considered a "hard" or *pathognomonic* sign of neurobehavioral disturbance and is usually invariably associated with central nervous system deficit. Pathognomonic signs include such signs as a markedly asymmetric motor or sensory pattern on half of the body (e.g., hemiplegia), dysarthria, abnormal reflexes, changes in pupillary size, and some visual field deficits. Evidence for these hard or pathognomonic signs has accumulated over the years and has been extensively documented to relate directly to underlying neurological dysfunction (see for instance DeJong, 1979). It is unclear exactly where the term "hard" sign began, but it probably had to do with the "hard evidence" of neurological dysfunction evidenced in these signs.

Measurement issues aside for now, some clinicians and investigators have found that during the course of a traditional examination, especially when assessing mildly disordered children, pathognomonic signs are not seen with the frequency or severity seen in cases where more obvious neurological disturbance is present. Sometimes the sign is irreproducible more than once, is apparently "minor" in relation to the traditional patho gnomonic sign, is nonpersisting over time, or gradually improves with development. Signs in these cases have been seen as different than the clearly pathognomonic signs in that they are not necessarily invariably associated with underlying disturbance (hence the numerous studies rehashing the same mixed findings), or they relate to different types of deficits (e.g., behavioral difficulties like an attention deficit disorder).

A variety of terms have been used for these signs including soft signs, soft neurological signs, minor neurological signs, equivocal signs, or nonfocal neurologic signs. Each of these terms was generated to emphasize one aspect of the sign. For example, the term "equivocal" sign emphasizes the fact that the meaning of the sign is not clear, whereas the term nonfocal neurologic sign emphasizes that the sign does not have the localizing power that the pathognomonic signs have. During ancillary procedures, most commonly electroencephalography, similar equivocal or nonspecific patterns have also been seen (Sharbrough, 1982) and have been recognized as perhaps another type of soft sign (see Chapter 6).

The existence of soft signs (as the more generic term used here) was known at the end of the last century and the begining of the present century (Kennard, 1960) but very little empirical work was done on these signs. At that early time, the signs were often termed equivocal signs and it is apparent that this term says as much about the state of the clinician's understanding at the time as it does about the signs themselves. Bender in 1947 was the first to actually use the term soft neurological signs during a neurologic investigation of 100 schizophrenic children. It was Bender's use of the term soft signs with its implications of minor cerebral damage and the growing climate of interest concerning minor behavioral and neurological disturbances in children (for instance, the introduction of the Strauss syndrome and the concept of "organicity") that catapulted soft neurological signs into a position of prominence (not necessarily deserved) in the diagnosis and classification of neurobehavioral disturbances ("minimal brain dysfunction").

Terminology has since been problematic with soft signs. What does "soft" mean? According to *Webster's Seventh New Collegiate Dictionary* (1971), "soft" can mean "unduly susceptible to influence" or "lacking in firmness, strength, or hardness." (One then needs to define soft in relation to hard?) Does the term soft describe, as mentioned above, the clinician's thinking (Ingram, 1973, said that reference to soft signs was "diagnostic of soft thinking"), their unreliability during an examination, or the presence of minor degrees of abnormality, to name just a few possibilities?

Of course, terminology can be expected to be problematic and variable with an issue like soft signs when the phenomena themselves are not clearly understood. With regard to terminology, there appear to be four terms commonly used in the literature to label these nonhard signs (see Table 1-1). Clearly, the most commonly used term is *soft signs*, or its equivalent, *soft neurological signs*. It has not only been used more frequently overall in the literature but has gained dramatically in popularity

Table 1-1
Number of Times Terms Related to "Soft Signs" Have Been Used in the Literature*

	Years			
Term†	**1945–1960**	**1961–1970**	**1971–1980**	**1981–1985**
Soft Signs or Soft Neurological Signs	3	8	38	25
Equivocal Signs	2	0	1	0
Nonfocal Neurologic Signs	0	0	1	6
Minor Neurological Signs	0	5	2	2

*Based upon a literature search conducted by the author.
†Terms were selected if used in the title or abstract of an article, chapter, or book. Passing references or citations were not included.

over the past 15 years. Almost all of this book's contributors used this term in reference to the signs they describe in their chapters, though there is, refreshingly, some variability in the terms and a noticeable attempt to be more specific. The term *equivocal signs*, while popular at the turn of the century, is clearly not popular now according to the table. One can only surmise why clinicians and researchers would be more comfortable with the term soft rather than equivocal (perhaps one would rather not hedge on findings although one would accept them if less hardness could be attributed to the signs themselves). The term *nonfocal neurologic signs* was first used in a study by Shapiro, Burkes, Petti, and Ranz (1978) to emphasize the nonspecificity or nonlocalizing power of these signs, in contrast to pathognomonic signs that often provide localizing data. The term nonfocal neurologic signs has much to recommend it in that it does seem to capture more specifically an attribute of at least a subclass of soft signs. The use of this term has been on the rise in the past few years primarily due to the work done at the New York Hospital-Cornell Medical Center by Margaret Hertzig, Theodore Shapiro, and their colleagues (see Chapter 4). The term signifies at least one attempt to assess the neurological significance of these signs. Finally, *minor neurological signs* is a term that does not seem to have caught on. The adjective minor implies at least two things; that the sign itself is somehow minor, and that the neurological underpinnings show minor deviation. Many people would have difficulty accepting either of these propositions without further research.

The terminology surrounding the study of soft signs therefore continues to be mixed. It appears that most investigators have chosen to stick to the original term proposed almost 40 years ago by Bender but that more recently attempts have been made to define more clearly the basis for their terminology regarding these signs. As the issues concerning classification, measurement, and the significance of these signs become resolved, one can expect the terminology to also become more clearly defined. Until then, researchers will need to describe more fully the phenomena they are studying so that even if the overall label doesn't fit, others can evaluate the signs they are using. The need for better (clearer) terminology still exists in the form it did when Bender first used the term soft signs 40 years ago.

CLASSIFICATION AND MEASUREMENT CONCERNS

It is predominantly clear that a good understanding of the appropriate classification and accurate measurement of soft signs is not the current state of the art. Chapters 2 through 6 of this book discuss classification issues related to soft sign measurement, describe commonly used soft and nonfocal signs, discuss the psychometric properties required of a soft sign item or examination, and more generally provide the current perspective on what is needed for future classification of soft signs. Before briefly summarizing these themes, it is useful to ask, "but what are the signs traditionally classified as soft?"

Many, many neurological items have been classified as soft neurological signs by a variety of authors. Clements in 1966 in fact presented a list of 99 different signs and symptoms of minimal brain dysfunction in children that could be called soft neurological signs. In a recent book by Small (1982), almost as many signs and symptoms were presented. More manageably, the Appendices to this volume show that most soft sign examinations include much fewer items and in fact there is a great deal of overlap and similarity among examinations. Table 1-2 provides a general listing of the variety of items that have been called "soft signs," listed according to a classification described previously by the present author (Tupper, 1986). As can be seen, the items included represent not only subtle manifestations of traditional pathognomonic signs (e.g., tone changes, minor reflexes) but also signs that appear to represent developmental processes gone awry and that lag behind (e.g., immature motor patterns and continued associated movements). The classification presented is a compilation of similar groupings proposed by other authors (Denckla,

Table 1-2
The Variety of Signs Called "Soft"*

Developmental Soft Signs

Associated (overflow or mirror) movements
Difficulty building with blocks
Immature grasp of pencil
Inability to catch a ball
Lateness in developmental milestones (e.g., standing, walking, talking)
Lateness in suppressing primitive signs (e.g., Babinski, tonic neck, reflexes)
Motor awkwardness; clumsiness for age
Motor impersistence
Poor gait, posture, stance
Slowness of gait, hand movements, opposing the fingers to the thumb, tapping
Speech articulation problems
Tactile extinction on double simultaneous stimulation

Soft Signs of Abnormality

Astereognosis
Asymmetries of associated movements
Auditory–visual integration difficulties
Choreiform movements
Diffuse EEG abnormalities
Dysarthria
Dysdiadochokinesis
Dysgraphesthesia
Hypokinesis
Labile affect
Motor impersistence
Nystagmus
Oromotor apraxia, drooling, active jaw jerk
Pathological reflex
Postural and gait abnormalities
Posturing of hands while walking
Reflex asymmetries
Reflex increase or decrease from normal
Significant incoordination
Tone increase or decrease from normal
Tremors
Word-finding difficulty

*From Tupper DE. Neuropsychological screening and soft signs. In Obrzut JE, & Hynd GW (Eds.). Child Neuropsychology, Vol. 2: Clinical Practice. Orlando, FL: Academic Press, pp 150–151. With permission.

1978; Gardner, 1979; Rapin, 1982; Rutter, Graham, & Yule, 1970) and includes most of the signs currently defined as soft signs.

It should be noted that traditionally most of the soft signs have been of the sensory-motor type. Slight motor abnormalities have been recognized by most authors as the more typical soft signs. Motor signs are discussed extensively in Chapter 5 and also in Chapter 11. Other slight abnormalities (e.g., nonspecific EEG findings) also seem to qualify as soft signs in the sense that they are not clearly pathognomonic of neurological dysfunction. Some authors, however, prefer to exclude ancillary findings like the EEG and keep the soft sign examination more purely neurobehavioral. Chapter 4 provides a thoughtful discussion of both exclusion and inclusion criteria in the assessment and classification of soft signs (see also Meehl, 1973, for a similar discussion of this need in defining soft signs in schizophrenia).

Rutter, Graham, and Yule (1970) during their Isle of Wight study (see also Chapter 2) provided the first subgrouping of soft signs in an attempt to define more clearly the nature of these signs. The authors proposed that we are not dealing with equally valid signs of disturbance but rather with three different groups of soft signs: (1) signs that indicate developmental delay and disappear with age, (2) signs that are difficult to elicit and have poor reliability during the neurological examination thus suggesting minor degrees of disturbance, and (3) signs that result not from pathological neurological conditions but from causes other than neurological damage. Many writers have since followed Rutter et al's (1970) lead and have continued to subgroup soft signs, though at present there is little empirical justification for the subgrouping. Most of the subgrouping has been done on the basis of clinical experience and theory rather than research. Both Denckla (1978) and Gardner (1979) have for example classified soft signs in much the same way as the present author, who borrowed heavily from Rutter et al's suggestions.

There are, of course, several advantages to the subgrouping of soft signs. As recognized by Rutter and colleagues, the first major advantage is for the exclusion of signs that are unreliable or due to nonneurological factors. Unfortunately, for most of the history of soft signs except for individual investigators, there has been little attempt to define or exclude unreliable items or exams — indeed, the issue is only now being evaluated (Shafer, Shaffer, O'Connor, & Stokman, 1983). A second advantage is that it may be useful to investigate the classes or subgroupings of soft signs separately; for example, signs that indicate motor disturbance might be examined in motorically-disordered or clumsy populations, signs that indicate developmental delay might be correlated with developmentally based disorders, and so on.

As Taylor describes in Chapter 14, such subgroupings — particularly of the motor items — may have quite specific implications for research in the subtyping of motor or learning disabilities. A further advantage is that if soft signs are subgrouped their specificity in relation to specific disorders may more easily be manifested.

Aside from classification and subgrouping issues, there are a multitude of measurement-related concerns that need to be satisfied with regard to soft signs. Until recently, few soft sign examinations or individual items have been evaluated critically for psychometrically sound reliability. In fact, few soft sign batteries report reliabilities (see the Appendices). Though very variable findings have been presented, a recent review of the reliability of soft signs by Shafer et al (1983) concludes that specific soft sign measures have adequate reliability when planned for in advance but that, more generally, few investigators have assessed this issue a priori. Goldstein and Tupper (Chapter 3) provide a review of some of the specific psychometric requirements that need to be met in the measurement of soft signs. Taylor (Chapter 14) also reviews briefly some of the necessary requirements.

Another issue requiring further research is whether individual soft sign items are more reliable and useful, or whether composite scores are better. Touwen (Chapter 13) touches on this issue in reference to neurological diagnosis where he identifies clusters of items seen in individual cases and describes briefly some of their characteristics. Nevertheless, this suggestion concerning composite scores requires further investigation.

The scaling of soft sign items and their dependence on developmental interpretations are crucial issues and recurrent themes in soft sign measurement (see Chapter 2). Unlike hard signs, which are usually either present or absent in a given individual, soft signs are more variable and can sometimes be measured along a continuum — for example, the number of thumb to index finger taps in 10 seconds. This creates the need for an identifiable scaling system with appropriate normative scores (Russell, 1986). Yule and Taylor discuss this need for developmentally-appropriate measures and norms, and Deuel and Robinson provide a nice review with concrete data of developmental-based norms for motor signs. Goldstein and Tupper consider the related issues regarding quantitative versus qualitative measurement approaches in their chapter. More attention paid to these issues will replace the need for examinations to caution that "only well trained individuals with experience can fully interpret the findings"; it would then be the case that soft signs can be objectively measured and documented as easily as other signs.

Finally, the incidence and prevalence of soft sign abnormalities would need to be determined to assist appropriate application of the soft sign batteries in clinical settings. Such data would provide needed information concerning the base rates of soft signs in various populations. For example, it would be expected that few soft signs would be seen in a population of mentally retarded children where hard signs would predominate, while a clinic-referred sample of learning disabled and emotionally disturbed children may show a high base rate of soft signs but very few hard signs.

The needs are great for better definition of the manifestations of soft signs in various populations, for more reliable and valid soft sign items and examinations, and for more detailed classification systems for grouping soft signs and relating the groupings to an appropriate set of disorders. Measurement concerns are the first order of business for those interested in understanding the relationship of various soft signs to other neurological or behavioral concepts.

NEUROLOGICAL SIGNIFICANCE

A sign is, of course, the basis for inference-making about a phenomenon not otherwise accessible directly. In the case of soft neurological signs, the phenomenon whose history is inextricably linked with the history of soft signs is the concept of minimal brain damage, minimal cerebral damage, or minimal brain dysfunction (MBD). The presence of soft signs has been used as one of the main bases to infer MBD in a given child in spite of those who state that using the term MBD is not to make a diagnosis, but to escape from making one (Ingram, 1973).

It appears that there are at least three main issues concerning the soft signs-MBD relationship. The first issue is, what would classify as MBD? That is, what is the usefulness of the MBD diagnosis itself? Many would argue that MBD is a wastebasket category (Ross, 1973). Certainly there is a large group of children out there who show minor deviations from the norm on a variety of neuropsychological or neurological measures, and who show no other signs of definite brain damage. The variety of children who have been suspected of having MBD have additionally been given various other labels. These labels include hyperactivity, dyslexia, specific developmental disorder, or more recently, attention deficit disorder. From the start, however, this heterogeneity was not acknowledged. In fact, there were very explicit attempts to group all of these children together into a large homogeneous category (e.g., Wender, 1971). Because much of the early history of the MBD concept grew out of Gestalt approaches (Strauss and colleagues) and simplistic beliefs concerning brain damage being manifested behaviorally as "organicity," which led to assessment with single tests, this global categorizing is understandable as an historical trend. More recently, however, the heterogeneity has been increasingly recognized and there has been a shift away from using MBD as a primary diagnosis (Weiss, 1980). In fact, a major problem with positing MBD in children is that the diagnosis of brain damage (intended or implicated) tends to turn into an end in itself and does not lead to further clinical action (Boll, 1983).

Clearly, as recognized back in 1962 by the Oxford International Child Study Group (MacKeith & Bax, 1963), the use of the categorical label MBD has more traditionally been made on the basis of behavioral, not neurological criteria so that, since there is heterogeneity in the behavioral symptoms so there is expected heterogeneity in the neurological correlates. Individual variation predominates. Current research therefore attempts to subclassify children with minor deviations in performance into distinct groups and the usefulness of the overall classification of MBD (as a behavioral concept) will most likely continue to decrease further. Taylor describes further (Chapter 14) the implications of the MBD concept in the history of soft signs research.

The second issue regarding MBD and soft signs relates to the suggestion that MBD be seen as a purely neurological concept (for instance, Spreen, Tupper, Risser, Tuokko, & Edgell, 1984) where minimal brain dysfunction represents only one point (or a delimited range) along a continuum of brain damage extending from none to a great deal of damage. This notion has historical precedents also (Taylor, 1983) and a great deal of intuitive appeal, particularly to those fond of speculating about the neurological basis of behavior. Towbin (Chapter 7) reviews some of the possible neuropathologic correlates of minimal brain injury discovered in some of his studies as a basis for treating MBD as a neurological concept. He clearly agrees with the brain damage continuum idea in suggesting that we all show a certain amount of variation and imperfection in our abilities and by implication our brains. In essence, one of the difficulties in this area is in defining neurological normalcy.

If we restrict discussion of MBD children to those shown to have proven evidence of slight damage to the nervous system through appropriate neurodiagnostic procedures, we obviate many of the behavioral classification difficulties but also see that the possible etiologies of MBD neurologically can be varied and could range through prenatal, perinatal, and postnatal factors. Nichols (Chapter 8) attempts to investigate some of the multitude of these factors as he reports findings from the National Collaborative Perinatal Project that bear on this MBD-soft signs issue. He has been able to find some interesting but nonspecific links in this association. Chapter 12 by Hertzig also presents a relatively focused neurological connection concerning low birthweight children and subtle neurological difficulties. Further studies along these lines using some of the newer neurodiagnostic procedures (CT, PETT, NMR imaging) as criteria for minor damage may prove to clarify this issue to an even greater extent.

The third issue relates more directly to the idea of soft signs as pathognomonic indicators of minimal neurological abnormalities. Even if we assume better neurological criteria, what is the nature of the evidence supporting the relationship between soft neurological signs and minor neurological deviation? It is interesting to note that very few textbooks on neurology or the neurological examination even index soft neurological signs (e.g., Bickerstaff, 1973; DeJong, 1979), let alone review this matter. Of course, this relationship is addressed throughout this volume, but it should be pointed out that our present understanding is based totally on *presumptive evidence* (Fletch & Taylor, 1984; Taylor,1983). That is, the research supporting the connection between soft sign measures and other neurological criteria is not substantial enough at present to indicate clear causal relationships, though the evidence is attractive and tempting to many. Hence, the true neurological basis for soft signs is not known and is probably influenced by a multitude of factors. As a predominant theme, many of the contributors to this book stress the need to use multifactorial methodology to elucidate the bases for soft signs since it is expected, given the heterogeneity of the children and the ambiguity in the phenomena studied thus far, that purely univariate research will neglect significant variables recognized only when numerous interactions are considered together.

BEHAVIORAL CORRELATIONS

From the start, the ambiguity in the MBD area as well as the intuitive appeal of soft signs as indicators of neurological dysfunction provided a rationale for correlating soft sign measures to behavioral or psychiatric symptomatology. Indeed, when Bender (1947) first introduced the term soft neurological signs it was during the investigation of a group of severely schizophrenic children. Of course, her approach can not be faulted retrospectively but it is abundantly apparent that the majority of studies investigating soft signs that have appeared since that time have included groups of children with primarily behavioral disorders. This trend may represent an enticing search for neurological deviations in a great variety of developmental disorders, some more thought out than others, but it also may represent a fruitless form of neuropathologizing when definite criteria for both the behaviors examined and the soft signs used are not provided, as has been the norm in many of the studies.

Investigators supportive of the soft signs concept who have searched for this indirect link suggesting biological factors in behavioral or psychiatric disorders contend that children with behavioral or learning disorders tend to have a greater number of soft signs than do normal children. Thus, a great many studies have been reported (see the reviews by Rie in Chapter 9 and Reeves & Werry in Chapter 10) that compare normal children with hyperactive, learning disordered, psychotic, or motor disordered children, all in search of that indirect link between neurological and behavioral status. Actually, most studies reported have been able to find an increased incidence of soft signs among a variety of exceptional children, though there have been some conflicting reports (see Tupper, 1986). In effect, some researchers have looked for biological marker variables (i.e., soft signs) for behavioral disorders. One of the overlooked factors in this association, however, is that even if there is an increased frequency or an increased number of soft signs in developmentally or behaviorally impaired children, it is unclear what exactly this increase would imply or whether it would aid in distinguishing neurologically impaired children from the larger classification of other childhood behavioral difficulties, or even help distinguish between various behavioral or psychiatric disorders (at least without greater use of individual item research). Overlap of soft signs in both abnormal and normal groups is also a significant cause for concern (Helper, 1980). Soft signs, therefore, would not serve as a specific neurological marker, but would be just another nonspecific factor in assessment of these children.

As was suggested earlier, though the relationship between soft signs as indicators of neurological status and behavioral disorders is at best presumptive and correlational, there is obviously a value in relating *precise* behavioral deficits to groups of specific soft sign items (see also Chapter 14 for a similar suggestion). For instance, measures of associated movements, because they involve motor functions, might be hypothesized to be increased in developmentally apraxic or clumsy children and thus be highly correlated (see Chapter 5). On the other hand, research between these same soft sign measures and more complex psychological functioning would be expected to show only modest correlations (see Badian & Wolff, 1977), thus identifying a more exclusive relationship between these variables.

Rather than emphasizing diagnosis by soft signs or the prediction of individual performance (which raises the issue of guilt by statistical association; Barlow, 1974), such research would clarify the relationship between specific soft signs and specific behavioral correlates by demonstrating dissociations between well-defined behavioral and soft sign categories. This would be an example of divergent validity.

Clinically, by sticking more closely to behavioral categories validly related to different soft sign measures, wild inferences about MBD can be held to a minimum and the children better served.

In researching behavioral, psychiatric, or learning disorders, which often have a varied etiologic basis, the need for truly multifactorial methodology becomes obvious. The same is true clinically when evaluating children for these types of disorders, particularly in a clinic-referred population. It then becomes the examiner's knowledge and expertise, more than any other factor, in integrating data concerning soft signs and giving them their proper weight and interpretation, in the context of other information about the child, that is truly useful in management or planning of effective interventions (Chapter 13 addresses the issue of neurological diagnosis using soft signs information in a context). Soft signs are rarely a causal factor in this type of integration.

OVERVIEW OF THE ISSUES

To summarize some of the themes and issues apparent throughout this book and the soft signs literature:

- There is a need for clearer definitions and terminology surrounding what one means by a "soft" neurological sign.
- There needs to be greater selectivity and more precision in defining and developing items that assess subtle neurobehavioral deficit. Both exclusion and inclusion criteria need to be established and met to define a true soft sign.
- Better classification systems and subgroupings of soft signs need further development and investigation in relation to a variety of neurological, developmental, and behavioral disorders in order to help establish their significance for these domains.
- More attention needs to be paid to the reported reliabilities of soft sign batteries both in evaluating past literature and especially in developing new examination instruments.

• The use of newer neurological technologies (e.g., CT scan, NMR imaging, PETT scan) is expected to yield greater precision in future validity studies, which should define clear criteria for minor neurological impairment.

• The use of imprecise behavioral categories (like MBD) should be discouraged in attempting to correlate soft signs to behavioral classifications. These global categories should be replaced with more objective, defineable performances.

• The need for a multifactorial perspective in evaluating the significance of soft signs is stressed by almost everyone working in this area.

These issues and themes will be discussed further in the remaining chapters of this book and it is hoped that the reader will come away with a clearer and much more secure knowledge base for understanding the limits of our knowledge about soft neurological signs. Unfortunately, the true significance of soft signs remains to be determined, but, fortunately, there are clearer and more identifiable directions to go in the future.

The bases of soft signs are bound to be complex, more so than for hard signs. It will probably evolve that our understanding will show that soft signs are multidetermined by a host of factors and do not have a simple unidimensional etiology. Thus, far from "soft thinking," this book provides a review for those determined to find hard evidence for these currently more ambiguous and probably multifactorial signs.

REFERENCES

Badian NA, & Wolff PH. Manual asymmetries of motor sequencing in boys with reading disability. Cortex, 1982, 13, 343-349

Barlow CF. "Soft signs" in children with learning disorders. American Journal of the Disabled Child, 1974, 128, 605-606

Bender L. Childhood schizophrenia: Clinical study of one hundred schizophrenic children. American Journal of Orthopsychiatry, 1947, 17, 40-46

Bickerstaff ER. Neurological Examination in Clinical Practice (Third ed.). Oxford: Blackwell Scientific, 1973

Boll TJ. Diagnosing brain impairment. In Wolman BB (Ed.). Clinical Diagnosis of Mental Disorders. New York: Plenum Press, pp 601-675, 1978

Boll TJ. Neuropsychological assessment of the child: Myths, current status, and future prospects. In Walker CE, & Roberts MC (Eds.). Handbook of Clinical Child Psychology. New York: John Wiley & Sons, 1983

Clements SD. Minimal Brain Dysfunction in Children — Terminology and Identification. Washington, D.C.: U.S. Public Health Services, 1966

DeJong R. The Neurological Examination (4th ed.). New York: Hoeber, 1979

Denckla MB. Minimal brain dysfunction. In Chall JS, & Mirsky AF (Eds.). Education and the Brain. Chicago: University of Chicago Press, 1978

Fletcher JM, & Taylor HG. Neuropsychological approaches to children: Towards a developmental neuropsychology. Journal of Clinical Neuropsychology, 1984, 6, 39-56

Gardner RA. The Objective Diagnosis of Minimal Brain Dysfunction. Cresskill, NJ: Creative Therapeutics, 1979

Helper MM. Follow-up of children with minimal brain dysfunctions: Outcomes and predictors. In Rie HD, & Rie ED (Eds.). Handbook of Minimal Brain Dysfunctions: A Critical View. New York: Wiley Interscience, pp 75-114, 1980

Ingram TTS. Soft signs. Developmental Medicine and Child Neurology, 1973, 15, 527-530

Kennard MA. Value of equivocal signs in neurologic diagnosis. Neurology, 1960, 10, 753-764

MacKeith R, & Bax M (Eds.). Minimal Cerebral Dysfunction (C.D.M. No. 10). London: Hienemann, 1963

Meehl PE. MAXCOV-HITMAX: A taxonomic search method for loose genetic syndromes. In Meehl PE (Ed.). Psychodiagnosis: Selected Papers. New York: W.W. Norton, pp 200-224, 1973

Rapin I. Children with Brain Dysfunction: Neurology, Cognition, Language, and Behavior. New York: Raven Press, 1982

Ross AO. Conceptual issues in the evaluation of brain damage. In Khama JL (Ed.). Brain Damage and Mental Retardation: A Psychological Evaluation (2nd ed.). Springfield, IL: Charles C. Thomas, pp 20-43, 1973

Russell EW. The psychometric foundation of clinical neuropsychology. In Filskov SB, Boll TJ (Eds.). Handbook of Clinical Neuropsychology (Vol. 2). New York: Wiley-Interscience, pp 45-80, 1986

Rutter M, Graham P, & Yule W. A Neuropsychiatric Study in Childhood (C.D.M. Nos. 35/36). London: Hienemann, 1970

Shafer SQ, Shaffer D, O'Connor PA, & Stokman CJ. Hard thoughts on neurological "soft signs." In Rutter M (Ed.). Developmental Neuropsychiatry. New York: Guilford Press, pp 133-143, 1983

Shapiro T, Burkes L, Petti TA, & Ranz J. Consistency of “nonfocal” neurological signs. Journal of the American Academy of Child Psychiatry, 1978, 17, 70-79

Sharbrough FW. Nonspecific abnormal EEG patterns. In Niedermeyer E, da Silva FL (Eds.). Electroencephalography. Baltimore: Urban & Schwarzenberg, pp 135-154, 1982

Small L. The Minimal Brain Dysfunctions. New York: The Free Press, 1982

Spreen O, Tupper D, Risser A, Tuokko H, & Edgell D. Human Developmental Neuropsychology. New York: Oxford University Press, 1984

Taber’s Cyclopedic Medical Dictionary. Thomas CL (Ed.). 12th ed. Philadelphia: Davis, 1973

Taylor HG. MBD: Meanings and misconceptions. Journal of Clinical Neuropsychology, 1983, 5, 271-287

Tupper DE. Neuropsychological screening and soft signs. In Obrzut JE, & Hynd GW (Eds.). Child Neuropsychology, Vol. 2: Clinical Practice. Orlando, FL: Academic Press, pp 139-186, 1986

Webster’s Seventh New Collegiate Dictionary. Gove PB (Ed.). Springfield, MA: G & C Merriam Co., 1971

Weiss G. MBD: Critical diagnostic issues. In Rie HD, Rie ED (Eds.). Handbook of Minimal Brain Dysfunctions: A Critical View. New York: Wiley-Interscience, pp 347-361, 1980

Wender PH. Minimal Brain Dysfunction in Children. New York: Wiley Interscience, 1971

Part I

Assessment

William Yule
Eric Taylor

2

Classification of Soft Signs

"...damage to the immature brain may lead to subtle distortions of development without any overt neurological condition of a textbook kind" (Rutter, Graham, & Yule, 1970). The textbooks referred to are those that stressed the importance of eliciting classical neurological signs. As Kennard (1960) put it, "The term equivocal neurologic sign has been in common use since the procedure for routine neurologic examination was first established by our clinical ancestors during the end of the last and the beginning of the present century." Hard signs were seen as providing unequivocal evidence of neuropathology. "Equivocal" or "soft" signs were seen to be suggestive of pathology but were "... either so slight as to be uncertain or only occasionally and not consistently present" (Kennard, 1960). Thus, this softness came from difficulty in eliciting them, or from them being less severe, or from being inconsistent and, as we will see, from difficulty in interpreting such signs when examining developing children. Little wonder that some clinicians become exasperated with controversies surrounding the measurement and meaning of soft signs. Ingram (1973) went as far as to state that "Soft signs are diagnostic of soft thinking," with his acerbic eye fixed on fellow clinicians rather than patients.

The purposes of this chapter are to describe neurodevelopmental examinations that yield measures of soft signs, to examine the reliability and validity of such measures, and to consider how such signs can be usefully classified. This will be done drawing on two sets of data that the authors have gathered. The chapter will conclude by posing questions about the relationship between such neurodevelopmental examinations, psychometric examinations, and newer types of neurophysiological examinations.

SOFT NEUROLOGICAL SIGNS
ISBN 0-8089-1841-9

CLASSIFICATION

The main purpose of any system of classification is to bring order into a given situation. As Quay (1980) put it:

> In many fields progress and increased scientific understanding have frequently been closely associated with the scientists' ability to describe entities or events and classify them into categories. The ability to set apart discriminable entities and events is a necessary precursor to the establishment of relationships among entities and events, and between them and other variables. Progess has also followed the advances in techniques for the measurement of phenomena under study. Accurate quantification is a particularly important requisite for the scientific study of human behavior.

The implications of this for developing a sound classification of soft neurological signs are that signs must be described clearly, that different signs must be discriminable, they must be measurable, and their relationship with other pertinent variables must be established.

The characteristics of good systems of classification have been fully discussed in relation to childhood psychopathology (Quay, 1980; Rutter, 1965; Yule, 1981). The main characteristics relevant to classifying soft signs are:

1. The classification must be based on signs that are operationally defined. Idiosyncratic interpretation should be reduced to the minimum.
2. Any classificatory system must be clinically relevant and convey prognostic information.
3. The classification must be reliable in the sense that different clinicians can agree to use the categories in the same way.
4. The categories must have demonstrable validity. Different patterns should be clearly discriminable and they should show coherent relationships with variables other than those used to place the sign in the category.
5. The system should be parsimonious, containing the minimum number of categories necessary to produce maximum reliability and validity.
6. There should be clear rules for using the system.
7. The system must be practicable within the limitations of a real life clinical setting. It should be based on information that is readily available and its use should quickly be seen as an aid to efficient clinical practice.

DEFINITION AND DESCRIPTION OF NEUROLOGICAL "SOFT SIGNS"

Most standard neurological examination of adults are based on tests developed from well confirmed views of the functioning of the central nervous system (Brain, 1955). Even so, the advent of computerized analyses of electroencephalographic measures, radioactive scanning of the brain, and positron emission tomography have all added greatly to the neurologist's diagnostic abilities. As far as the neurological examination of the child is concerned, the child's developmental level is an important variable that must be taken into account both in the examination and in the interpretation of any results. Over the past 25 years, it has been accepted that the neurological examination of the child must include a variety of developmental assessments that are not usually part of the adult examination (Paine & Oppe, 1966; Prechtl & Beintema, 1964; Rutter et al, 1970). These modifications owe much to the work of child psychologists (Bayley, 1968; Griffiths, 1954). In psychometric testing, it is well recognized that the age and developmental level of the child must be taken into account in interpreting scores. This is not so well appreciated by clinicans trained in classical neurological examinations. The failure to appreciate individual differences in response to tests lies behind much of the muddled thinking epitomized in the portmanteau concept of "minimal cerebral dysfunction" (MacKeith & Bax, 1963; Rutter et al, 1970; Yule, 1978).

There are now a number of detailed descriptions of neuropsychological examinations suitable for children of different ages. More recent ones are notable for the detailed prescription of the way the examiner should prepare the child, precisely what should be done, and how the results should be rated (Baird & Gordon, 1983; Drillien & Drummond, 1983; Rutter, et al, 1970; Touwen, 1976, 1979). Roughly speaking, the developmental examination covers four major areas: examination of the head and cranial nerves; assessment of movement, power, tone, and reflexes; examination of the trunk, posture, and gait; and assessment of higher cortical functions such as speech, language, and cognitive level. Readers are referred to the above sources for detailed descriptions of the assessments. Rather than reprint a comprehensive list here, we will briefly describe one set of tests used in one study.

THE ISLE OF WIGHT NEUROLOGICAL ASSESSMENT

In the early 1960s, a number of epidemiologic studies were undertaken on the Isle of Wight, a small island off the south coast of Britain. At that time, the total population was approximately 100,000, with about 1000 children in each year group. The aim of the studies was to provide evidence on the nature and interrelationships of handicapping conditions in childhood, which would be of value in planning services as well as in illuminating the nature of the problems. One focus of interest was the relationship between neuropsychological status and psychiatric disorder. All children with known neurological problems in the 5-15 year age range were available for study. The neurological assessment was chosen with this age range in mind. As it was part of a wider set of assessments, the neurological examination was so developed as to be completed in 20 minutes, following a 30 minute psychiatric interview with the same examiner. Thus, the children were relaxed and familiar with the examiner. Samples of speech and language were easily obtained. Children were examined in their schools and the only undressing necessary was the removal of shoes and socks. Potentially distressing aspects of the examination such as examining plantar responses were left to the end.

The items included in the neurological examination were:

Eyes
- Ptosis (drooping lids)
- Nystagmus (involuntary movements)
- Strabismus (squint)

Face
- Facial Symmetry
- Facial Power
- Tongue Movements

Fine Motor Coordination
- Threading beads
- Holding pencil
- Touching finger with thumb
- (Overall rating of limb "dyspraxia")

Gross Motor Coordination
- Gait
- Kicking ball
- Throwing ball
- Hopping on one foot

Walking and turning
(Overall rating of cerebellar dysfunction)
Constructional abilities
Children copy five shapes with matchsticks
Stereognosis
Four objects to be recognized by feel
Tremor
Rated during fine and gross motor testing
Speech and Language
Articulation defect
Speech syntax rating
Overall speech complexity
Adequacy of description
Laterality
Hand, foot, and eye laterality separately assessed
Mirror Movements
Tested in each hand, squeezing clothes peg and then bulldog clip
Muscle Tone
Tested separately for right and left,
upper and lower limbs
Muscle Power
Rated separately for right and left,
upper and lower limbs
Reflexes
Supinator
Biceps
Triceps
Knee
Ankles
Plantar

In every case, the procedure to be followed was described in detail. For example, in rating Nystagmus, “external occular movements were tested for each eye separately and the presence of or absence of nystagmus was noted. Nystagmus was regarded as present only if there were four or more beats occurring after the eye had reached a position of rest when fixating a finger 18 inches away and 60° from the middle. It was coded as 'none', 'slight', or 'marked', but a full description was recorded whenever it was present” (Rutter et al, 1970, p. 25).

"Hand laterality was assessed on the hand used in drawing ..., in throwing a rolled up piece of paper ..., and to knock on the door" (p. 35).

Examiners had to check off the appropriate point on a three point rating scale for most items. They also had to record details of detected abnormalities. This made it easy to get a variety of composite scores and to compare ratings on a reliability study. Finally, the examiner had to make a final rating on the presence and severity of neurological disorder (none, dubious, slight, or marked).

Schedules, such as that used on the Isle of Wight, give detailed advice on undertaking a developmental neurological examination and recording the results. Do they help different clinicians agree on the presence and absence of soft signs?

RELIABILITY OF SOFT SIGNS

As Shafer, Shaffer, O'Connor, and Stokman (1983) point out in a thoughtful review of the area, one has to differentiate a number of aspects of reliability. Notably, the question of whether two examiners agree must be separated from the question of whether the child shows evidence of the same sign at two different points in time.

In the Isle of Wight studies, two reliability exercises were undertaken. Eighty nine children ages 10-11 years were seen by each of 2 examiners from 1 to 30 days apart. A further 27 physically handicapped children aged 7-13 years were similarly assessed 1-14 days apart. The agreement between examiners varied according to the sign being tested and whether the child was normal or physically handicapped. Expressing agreement in terms of product-moment correlations, reliability on developmental items ranged from 0.56 for testing mirror movements in normal children to 0.93 for testing constructional difficulties. For cranial signs, percentage agreement ranged from 59 percent for tongue movements in the physically handicapped to 92 percent on nystagmus in normal children. Agreements on fine and gross motor coordination were modest (r = 0.58-0.89), but tended to be better on the rating of power and tone of limbs. Agreement on rating reflexes was very variable — r = 0.20 for supinator to r = 0.86 for knee.

Overall, the global ratings agreed well — r = 0.88 in normals and r = 0.80 in physically handicapped children. However, as Rutter, Graham, and Yule (1970) point out, high correlations can conceal differences in threshold for abnormality between examiners. As long as one examiner is consistently more severe (or less severe) in his or her judgment, it is possible for two examiners to agree well in rank ordering individuals but to disagree on which individuals are placed beyond a cut-off point for abnormality. Shafer, Shaffer, O'Connor, and Stokman (1983) suggest that a number of statistics be presented to safeguard against this possibility. Indeed, in the Collaborative Perinatal Project across 14 institutions in the US, there was good interrater agreement within institutions but very discrepant rates of soft signs between them (Nichols & Chen, 1981).

The results from these large studies and several small, clinic based ones, suggest that good interrater agreement can be achieved, but that it must be planned for. Methods must be adequately standardized and examiners must be properly trained. However, it must also be noted that agreement was far from perfect even on the "hardest" of the soft signs. Agreement was poor on slight deviations from normality.

STABILITY OF SOFT SIGNS

Shafer et al (1983) reviewed a number of small studies — either small in terms of the numbers of children retested or the number of signs examined — and concluded that "... some signs elicited in certain ways are not ephemeral ... [and] ... that short-term within subject or within-rater variability may contribute more to total variance than does interrater variability" (p. 137).

This should not come as a surprise to psychologists who are used to considering the problems of short-term retest effects in children. While the reliability of a composite score may be acceptably high, the stability of response to any single test item may be very low. Once exposed to test items, practice effects are not uncommon. Thus, Foster, Margolin, Alexander, Benitez, and Carr (1978) found considerable improvement on 5 soft signs — finger approximation, tandem gait, one-eyed winking, nystagmus, and plantar response — when 10 inpatients aged 7-12 years were tested on 6 occasions over 37 days. Foster et al make the illogical recommendation that because children's performances improve with testing, the items should be eliminated from examination for "minimal brain damage," thereby betraying the deeply imbedded view of neurological signs as being related to CNS functioning in an absolute way. Rather than drop these signs, the examiner must know how performance is affected by exposure.

Hertzig (1982) followed up 53 children, approximately one-third of a group first seen at age 10 ½ years. At first testing, there was a clear relationship between the number of soft signs elicited and the age of the children — older children showing fewer signs. At 10 ½ years, the average number of signs for the reduced sample had been 4.47. Four years later, the average dropped to 2.70. The number of children who showed two or more soft signs on each occasion remained constant — the lower the IQ of the children, the more signs they showed. Children with lower IQs, however, were found to have less consistency over the 4 years.

Hertzig (1982) interprets her results as providing partial support for the view put forward by Rutter (1977) that soft signs mainly indicate developmental delays rather than provide prima facie evidence of CNS dysfunction. This argument is strongest where signs show clear age trends, but not all those she examined do so.

Thus, the evidence from interrater reliability studies and from retest, follow-up studies suggest that signs *can* be elicited reliably, that different raters *can* agree on their presence, that many signs persist across time, that some signs decline with age, and that many are correlated with overall measures of intelligence. In other words, these are *real* phenomena. The next stage in attempting to classify them is to examine how they cluster together.

Empirical Classifications of Supposed Minor Signs of Brain Dysfunction

If brain damage or MBD were to account for any significant number of psychologically disordered children, then there should be a number of syndromes — perhaps an extremely large number. Some kinds of mild brain damage will be localized, and so give rise to a relatively specific pattern of dysfunction. On these assumptions, there should be several different patterns of perceptual deficit: different sorts of motor impairment and some abnormalities of behavior or learning with no other accompaniment.

Accordingly, the simplest sort of classification of the results of brain damage is according to the domain in which problems are chiefly presenting. "The clumsy child," "the learning-disabled child," and the "hyperactive" or "unregulated" child have all been the subjects of monographs and intervention programs. Such a classification, however, has little purpose except to delineate areas of study. These are in no sense alternative categories. Clumsy children may very well have perceptual and behavioral disorders too. Indeed, the link between learning disorder and conduct disorder (for which no brain etiology necessarily contributes) is just as strong as that with hyperactivity (traditionally regarded as a more neurological pattern).

Some approaches to classification have tried to include data from several domains, and identify patterns that will be made up of different kinds of sign. Clinical and statistical lines have both been followed, and both have advantages and disadvantages.

Denckla's (1977) report is a good instance of a clinician's attempt to order the problems of referred cases. Her classification was initially based upon a sizeable series (190 children referred for private neurological assessment) and upon a lengthy neurologic evaluation lasting for 2 hours. The majority of the children (70 percent) fell into no clear category: they had an unclassifiable mixture of problems. The remaing 30 percent showed 1 of 3 defined clusters. Those in the first cluster (making up 15 percent of the series) were failing in reading and spelling, and performed poorly on various tests, including those believed to assess memory, language, and coordination and sequencing. They were labeled as showing specific language disablity and, very speculatively, considered to have poor rote-functioning. A second subgroup (specific visuospatial disability) comprised 5 percent of cases, who were impaired in arithmetic and writing; and they were also emotionally maladjusted. A third group (dyscontrol syndrome) were impulsive and immature in their behavior, normal in language and perceptual function, and said to respond well to amphetamine-type drugs. Indeed, one may doubt whether this last group represents anything more specific than being oppositional or defiant. It may well relate to the processes of socialization rather than neuronal regulation.

There was no suggestion that the signs addressed by this study were in fact pathognomonic of brain disorder. Simple disturbances of motor function, reflexes, or primitive sensation were not reported in detail, and apparently no clusterings of those signs had been noted. Most of the clinical features were descriptions of psychological functions, that are best assessed by standardized psychometric tests of known reliability.

Standardized tests and a neurological examination were the basis of Mattis, French, and Rapin's (1975) attempt at classification. They subdivided a group of children, adolescents, and young adults who had been referred with problems of learning, behavior, or both. One group had abnormalities of neurological examination but not of reading; one group read poorly but had normal examinations; and a third group had both kinds of abnormality. This is not of course in any way surprising, nor in itself very helpful.

However, the authors felt able to recognize three patterns among the poor readers: those with language disorder, those with poor articulation and writing, and those with visuospatial perceptual difficulties.

A classification such as this has some limited face validity but little else to recommend it in present knowledge. The study did not establish the replicability or validity of the subdivision. For the purpose of this chapter, however, it contained a useful negative lesson. The various kinds of abnormality of sensorimotor coordination that were tested by the neurological examination did not associate in any regular way with the different patterns of psychometric test performance.

Attempts by clinicians to decide intuitively about the presence of subgroups could be scientifically valuable. The human brain is a most effective instrument for recognizing patterns. It is particularly likely to recognize a clustering of rare and salient problems. One must face the fact, however, that none of the skilled and experienced clinicians who have addressed themselves to this area of children's problems has yet produced a powerful subgrouping of signs (see below). It is therefore necessary to turn to statistical attempts at classification. These seek patterns of correlations between signs or clustering of cases on the basis of their signs.

One thorough and frequently cited study was reported by Werry (1968). Factor analysis was applied to sets of measures from questionnaires, tests, neurologic examinations, and EEG records. The analysis was rather clear — each source of data was separate from the others. Abnormalities on the EEG record or the neurological examination, for example, could not be taken as a good index of overall cerebral dysfunction because they were not associated with one another into any larger dimension.

Werry's predominantly negative results have been rightly interpreted as an argument against a common unitary syndrome of brain dysfunction. They would be compatible with the presence of many small syndromes, but no evidence yet indicates what those minisyndromes should be. The findings are an example of the frequent tendency of factor analytic studies to produce factors restricted to one data source. More recent analytic techniques are available to counteract this tendency, but have not yet been applied to indicators of cerebral dysfunction. Nor, if such techniques were applied, would they prove that an overarching dimension reflects any natural ordering. Techniques of numerical taxonomy do not demonstrate the validity of the assumptions that underlie them, but only their results.

The lack of any clear, single dimension of brain dysfunction has been argued by several other studies. Behavioral, psychometic, and neurologic abnormalities are not accurate predictors of one another (Rutter, 1983). Accordingly, the research strategy needs to shift. It becomes more fruitful to concentrate upon one or two domains (psychometric, behavioral, neurological, pharmacologic, or physiologic); to idenfity patterns within those domains; and to examine the possibility that individual patterns have a specific link to disorder in another domain.

Ordering of Cases By Test Performance

Conners (1973) reported a statistical approach within this strategy. He applied a battery of psychological tests and behavior ratings to 90 children referred to research clinics. The result was a set of groups, each with a characteristic profile of test scores. One group, for instance, was notable for normal scores on information-processing tests and mild degrees of behavioral problems.

The possibility of identifying separate groups in this way is encouraging. On the other hand, the groups did not correspond to clinically recognized categories, and so did not have any immediate validity. The next step of Conners' investigation was therefore very necessary: to examine any neurophysiological distinctions between the groups. It turned out that there were significant differences between his groups on measures of the averaged visual evoked response of the EEG, and also in their responsiveness to stimulant medication.

There have, of course, been very many attempts to generate a stable classification of the disorders of learning. They are, for the most part, outside the scope of this chapter since they are not intended to provide different categories of neurological dysfunction. The study described by Petrauskas and Rourke (1979) does however need to be considered in this context. They used the Q-factor analysis approach to generate three reliable subtypes of reading-disabled children on the basis of test scores. The largest group (1) had poorer verbal than performance IQ scores; and worse reading than arithmetic. The second group (2) had small V-P discrepancies, poor arithmetic, finger agnosia, and poor short-term memory in a test requiring the recall of visual sequences. The third group (3) was less clearly characterized: they did not show the specific disabilities of the former two groups and they had better psychomotor performance on the left side than on the right.

The first two groups had some similarity to the "language disorder" and "visuospatial" groups of Mattis et al's (1975) poor readers (see above). Finger agnosia is traditionally a neurologist's sign and poor arithmetic performance a psychologist's: the coexistence of the two in one group emphasizes the logical similarity of these different sorts of sign. Petrauskas and Rourke related their group 1 to temporal lobe dysfunction, group 2 to dysfunction of posterior parts of the left cerebral hemisphere, and group 3 to anterior left-sided cerebral dysfunction. These neurological links are entirely speculative. They do not validate the classification. Different patterns of brain function have not been established. The meaning of the different patterns of test performance will need more research.

Ordering of Cases by Psychological Symptoms

Within the domain of behavioral problems, there have also been many statistical and clinical attempts to generate a useful classification. Diagnostic schemes have very many purposes besides the establishment of signs of minor neurological dysfunction, and it is not our purpose to review them. The major conclusion from many reviews is that behavioral problems (such as overactivity and inattention) are not pointers to organic cerebral problems (Taylor, 1983).

A recent cluster-analytic study of boys aged 6-10, referred to a psychiatric hospital because of behavior problems, is relevant here (Taylor, 1985). One cluster comprised boys with pervasive hyperactivity and poor concentration, one cluster was characterized by high levels of emotional disturbance, while a third had conduct problems only in the classroom. These groups proved to be significantly different in neuropsychological abilities. The first, hyperkinetic group had frequent histories of language and motor delays and high rates of neurological soft signs. The third group, classroom-specific conduct disorder, was more likely to show specific reading retardation. The first group was most likely to respond to stimulation medication.

While this distinction may yet be useful for psychiatric classification, it still falls short of providing signs of brain dysfunction; let alone demonstrating different patterns. Nonorganic factors could have given rise to the different patterns.

Ordering of Cases by Physiologic Measures

Neurophysiologic measures have often been considered as soft signs, especially recordings of the EEG. EEG abnormalities are "soft" when they are not clearly shown to be the result of brain pathology. It does not, of course, follow that they must be the result of minor brain dysfunction. The electrical function of the brain can be explained by psychologic concepts, just as much as the other way around. Abnormal evoked potentials can be the result of altered attention — just as physiologically recorded lachrymation may better be explained by misery than by overactivity of tear centers. Nevertheless, minor EEG abnormalities have to be classsified before they can be explained.

John et al (1977) have described the application of numerical taxonomy to identifying different patterns of abnormality of the large number of EEG measures that are used for a neurometric data base. So far, their multivariate analyses have not been fruitfully applied to children's neurological disorders. Localization has been explored, with the simple but suggestive finding of smaller EPs on the left side of the brain in children with reading disabilities and on the right side in arithmetic disability. This evidently falls short of generating a useful classification.

A welcome feature of this program of study has been the inclusion of a distinction between delays of development and abnormalities of development of the EEG (Prichep, John, Ahn, & Kaye, 1983). Sets of equations have been derived to model the age changes in different parts of the brain. It is therefore possible to describe any given abnormality of function either in terms of the age at which it would be normal or as a change that would not be normal at any age.

Some aspects of neurometric analysis are therefore well advanced, but others are not. It is not yet clear that it is valid as an index of organic cerebral abnormality; nor that it is of educational or prognostic value. At this stage it is of interest as a research technique that may yet prove to be of considerable value to the classifier, not yet a classification good enough to guide practice.

Ordering of Cases by Neuromuscular Coordination

Clumsiness has usually been considered as one problem, not many. It can, of course, be caused by mild forms of cerebral palsy or other neurological diseases — but then the signs are in no sense soft but explicit and localizing.

A few individual patterns have been suggested. A choreiform syndrome, for example, was proposed by Prechtl (1965). Involuntary spasmodic contractions of different muscle groups were suggested to be a motor manifestation of the same neural abnormality that produced learning disabilities and hyperactivity. The suggestion did not, in fact, stand the test of empirical studies. Choreiform movements may possibly be more common in psychiatric disorder, but they do not associate with any particular pattern of psychological problems (Rutter et al, 1970).

A minor syndrome of right hemisphere dysfunction has been argued by Denckla (1983). For instance, Rudel et al (1974) noted a combination of arithmetic disability, visuospatial deficit, left-sided motor signs, and oculomotor impairment. Weintraub and Mesulam (1983) described 14 patients (many of them young adults) with "nondyslexic learning disabilities and difficulties in interpersonal skills." They had, as a group, performance IQs lower than verbal; they were shy or isolated; and they showed left-sided motor incoordination or abnormal reflexes. As already noted, localizing signs such as these are not soft in any helpful meaning: they should be replicable and persistent and lose their evidential value if they are not.

On this kind of evidence it is not even demonstrated that right hemisphere dysfunction causes particular psychological deficits. The weakness is the lack of suitable controls. No doubt it is possible to recognize some cases that combine learning disabilities with shyness and left-sided incoordination. But might not the same clinical population contain individuals with similar interpersonal problems and right-sided weakness: or signs of right hemisphere dysfunction combined with a quite different psychiatric pattern such as hyperkinesis? We have seen examples of both such "anomalous" combinations. Perhaps a series could be accumulated in the same way and yet another "syndrome" described.

Another distinct pattern of minor cerebral dysfunction has been suggested by the Fog tests of primitive postural reflexes (Fog & Fog, 1963). These elicit "overflow" movements when difficult actions are carried out. They are less noticeable as children mature, and are therefore usually regarded as truly "developmental" abnormalities. Szatmari and Taylor (1984) found that the uninvolved arms and hands took up standard positions in response to specific foot postures — even in some children who could not carry out the foot movements but only "intended them." The arm movements could, for the most part, be voluntarily suppressed. These immature responses were more frequent in children with psychiatric disorders.

It is not yet clear whether there is any specificity in this test, or whether it measures anything different from other kinds of soft signs. Abnormalities such as these cannot, in present knowledge, be taken to amount to a minor syndrome.

We are not seeking to deny the possibility — even the likelihood — that recognizably different forms of minor brain impairment exist. We are, however, constrained to remark that the search for separate syndromes has, so far, been rather unrewarding. Accordingly, most neurologists conceive of different sorts of clumsiness (if at all) as alternative pointers to a common pathology of delay in cerebral maturation. The developers of scorable versions of the neurological examination have followed this model and assigned an overall score to each patient on the basis of an unweighted sum of abnormalities noted. Individual signs would therefore need to be listed rather than classified.

Nevertheless, there might be an order in such signs. Theoretically, at least, there could be a classification according to the brain processes that have been affected. This, however, may well require a much more experimental analysis of the processes involved than has yet been given. A boy who has been asked to put his finger on his nose must have many abilities, including those of hearing and understanding the request; of planning the action and willingness to do it; of monitoring and feedback of the action as it proceeds; and of finely regulating movement in accordance with the previous monitoring. Clinicians often do form an opinion about the processes involved, but their means of doing so is neither explicit nor shown to be reliable.

Numerical taxonomy can, of course, be applied to items from a scored neurological examination as readily as to psychometric tests. It is much less often used in this domain. If replicable dimensions are found, they might relate to different parts of the body; or to abilities transcending the system tested. One might, for instance, need to use a construct of accuracy of movement if there were a coherent dimension of accuracy (as distinct from speed or smoothness) involving different parts of the body.

We shall therefore briefly describe the patterns of relationship between different signs in data from two separate investigations. The first entailed the intensive study of 64 boys aged 6-10 years referred from normal schools to psychiatric clinics because of severe behavior problems. The series has been separately described (Taylor, 1985). The second investigation involved the screening of a whole borough in East London to detect 6- to 7-year-old boys with conduct disorders and/or hyperactivity. One hundred and seventy-one cases were chosen in this way for further study — which included the same scored neurological examination (normal controls were also examined, but not reported here). Both series are therefore made up of boys showing disruptive conduct for any of several different reasons.

The same brief, scored neurological examination was applied in both studies (Taylor, 1985). It consisted of 15 items, all concerned with the control of different sorts of movement. The development of this examination was by selection of items from a lengthy examination culled from several printed sources (especially Touwen, 1979). Items were chosen if they proved to have adequate interrater reliability and test-retest stability in preliminary studies, and if they yielded a positive (abnormal) score in at least 10 percent of children referred because of learning and/or behavior problems. The aim was an easily administered test that would be more psychometrically satisfactory than any existing schemes of examination (Werry, 1968). It was not intended to cover every area of possible impairment, so it would not be a suitable instrument for generating a comprehensive classification.

Each series of cases was submitted to factor analysis with varimax rotation. The results are set out in Tables 2-1 and 2-2. In the clinic series, five factors were extracted with eigenvalues greater than unity. Together they accounted for 70 percent of the total variance. The item loadings are given in Table 2-1. In the community-based series, 6 factors were extracted, that together accounted for 74 percent of the total variance. Table 2-2 shows the loadings of items on the factors.

No clear factor structure is replicated across the two series. In the epidemiologically based study, the largest factor was loaded chiefly with three measures of lower limb coordination (standing, hopping, and heel-toe walking). These three measures also formed a factor in the analysis of the clinic series (this time in combination with upper limb coordination when eyes are closed).

In the clinic series, the largest factor comprised the measures of fine finger coordination and mirror movements; together with athetosis (and, to a lesser extent, steadiness in heel-toe walking). Fine finger coordination and mirror movements also emerged as a factor from the epidemiologic study, but athetosis and gait were distributed on other dimensions.

No general factor of inaccuracy or jerkiness of movement appeared; and there is not a replicated factor of involuntary movements as opposed to impaired voluntary movements. Insofar as any subclassification is supported at all, it would only be one in which each system tested (e.g., lower limb movements) yielded several, positively intercorrelated scores. This could reflect examiner bias as much as any more substantive reason for association.

The internal consistency of the scales was not very impressive either. There were significant but modest correlations between nearly every item and the total scale scores, varying from 0.24 (for choreiform movements) to

Table 2-1
Principal Factor Analysis of Neurological Examination in Clinic Series of 64 Boys

Item	Factor I	II	III	IV	V
Involuntary movements:					
Chorea	.12	.04	-.06	*.67*	-.03
Athetosis	*.70*	.10	-.09	-.13	-.23
Tremor	.18	.15	*.54*	.09	.12
Upper limb:					
Impersistence	.01	.12	.06	.10	*.85*
Finger-nose (smoothness, eyes open)	- 11	-.07	*.94*	-.09	-.02
Finger-nose (accuracy, eyes open)	.05	-.06	*.91*	-.12	-.07
Finger-nose (smoothness, eyes shut)	.26	*.55*	-.11	-.41	.43
Finger-nose (accuracy, eyes shut)	.09	*.80*	-.08	-.12	.30
Fingers:					
Finger-thumb (smoothness)	*.81*	.15	.12	.13	.31
Finger-thumb (accuracy)	*.81*	.11	.19	.20	.14
Mirror movements	*.75*	.24	-.02	.16	-.07
Eye movements:	.13	.32	-.04	*.75*	.18
Lower limbs:					
Balancing	.22	*.79*	.03	.31	-.01
Hopping	.33	*.58*	.19	.27	-.35
Heel–toe gait	.48	*.50*	.36	.29	-.01

0.65 (for fine finger movements). The exception was tremor, which did not significantly correlate in the epidemiologic study (r = -.02). Cronbach's alpha, a commonly used reliability coefficient was only 0.69 for the community-based series. For the clinic series, which was probably more homogeneous in being composed mostly of quite severely disturbed children, the alpha coefficient was a little better, at 0.80, but still not high enough to be confident that all the measures tap a single ability.

It seems probable that current schemes of examination do not yield sufficiently detailed information to allow for descriptions of underlying processes. The developmental neurological examination is more of a rough-and-

Table 2-2
Principal Factor Analysis of Neurological Examination in 174 Cases Identified from General Population

	Factor					
Item	**I**	**II**	**III**	**IV**	**V**	**VI**
Involuntary movements:						
Chorea	.14	.04	.13	.00	*.80*	-.07
Athetosis	*.41*	.10	.03	.07	*.52*	.21
Tremor	-.25	.14	-.16	-.05	.50	.09
Upper limb:						
Impersistence	.17	-.04	.02	.12	.22	*.84*
Finger-nose (smoothness, eyes open)	.02	-.08	.07	*.81*	-.03	.21
Finger-nose (accuracy eyesopen)	.00	.03	*.92*	.14	.00	.08
Finger-nose (smoothness, eyes shut	-.01	.14	.15	*.83*	-.01	-.12
Finger-nose (accuracy, eyes shut)	.14	-.01	*.91*	.09	.06	.09
Fingers:						
Finger-thumb (smoothness)	.21	*.83*	-.09	.05	.02	.06
Finger-thumb (accuracy)	.23	*.82*	.04	.12	.13	.10
Mirror movements	.07	*.51*	.16	-.18	.39	.01
Eye movements:	.06	.38	.27	-.05	-.17	*.66*
Lower limbs:						
Balancing	.80	.18	-.02	-.07	.10	.09
Hopping	*.77*	.15	.17	.15	.14	-.03
Heel–toe gait	*.80*	.17	.03	-.07	-.12	.17

ready scale for estimating degrees of incoordination, however they may be caused. Perhaps it should give way to much more standardized tests that can be more satisfactorily analyzed.

This review of some empirical attempts at classifying soft signs had to end with a negative conclusion. No scheme of categorization has been demonstrated, replicated, and validated. There may be different types of learning disorder (e.g., reading backwardness versus specific reading retardation; or reading disability versus arithmetic disability), but they have not yet been shown to be rooted in different kinds of organic brain dysfunction. Further progress is likely to require a much more experimental approach to identifying the developmental processes involved in the control of skilled movements and the processing of information.

PRELIMINARY CONCLUSIONS

We are not denying that children may have many varieties of CNS dysfunction. The very fact that it has proven so difficult to discern order within the heterogeneous problems presented to clinics means that we are not yet very good at describing and measuring the phenomena, let alone classifying them. If we are to help the children who present with real difficulties, we must improve our diagnostic procedures, not jettison all standards with respect to establishing the reliability and validity of soft signs.

Rutter, Graham, and Yule (1970) noted that the poor interrater reliability on some items meant that it would be unwise to place too much emphasis on the presence of slight isolated abnormalities when considering the presence of an organic brain disorder. Hertzig's (1982) and Shaffer, O'Connor, Shafer, and Prupis's (1983) findings serve to reinforce this view.

The Isle of Wight findings pointed up another apparent paradox. It was found that the greatest problems in reliability involved items from the so-called "harder," traditional neurological examination rather than from developmental assessment of higher function. The latter were assessed by methods that have more in keeping with psychological assessments.

An attempt was made in the Isle of Wight study to look at the validity of soft signs by comparing the assessment of children with unequivocal neurological conditions with normal children and other groups with epilepsy, reading retardation, and intellectual retardation. In most instances, soft signs were clearly associated with conditions involving the CNS. But many normal children showed evidence of isolated signs. Where a total composite summation of signs was performed for each child, children in the neurological cohort scored significantly higher than did normal controls and other groups. Even so, a substantial minority of children with neurological disorders were found to have low scores.

More problematic was the finding that the composite score did not differentiate children with epilepsy, mental retardation, or reading retardation from the normal controls. This argues against the use of a crude summation of signs as a screening instrument. As Rutter, Graham, and Yule (1970) concluded:

A very high number of minor neurological signs makes it likely that the

> child has some kind of neurological disorder, but a moderate number of minor signs is quite compatible with normality. It is more important to distinguish which signs are abnormal and in this connection neurological judgement based on the knowledge of the significance of each type of abnormality is more important than a single sum of the number of abnormalities (p. 77).

It would be most unfortunate if the testing of soft signs went the same way as intelligence testing, where isolated but related items were summated to produce scores that had some useful purpose but often concealed more than they revealed. Rather it is worth considering a strategy whereby the sort of *brief* testing of soft signs, used in the Isle of Wight, Newham, and the Collaborative Perinatal projects, would be seen as *screening* tests to be followed up by more elaborate and precise tests.

It is notable that those items on the Isle of Wight screening that most resembled psychometric tests proved most reliable. Testing of motor function has been elaborated into a number of detailed tests, often based on the original Oseretsky (1931) test. Even an age-specific shortened version of this takes about 20 minutes and has only modest test-retest reliability ($r = 0.69$) over an average of 8 days. Tests of language function can likewise take 20 minutes to administer, and longer to score if detailed analyses of syntax and pragmatics are necessary. The point is that it is possible to develop standardized tests of different functions, but they are time consuming.

Recently, with the availability of inexpensive microcomputers, there is widespread interest in developing automated tests of many neuropsychological functions. Some test batteries are little more imaginative than computer presented versions of existing tests, others utilize the microprocessor's capacities to give multiple trials and obtain information on speed of intellectual processing, strategy etc. So far, the most promising of these developments center around a variety of measures of aspects of attention — various measures of reaction time, vigilance, continuous performance, and the like. Should these methods prove as valuable, as is hoped, they will revolutionize the assessment of some of these "softer" psychological functions.

In parallel, there have been considerable developments in neurophysiologic measures. The use of computers to analyze power-spectra from EEGs, laboratory EEG changes during passive conditioning (Otto, Benignus, Miller, & Barton, 1981), auditory and visual evoked potentials, CT scans, and, above all, Positron Emission Tomography (PET) scans of the working brain may all revolutionize the way in which developmental neuropsychological assessments are undertaken. Certainly, they will replace the out-moded, old-fashioned static battery approach of older generations (Rourke, Bakker, Fisk, & Strang, 1983).

A PRELIMINARY CLASSIFICATION OF SOFT SIGNS

Whatever these developments, there will still be a need for a quick screening examination of soft signs. Given the multitude of functions that can be examined, there is a need to classify them in some meaningful way. The signs do not fall into obviously meaningful clusters when contrasting diagnostic groups are compared (see below). How, then, can order be improved?

Rutter, Graham, and Yule (1970) proposed a preliminary classification that still seems to have heuristic value. From clinical experience and on the basis of the epidemiologic data, they argued that the signs fell into three distinct groups. They argued that pooling signs across groups was likely to lead to confusion.

(i) Signs Of Developmental Delay

This group consists of signs that can be reliably elicited and scored. They are not "minor" signs in that they include ratings of speech where absence is clearly a major problem. Other such signs are motor-coordination, perception, right-left differentiation, mirror movements. In each case, the interpretation of the sign depends on assessing the degree of impairment in relation to the child's chronologic and mental age. In other words, the function tested by each sign follows a characteristic course of development in normal children.

(ii) Signs Due to Both Neurological and Other Factors

Nystagmus and strabismus were cited as signs that are usually due to neurological disorder, but may have other causes. The significance of each sign has to be determined separately for each child on the basis of the detailed characteristics of the sign and its known association with other characteristics.

(iii) Slight Abnormalities That are Difficult to Detect

Usually, these are minor examples of classical neurological signs, such as slight asymmetry of tone, or slight asymmetry of the skull. Here the "softness" lies in the demonstrated unreliability of judgment concerning their presence. Repeated elicitation of such a minor abnormality increases the probability that some abnormality is truly present. However, little significance can be attached to the presence of isolated soft signs that have only been elicited on one occasion.

Beyond this preliminary and very broad classification, it is difficult to see how soft signs could reliably be categorized, especially in relation to children. Increasing use of sophisticated neurophysiological assessment, combined with better observation and neuropsychological testing, may enhance our understanding of the significance of soft signs. More precise brain-behavior relationships may yet be established. But that day is not yet here. It will be doing our children a great disservice if we prematurely adopt any classification system that will impede scientific and clinical progress.

REFERENCES

Baird NW, & Gordon EC. Neurological Evaluation of Infants and Children. Clinics in Developmental Medicine Nos. 84/85. London: SIMP/Heinemann, 1983

Bayley N. Infant Scales of Development. New York: Psychological Corporation, 1968

Brain WR. Diseases of the Nervous System (5th Ed.). London: Oxford University Press, 1955

Conners CR. Psychological assessment of children with minimal brain dysfunction. In de la Cruz FF, Fox BH, & Roberts H (Eds.). Miminal Brain Dysfunction. New York: New York Academy of Sciences, 1973

Denckla MB. Minimal brain dysfunction and dyslexia: Beyond diagnosis by exclusion. In Blau ME, Rapin I, & Kinsbourne M (Eds.). Topics in Child Neurology. New York: Spectrum, 1977

Denckla MB. The neuropsychology of social-emotional learning disabilities. Archives of Neurology, 1983, 430, 461-462

Drillien C, & Drummond M. Development Screening and the Child With Special Needs: A population study of 5000 children. Clinics in Developmental Medicine No. 86. London: SIMP/Heinemann, 1983

Fog E, & Fog M. Cerebral inhibition examined by associated movements. In MacKeith R, & Bax M (Eds.). Minimal Cerebral Dysfunction. Clinics in Developmental Medicine No. 10. London: SIMP/ Heinemann, 1963

Foster RM, Margolin L, Alexander C, et al. Equivocal neurological signs, child development and learned behavior. Child Psychiatry and Human Development, 1978, 9, 28-32

Griffiths R. The Abilities of Babies. London: University of London Press, 1954

Hertzig ME. Stability and change in non-focal neurological signs. Journal of the American Acadamy of Child Psychiatry, 1982, 21, 231-236

Ingram TTT. Soft signs. Developmental Medicine and Child Neurology, 1973, 15, 522-530

John ER, Karmel BZ, Corning WC, et al. Neurometrics. Science, 1977, 196, 1393-1410

Kennard MA. Value of equivocal signs in neurological diagnosis. Neurology, 1960, 10, 753-764

MacKeith R, & Bax M (Eds.). Minimal Cerebral Dysfunction. Clinics in Developmental Medicine No. 10. London: SIMP/Heinemann, 1963

Mattis S, French JH, & Rapin I. Dyslexia in children and young adults: three independent neuropsychological syndromes. Developmental Medicine and Child Neurology, 1975, 17, 150-163

Nichols P, & Chen T. Minimal Brain Dysfunction: A Prospective Study. Hillsdale, NJ: Erlbaum, 1981

Oseretsky N. Psychomotorik Methoden zur untersuchung der Motorik. Zeitschrift angewandt Psychologie, 1931, 17, 1-58

Otto D, Benignus V, Miller K, & Barton C. Effects of age and body lead burden on CNS function in young children. I. Slow cortical potentials. Electroencephalography and Clinical Neurophysiology, 1981, 52, 229-239

Paine RS, & Oppe TE. Neurological Examination of Children. Clinics in Developmental Medicine No. 20/21. London: SIMP/Heinemann, 1966

Petrauskas RJ, & Rourke BP. Identification of subtypes of retarded readers: A neuropsychological multivariate approach. Journal of Clinical Neuropsychology, 1979, 1, 17-37

Prechtl HFR. Nuerologische afukingen na pre-en paranatale hypoxie. Nederlands Tidjschrift Voor Geneeskunde, 1965, 109, 1991

Prechtl HFR, & Beintema DJ. Neurological Examination of the Full Term Newborn Infant. Clinics in Developmental Medicine No. 12. London: SIMP/Heinemann, 1964

Prichep L, John ER, Ahn H, & Kaye H. Neurometrics: Quantitative evaluation of brain dysfunction of children. In Rutter M (Ed.). Developmental Neuropsychiatry. New York: Guilford, 1983

Quay HC. Classification. In Quay HC, & Werry JS (Eds.). Psychopathological disorders of childhood (2nd ed.) New York: Wiley, 1980

Rourke BP, Bakker DJ, Fisk JL, & Strang JD. Child Neuropsychology. New York: Guilford Press, 1983

Rudel RG, Teuber H-L, & Twitchell TE. Levels of impairment of sensorimotor functions in children with early brain damage. Neuropsychologia, 1974, 12, 95-108

Rutter M. Classification and categorization in child psychiatry. Journal of Child Psychology and Psychiatry,1965, 6, 71-83

Rutter M. Brain damage syndromes in childhood: concepts and findings. Journal of Child Psychology and Psychiatry, 1977, 18, 1-21

Rutter M. Introduction: Concepts of brain dysfunction syndromes. In Rutter M (Ed.). Developmental Neuropsychiatry. New York: Guilford, 1983

Rutter M, Graham P, & Yule W. A Neuropsychiatric Study in Childhood. Clinics in Developmental Medicine Nos. 35/36. London: Heinemann Medical Books, 1970

Shafer SQ, Shaffer D, O'Connor PA, & Stokman CJ. Hard thoughts on neurological "soft signs." In Rutter M (Ed.). Developmental Neuropsychiatry. New York: Guilford Press, 1983

Shaffer D, O'Connor PA, Shafer SP, & Prupis S. Neurological "soft signs:" Their origins and significance for behaviour. In Rutter M (Ed.). Developmental Neuropsychiatry. New York: Guilford, 1983

Szatmari P, & Taylor DC. Overflow movements and behaviour problems scoring and using a modificaton of Fog's test. Developmental Medicine and Child Neurology, 1984, 26, 297-310

Taylor EA. Measurement issues. In Rutter M (Ed.). Developmental Neuropsychiatry. New York: Guilford, 1983

Taylor EA. Subclassification and diagnosis. In Taylor EA (Ed.). The Overactive Child. Oxford: SIMP/Blackwell, 1985

Touwen B. Neurological Development in Infancy. Clinics in Developmental Medicine No. 58. London: SIMP/Heinemann, 1976

Touwen B. Examination of the Child with Minor Neurological Dysfunction (2nd Ed.). Clinics in Developmental Medicine No. 71. London: SIMP/Heinemann, 1979

Weintraub S, & Mesulam M-M. Developmental learning disabilities of the right hemisphere: emotional, interpersonal and cognitive components. Archives of Neurology, 1983, 40, 463-468

Werry JS. Studies on the hyperative child: IV. An empirical analysis of the minimal brain dysfunction syndrome. Archives of General Psychiatry, 1968, 19, 9-16

Yule W. Developmental psychological assessment. Advances in Biological Psychiatry, 1978, 1, 35-45

Yule W. The epidemiology of child psychopathology. In Lahey BB, & Kazdin AE (Eds.). Advances in Clinical Child Psychology (Vol. 4). New York: Plenum, 1981

Perry C. Goldstein
David E. Tupper

3

Quantitative and Qualitative Measurement of Subtle Neurobehavioral Deficit

The topic of soft neurological signs has generated a plethora of debate, and studies supporting or rejecting varying hypotheses concerning their significance. This chapter will review some basic issues concerning recurrent difficulties in the measurement and definition of soft signs, as well as problems in determining the relationship of "soft signs" to other objective external criteria.

Many of the controversies surrounding the study of soft signs frequently involve criteria for diagnosis; what constitutes the presence or absence of a soft sign? Diagnosis of any disease or trait usually assumes unique, separate, and orthogonal categories (Skinner, 1981). Rutter, Graham, and Yule (1970) define the presence or absence of neurological abnormalities based upon specific performance on a variety of neurological and psychometric measures. The Rutter et al (1970) study was the first attempt to more clearly define what was then referred to as minimal brain dysfunction (MBD). These authors demonstrated the great heterogeneity of soft or ambiguous neurological findings in children. Rutter et al (1970) suggested three distinct types of soft neurological signs:

1. Signs associated with developmental immaturity or delay, which dissipate with age (e.g., motor incoordination, speech, and language delays). These signs are typically defined in relation to chronological age norms.

SOFT NEUROLOGICAL SIGNS
ISBN 0-8089-1841-9

2. Unusual or irregular findings from the clinical neurological examination (e.g., mild asymmetries in muscle tone or reflexes). These signs are not severe enough to warrant consideration as a definite abnormality.
3. Finally, there are signs, such as strabismus, which result from physical causes *other than* cortical damage.

The heterogeneity and ambiguity of soft signs led a United States task force to criticize their use as a diagnostic entity (Clements, 1966). The ascribed significance of soft signs is often based upon the assumption that these findings are the *direct* result of damage (e.g., structural, chemical, metabolic, or electrophysiologic) to the central nervous system.

DIAGNOSTIC ISSUES

Certain types of diagnostic enterprises more readily lend themselves to standard assessment techniques, development of cut-off scores, and standard criteria; these usually involve physical diseases. For example, a symptom cluster consisting of headache, fever, swollen lymph glands, general malaise, and hoarseness strongly suggest a streptococcal throat infection. This is easily testable by microscopic evaluation of throat cultures. The presence of specific, unique, well-defined organisms confirms the diagnosis and suggests a specific treatment strategy. In this case, a specific set of symptoms predict the presence of a unique disease entity. These symptoms may be considered *pathognomonic signs* of this infection. Pathognomonic signs are simple, specific, observable and replicable findings that indicate the presence of a specific disease in nearly 100 percent of cases. Another example of a pathognomonic sign is the presence of an expressive aphasia in a right-handed adult. This sign will predict the presence of an anterior, left hemisphere cortical brain lesion in 90-95 percent of all people. Further examination by CT scan, magnetic resonance imaging, angiography, or brain electrical activity mapping may reveal the specific etiology of this behavioral sign. In general, discrete disease entities produce specific pathognomonic signs.

Syndromes are different from disease states, although they too represent clusters of observations or test findings that occur together. A syndrome, unlike a disease, may result from a variety of different causes. Hence, syndromes are nonspecific and generally diagnosed by behavioral criteria, while pathognomonic signs are highly specific in predicting individual disease states. Additional discussions of the specificity of test measures will follow in sections on measurement.

A common syndrome often diagnosed by many health care professionals is Organic Brain Syndrome. According to the Third Edition of the *Diagnostic and Statistical Manual* (DSM-III) of the American Psychiatric Association, this syndrome requires the presence of a cluster of symptoms including disorganization in thinking and memory and alterations in sensory-perceptual processes not associated with psychiatric disorder (APA, 1980). These symptoms may result from a variety of etiologies including tumor, trauma, infection, vascular disease, or metabolic disorder. Hence, this symptom cluster is not specific for a unique disease state. We may also consider soft signs or MBD as a group of syndromes or clusters of behaviors that tend to occur together. Soft signs measure a multifactorial and heterogeneous neurobehavioral syndrome, rather than a specific or unique disease state. Consequently, we suggest that the most parsimonious strategy for the scientific study of soft signs involves a multivariate approach to data collection and analysis. Further, a taxonomy of soft sign findings with subtyping of clusters and identification of relationships to external criteria could allow for significant advances in this area. Adams (1985) presents a model for taxonomic approaches relevant for soft signs. Before attempting data analysis for any classification system, Adams (1985) suggests careful evaluation of all measures in terms of quantitative and qualitative aspects of the following parameters:

1. Relationship of the variable to known effects of brain damage or injury.
2. Relationship of the measure to known paths of development or theoretical developmental frameworks.
3. Relationship of the variable to more general experimental psychology concepts of the construct being measured.
4. Evidence for the reliability of the measure in the broadest sense.
5. Evidence for the validity of the variable in the widest sense.

A taxonomic approach provides some advantages. Rather than seeking a unitary or homogeneous set of soft signs (which appears quite unlikely), this methodology provides a system by which specific patterns of findings may be related to specific patterns of neurodiagnostic findings or outcome measures. A more detailed description of this methodology is beyond the scope of this chapter. However, such an approach relies upon an understanding and applications of traditional assessment and measurement techniques.

GENERAL ASSESSMENT AND MEASUREMENT ISSUES

Assessment involves the collection of data across a variety of domains; in the case of soft signs, these are neurobehavioral domains. As previously described, soft signs can include a variety of behaviors characterized by motor, sensory, cognitive, attention, language, memory, and other deficits. In addition, as the following chapters demonstrate, soft signs are also associated with a variety of concurrent neurological, psychiatric or emotional disorders. Therefore, in order to completely *assess* subtle deficits, one should include measures representing at least those domains listed above. This corresponds to criteria #1 and #2 listed by Adams (1985) for taxonomic approaches. This information may be collected by a combination of qualitative and quantitative measures. In fact, there is ample evidence that standard, statistical analyses of information obtained by both *clinical techniques* and *objective test data* significantly improve predictive validity over the exclusive use of either data collection technique alone (Sawyer, 1966). It is therefore important to collect clinical and objective data across a variety of neurobehavioral domains included under the rubric of soft signs.

QUANTITATIVE ASSESSMENT

Reliability

The importance of adequate assessment across all relevant domains is the foundation for traditional measurement theory; including reliability. Reliability is largely a function of sampling. When we speak of measuring traits or constructs such as soft signs or neurobehavioral dysfunction, there are two primary sampling domains that should be considered. The sampling of test items or content areas is generally associated with the reliability of a given test instrument. This is sometimes confused with the term *internal validity*, which is a misnomer, since validity largely depends upon adequate sampling of the population(s) to which test results will be applied. In other words, reliability concerns the sampling characteristics of the measure itself. Conversely, validity concerns the ability to generalize predictions or classifications made with a given test instrument from one population to other populations (Nunnally, 1978). Although reliability and validity appear independent, they are also closely interwoven. A necessary condition for high validity involves high reliability. For reasons to be discussed later, a measure having a low reliability coefficient will insure poor validity when attempting to utilize test measures for diagnosis and prediction.

Reliability concerns the relationship between scores actually made on a test and hypothetical "true" scores that would be made if all possible test items in the domain(s) of interest had been administered. Statistically, reliability represents the correlation of obtained scores with "true" scores, usually described as a Pearson moment correlation.

The *domain sampling model* postulates an infinite number of possible test scores or items within any domain. The model predicts that the greatest reliability estimates may be obtained by randomly selecting smaller subsets of items from the domain of interest. In actual practice, tests or test items are rarely selected randomly; they are usually selected for use based upon prior qualitative observations. However, high reliability estimates may still be obtained in actual practice if: (1) there are a wide variety of items used to assess each domain and (2) multiple attributes or domains are equally represented in number of test items, within larger test batteries (Nunnally, 1978).

Soft signs represent a variety of neurobehavioral domains including motor, sensory, cognitive, language, and other functions. Measurement theory would predict that the most reliable test of soft signs should include a random sample of items measuring each domain of behavior associated with soft signs. The domain sampling model views a test as a random sample of items and a test battery as a sample of tests. We may view a test battery as a series of unique, homogeneous tests constructed to assess a variety of heterogeneous abilities. Test batteries do not usually represent random samples of items; they are selected on the basis of desired application and generalizations (validity). It follows that a reliable measure of motor strength *alone* or coordination *alone* may not be a reliable measure of subtle neurobehavioral deficit, since we have already determined that soft signs represent a heterogeneous syndrome of behavioral findings. However, clusters of coordination measures taken together may be reliable measures for that particular behavioral category. To review, a convenient method to increase reliability of soft sign measures involves adequate sampling of test items across all relevant domains of interest.

In clinical practice, there is frequently a need to sacrifice reliability for brevity and economy of test administration. Clinicians should be weary of the reliability of abbreviated or shortened versions of standard test measures. The reliability of any test (including rating scales) *declines* when the number of test items is decreased. Similarly, reliability will invariably increase when test items are added. The quantitative effect, on reliability, of lengthening or shortening tests may be obtained from the Spearman-Brown formula (Anastasi, 1982; Nunnally, 1978).

In cases where brief tests or test batteries are essential, *factor analysis* provides a standard method for obtaining a smaller set of items that are representative of the domain of interest. Factor analysis is a correlation technique that groups items according to their shared or common variance. A standard procedure during new test construction involves factor analyzing scores of a large set of potential test items. These items are then examined for their loadings (shared variance) across the derived factors (groups of interrelated items). Only items with the highest factor loadings are then selected from each factor, thereby condensing the total item pool, while maintaining a representative sample of items. This standard procedure is far superior to the common practice of simply shortening longer tests or rating scales for rapid clinical applications. Rie, Rie, Stewart, and Rettemnier (1978) have provided the first known factor analysis of soft sign items (see also Chapters 2 and 8). Using a group of 80 children with learning difficulties, the authors identified 6 different factors in a soft sign battery; these included a general broad-range ability factor, verbal-motor and visuo-motor integration factors, and age, sex, and hyperactivity factors. While these factors may not be replicated in other populations, this is the type of study that is sorely needed, but often absent in the soft sign literature.

Increasing the number of test items is sometimes confused with increasing the number of persons assessed with a test instrument. While increasing test items will increase reliability, administering the same set of test items to a greater number of people will have no effect upon the reliability. We can demonstrate this point through the use of a standard pair of dice. The probability of occurrence of a given number may be considered equivalent to the reliability estimate of obtaining that score. The probability of obtaining any number on any given roll of the dice always remains constant, as long as the same set of die (test items) are used, independent of the number of throws or the number of people (tests) throwing the die. However, if the die are altered to include only one, two, and three, the probability (or reliability) increases significantly for the numbers two, three, four, five, and six. However, this increased probability will remain constant across all who may role the die. Hence, administering a test of low reliability to a large group of people will not increase the statistical significance of the test itself or its ability to predict external correlates.

Reliability is also increased when a wide distribution of difficulty levels (probability of a scorable response) are included among the test items. Simply put, there should be an equivalent number of easy and difficult test items within each test and between tests in any soft signs battery. Without a wide range of test difficulty, a condition known as *restriction of range* occurs. Restriction of range decreases reliability and validity by reducing the available true variance of a test (Nunnally, 1978).

Compiling test items or batteries that are objective and easily quantified is also essential for reliable tests by reducing *measurement* or *random error*. While quantification is important, direct observation is not always essential and at times may be impractical. For example, what do we quantify when measuring temperature? Temperature is a *hypothetical construct*; we cannot observe it directly. We observe the effect of temperature upon an *intervening variable*, namely mercury placed inside a thermometer. Prior observations suggested that "heat" or increased temperature causes many materials to expand. Mercury was chosen as an intervening variable for temperature because it expands in a regular and consistent manner. A rise or fall of one degree (or one kilocalorie of heat) consistently results in a one millimeter rise or fall in a thermometer, assuming the altitude of measurement remains constant (we will address the importance of altitude later). Neurological dysfunction measured by soft signs may similarly be considered a hypothetical construct, characterized by a variety of unusual or "abnormal" behaviors (intervening variable) (MacCorquodale & Meehl, 1948). We do not measure neurological dysfunction directly with soft signs; various motor, sensory, and congnitive functions are measured and said to reflect neurobehavioral status.

An important characteristic of all intervening variables is that they can be accurately and reliably measured. Once reliability is established, a valid and predictive measure of other external events can be constructed. For example, a temperature of 32° F or 0° C (at sea level) consistently predicts *certain* external events, such as water freezing. If the temperature, as measured by mercury, were not reliable, we could not safely say that water would freeze or snow would fall at 0° C; sometimes these events might occur, while at other times they might not. It is for this reason that the reliability of any measure sets the upper limit of validity for that same measure (Anastasi, 1982; Nunnally, 1978). It should also be noted that while a highly reliable measure may have high validity for predicting certain external criteria, it will not be uniformly valid for all purposes. The thermometer may be able to predict when water will freeze but the relative height of mercury cannot predict the likelihood of future cold weather. Altitude, in this case, may be considered a moderating variable (discussed in later sections) that alters the rate at which temperature change occurs due to decreased density of air at higher altitudes and increased density at lower altitudes. However, while the energy required to cause a one degree change may increase at higher altitudes, a one degree change at high or low altitudes represents the same change in temperature. The analogy used above represents an ideal case of a perfectly reliable and valid measure.

Unfortunately, behavioral measures are much less precise and reliable. As a result, consumers of behavioral measures or psychometric tests should be specific in determining the type of reliability or validity that is necessary to accomplish their desired goal. Cronbach (1970) suggests that we ask the following questions: "How valid is this test for the decision I wish to make or how valid is the interpretation I propose for the test?" The same questions may be posed for the use of reliability indexes.

Types of Reliability

Test-retest reliability is the correlation between the scores obtained by the same persons on two administrations of the same test. When test-retest reliability is reported, a crucial aspect that needs to be considered is the interval between test administration, since correlations tend to decrease progressively as this interval lengthens. There are a number of possible retest reliability estimates for any test, varying by the retest interval. The types of intervening experiences between test administrations need to be reported for persons participating in the initial reliability study. Most retest reliabilities reported for soft sign assessments usually involve intervals of days to weeks, since longer intervals will likely involve significant developmental changes that will lower the reliability estimate. In fact, the stability or reliability of soft signs over an 8 week period appeared questionable in 1 prior study (McMahon & Greenberg, 1977). However, the likelihood of significant practice effects is higher with shorter test-retest intervals, especially on cognitive tests of reasoning, comprehension, or problem solving requiring a single answer. Of all abilities, sensory discrimination and motor tests are typically least affected by practice effects from repeated test administration. Finally, in addition to specifying intervals between administrations, if two or more retests are planned the intervals should be identical in order to control for the same degree of maturational changes and intervening events between tests (Anastasi, 1982). This is especially important when performing longitudinal studies of soft signs in young children. While significant cognitive and sensory-motor changes are likely to occur over a 10-year period, these changes reflect a variety of other factors unrelated to the test characteristics. Retest reliability estimates on the order of 1 or 2 weeks generally provide a good index of measurement error related to the test itself. The issue of error due to examiner variability must also be considered when rating scales are used as measures.

Alternate form reliability is the correlation between scores obtained on parallel forms of a given test. Alternate forms of tests provide one means of avoiding the confound of practice effects in longitudinal studies. However, this reliability coefficient is influenced by both temporal and item sampling factors. As discussed above, time between alternate form administrations will affect reliability. More importantly, adequate item or content sampling will insure higher reliability estimates (Anastasi, 1982). This type of reliability is most important in aptitude and achievement testing, although it is also relevant for assessment of soft signs.

Split-half reliability is obtained by computing the correlation between two-halves (odd versus even items) of a single test administration, corrected for the number of items. Since test-retest and alternate form reliabilities are calculated on all test items, lower split-half reliabilities would consistently be obtained without an adjustment for the number of total items, as outlined in our prior discussion. The Spearman-Brown formula may also be used to compute split-half reliability (Anastasi, 1982).

Interitem consistency is another method for determining reliability from a single test administration. Use of this method assumes that the test measures a unitary or homogeneous construct. The greater the homogeneity of test items, the greater will be the internal consistency estimates. For tests with dichotomous responses (right or wrong) the "Kuder-Richardson formula 20" may be used to calculate this index. For tests with multiple choice or multiple rating alternatives, internal consistency is determined by coefficient alpha (Anastasi, 1982; Ebel, 1965). This type of reliability is probably most important in evaluating individual components of soft signs batteries, but not the entire heterogeneous battery.

Due to a heavy reliance upon rating scales for assessment of soft signs, *interrater* or *scorer reliability* is an extremely important form of reliability. The most common form of rating scale used for soft signs are Likert-type ratings. For these types of rating scales, items are selected on the basis of internal consistency (to assess homogeneous traits and applications to external criteria). Individual ratings are usually expressed in terms of degree of deficit along the behavior of interest. A typical Likert scale uses ratings from 1 to 5, although scales with 3 or 4 possible ratings may yield higher reliability estimates due to decreased potential for confusion between points. Frequent problems encountered when using rating scales include the following: (1) *error of central tendency*, the tendency to place persons in the middle of the scale in order to avoid extreme positions; (2) *leniency error* is the reluctance of raters to assign impaired ratings; and (3) the *halo effect* is the tendency for raters to be strongly influenced by a superior score on one trait or item resulting in similar ratings across unrelated items (Wiggins, 1980). Many of these difficulties can be minimized by providing easily defined *anchor points.* Anchors are criteria needed in order to achieve a given rating (e.g., no abnormality = 0). Significant improvements in reliability are typically associated with anchors provided for each rating point, rather than only two anchors typically found at the extreme ends of rating scales.

An additional consideration in developing or using soft sign rating scales is whether *time sampling* or *event sampling* is the method of observation. Time sampling involves recording of specific behaviors at predetermined times and specific interval lengths. Event sampling emphasizes elicitation of the behavior of interest in a controlled setting. Event sampling approaches appear best suited for soft sign assessment. Time sampling techniques are likely to ignore natural sequences of ongoing behavior and often provide limited observation periods. Time sampling techniques may not provide adequate samples of behavior for assessment of soft signs.

Soft sign ratings can be significantly improved by training raters. A number of studies have demonstrated marked increases in reliability and validity of ratings following training programs (Landy & Farr, 1980). A convenient training method involves the production of a series of videotapes (we suggest 20-30), as a means of providing standardized situations for groups of raters. Trainees may compare ratings to a "master" key, discuss disagreements together, and review specific aspects of the evaluation where disagreements occurred. Review and ratings of ten assessments should provide ample training experience. Additional interviews, independent of the training sessions, should then be used to compute interrater reliability estimates. In order to maintain strong agreement between raters, periodic retraining or probe sessions should be scheduled on a regular basis. A common phenomenon is called *rating drift*, when raters slowly alter criteria for specific scores due to fading memories of anchors learned in training sessions. Three-month intervals between probe sessions are usually sufficient to prevent significant drift. Yet, the effects of drift and use of unstable anchor points have not been reported in soft signs literature.

The *kappa coefficient* (Cohen, 1960; 1968) is the best known index of agreement (reliability) for use with nominal or ordinal rating scales. This correlation coefficient represents an equivalent to alternate-form reliability for magnitude-scaled data. Kappa is computed for agreement between *two* observers. The *intraclass correlation* is used to calculate degree of correspondence between multiple raters or ratings (Cronbach, Gleser, Nanda, & Rajaratnam, 1972; Lahey, Downey, & Saal, 1983). Unfortunately, a recent review (Shafer, Shaffer, O'Conner, & Stokman, 1983) indicated that only *one* soft sign study was found reporting a kappa coefficient. In this study, Quitkin, Rifkin, and Klein (1976) found perfect agreement on 9 of 16 signs, across 25 patients, with a significant kappa in 10 of 11 signs reported by at least 1 examiner. This study suggested that high levels of agreement are possible, but need to be documented. While high interrater reliability is necessary for valid generalizations from data, it is not sufficient in and of itself.

Percentage of agreement measures, such as those above, depend upon the frequency, or *base rate* of the measured behavior in the sample assessed, as well as the congruence between raters (Meehl, 1973). Base rate or the prevalence of any sign or symptom within a population tends to cause *threshold changes* between institutions or clinical populations. Threshold differences are similar to rater differences, except they represent interinstitution differences. For example, all raters within clinic A and clinic B may demonstrate high interrater reliabilities, as measured by kappa. Let us suppose, however, that clinic A has a soft sign prevalence of only 20 percent, while clinic B has a prevalence of 80 percent. The rating criteria within clinic B may be less conservative or more liberal relative to clinic A.

In other words, incidence and prevalence data of *rated* symptoms may vary significantly between institution due to variance in population, training, expertise or experience between the two staffs, but not due to low interrater reliability (Fleiss, 1981; Meehl, 1954). Such problems were clearly illustrated in the Collaborative Perinatal Project (Nichols & Chen, 1981). The incidence of soft signs across 14 different institutions showed great variability, while consistently high levels of agreement were found within each institution. Just as improved training increases interrater reliability, the use of standard rating criteria, standard assessment batteries, and training videotapes *across* institutions could serve to reduce this problem in the future. At present, this likely accounts for the great deal of variability reported across soft sign studies. For this reason, we suggest that rating scales be reserved for assessment of emotional or psychiatric status, rather than neurological signs that are better measured by objective or psychometric tests.

Application of Test Reliability

As mentioned previously, the most important type of reliability for clinical or research applications depends upon the intended use of the measure. For example, a soft sign assessment battery may have low split-half reliability or a nonsignificant coefficient alpha. This situation may be acceptable, especially since soft signs represent a set of heterogeneous behaviors. However, test-retest and interrater reliability may be crucial if repeated measures of rating scales are being considered.

It should now be clear to the reader that a 10-15 minute "quick and dirty" soft sign assessment battery may be economical, but will likely "muddy" the waters. It is unlikely that such limited or abbreviated batteries can adequately assess most behaviors, in a reliable fashion, considered under the heading of soft signs. If such batteries were redefined as measures of the behavior they assess, rather than tests of subtle neurobehavioral deficit, much potential confusion could be avoided in both clinical and research settings.

Validity

Insuring that a test measures what it is supposed to measure involves the general notion of validity. Inferences, predictions, and generalizations made from test scores generally fall under this heading. Clinically, validity refers to the *meaningfulness* of test results in relation to diagnosis and treatment. As with reliability, validity should not be reported in global terms; validity must be established for the particular application of a test. Hence, one measure may have a number of validity coefficients associated with its use. In principal, procedures for establishing validity determine correlations between test scores and other *independently observable* events or behaviors assumed to be related to test performances. Validity coefficients can also be expressed in the form of expectancy tables giving probabilities for criterion performance, based upon a test score (Anastasi, 1982).

In order to improve the validity of tests (assuming high reliability) adequate sampling of people or populations is required. If this is not possible, it is important to qualify the reported validity estimates by carefully documenting the characteristics of the validation sample. Restriction of range is one effect of inadequate sampling techniques. This is similar to the case where a homogeneous item pool is used to assess a heterogeneous trait. For validity, restriction of range involves preselected or narrow groups of subjects on which a test may be used for selection or predicitive purposes. For example, it is well known that many aptitude tests cannot predict success of medical students or graduate students of post-bachelor programs. However, these aptitude tests continue to be successfully administered as selection tools. While they may be efficient at selecting successful candidates from the general population, they are not equally valid for predicting success within a preselected population of persons already admitted to these programs. The general population represents a heterogeneous group with a wide range of variability (on tests), while the admitted sample is quite homogeneous, with similar aptitude test scores and little interindividual variation. A different test would be needed, with greater variability between subjects, in order to predict success among those admitted.

Similar difficulties may arise in developing a general soft sign *screening* battery, versus assessment of soft signs among a preselected clinic population. Correlations between soft signs and other criteria (e.g., psychiatric disturbance, school achievement, social skills) are likely to be small and nonsignificant in a clinic population, but large and highly significant from an unselected elementary school sample (Nunnally, 1978). Restriction of range is also related to the issue of base rates discussed previously. An extremely high (90 percent) or extremely low (10 percent) base rate of any given symptom or diagnosis among a population is equivalent to a homogeneous, restricted range of potential scores on a test. Therefore, in these situations, validity coefficients (correlations between test scores and external criteria) will be low. In practical terms, the use of tests in such situations may not be helpful for either diagnostic or treatment purposes. It might be just as efficient and accurate to diagnose all cases as having the trait with a 90 percent base rate and never diagnosing a trait when the base rate is 10 percent.

The degree to which tests improve prediction is called *incremental validity* and is greatest when the base rate is near 50 percent. Incremental validity can be calculated when the base rate, selection ratio, and validity coefficient are known (Anastasi, 1982). Incremental validity and the efficiency of tests are also related to sensitivity and specificity (discussed in following sections).

The form of the relationship between a test and external criterion will also influence the validity coefficient. The Pearson correlation coefficient assumes a linear, uniform relationship or homoscedasticity throughout the range of scores. In certain situations, it is possible that variability in the criterion will be greater in some ranges and smaller in other ranges; this is referred to as heteroscedasticity. For example, low scores on an aptitude test may uniformly predict poor school achievement. High scores may not predict high achievement if students achieving high scores are divided into motivated and unmotivated groups.

Motivation is one type of *moderator variable* that can influence the validity of any test. Moderator variables are considered personal characteristics that decrease validity coefficients among subgroups of the population. For example, a given test may be a better predictor for men versus women or lower versus higher socioeconomic subjects. A relatively simple means of avoiding the influence of a moderator variable is the use of tests validated on similar populations (e.g., male versus female; low versus high SES).

Whereas moderator variables may decrease validity, *criterion contamination* artificially inflates validity coefficients. Criterion contamination is the case where test scores (independent variable) are part of or influence position on the criterion (dependent variable) directly. For example, if we wished to shorten an extensive soft signs battery, one approach might include selecting the hypothesized "crucial" items from the large battery. We might then attempt to correlate scores from our smaller set of critical items with the scores from the initial, larger battery. High correlations would be obtained, suggesting that our subset of items are valid in predicting scores from the larger battery. We have apparently saved hours of valuable time and created a highly valid soft signs battery; but this may not be the case. The abbreviated test is contaminated because it contains *identical* items in the criterion (larger test) that we are attempting to predict, producing spuriously high correlations. A more appropriate method would involve construction of an abbreviated measure totally independent from the criterion test we are attempting to predict and evaluating it in a new sample.

In all cases, *cross-validation* studies should be reported, confirming the stability of the reported validity for any test. Cross-validation simply involves applying a test to predict the same criterion in populations independent from the initial validation study. A significant degree of *shrinkage* usually occurs with cross-validation. Shrinkage refers to the decline in correlation coefficients due to multiple correlations performed on scores from preselected subject samples (Nunnally, 1978).

In addition to test characteristics, the nature of the criterion strongly influences the validity coefficient, especially in concurrent and predictive validity. For example, many soft sign findings have shown no consistent abnormalities on standard neurodiagnostic tests in the past. However, with current technological advances, including electrical brain mapping, regional cerebral blood flow, positron emission tomography, and magnetic resonance imaging, the neurological criterion has improved and thus changed. Future studies will likely produce more significant relationships between behavioral abnormalities and diagnostic tests due to increased sensitivity of the criterion. Finally, while sample size was irrelevant for reliability, larger validation samples increase the predictive power and ultimate validity of most tests.

Types of Validity

Criterion-related validation involves the effectiveness of tests in predicting behavior or traits in specified situations. Concurrent and predictive validity are two types of criterion-related validity important in measurement of soft signs. Concurrent validity usually involves the use of tests for diagnosis of present conditions, and is most relevant for psychiatric and neurological studies. The ability of neuropsychological or behavioral neurology tests to predict the location of brain damage (as assessed by CT scan) is one example of a concurrent validity study. Predictive validity refers to prediction of some future criterion over a time interval. Attempting to predict future psychopathology based upon the incidence of early soft neurological signs is an example of predictive validity. Criterion-related validity should be evaluated on well-defined samples of subjects in which tests are used to predict diagnosis or longitudinal outcome. This form of validity is probably most important when evaluating the clinical usefulness of soft sign assessment.

Content validity examines the test content to insure it adequately samples the behavioral domain of interest. This is more relevant for academic achievement tests. Soft sign batteries, by definition, define their content in relation to traditional neurological signs. However, the issue of what constitutes "soft" neurological signs is another problem related to construct validity.

Construct validity is the degree to which a test measures a theoretical construct or trait. Soft signs present a difficult problem in this respect since they are characterized by a heterogeneous set of symptoms *not necessarily related* to each other. In addition, it is unclear that developmental changes and other requirements for a taxonomic approach to study soft signs have been defined. This is important, since age differentiation, correlations with other hypothetically similar measures, and factor analysis are methods used to demonstrate construct validity. A factor analysis of a soft sign battery will likely yield multiple independent factors, rather than one factor representing soft signs (e.g., Rie et al, 1978). In fact, further study of this issue appears necessary.

A method by which relative interrelatedness of soft signs may be evaluated further is the *multitrait — multimethod matrix* (Campbell & Fiske, 1959). In this model, *convergent validity* is defined as the correlations betwen hypothetically related measures. *Discriminant validity* refers to nonsignificant correlations between hypothetically unrelated or irrelevant measures. Construct validity may be demonstrated by high convergent and discriminant validity. Hence, while certain soft sign measures are likely to correlate with each other, if they also correlate with irrelevant measures they are said to have little discriminant validity. To our knowledge, studies of convergent and discriminant validity of soft signs test batteries have yet to be reported. Criterion-related validity is similar in many ways to the issues of test sensitivity and specificity.

Sensitivity and Specificity

Sensitivity of a test refers to the proportion of individuals with a disorder who show a positive test result. The *specificity* of a test refers to the proportion of people without a disorder who show a negative test result. A related issue is prevalence estimates or base rates, as discussed in prior sections. Prevalence represents all those having a trait, from all persons evaluated. Sensitivity and specificity are stable properties of tests (Buchsbaum & Haier, 1983). As a test becomes less stringent it becomes more likely to pick up more of the disease population (increased sensitivity) but at a cost of greater false positives (decreased specificity). The usefulness of a test result in diagnosis is termed its *predictive value*. The likelihood that a patient with a positive test actually has a disease or trait is the *positive predictive value*. False positives decrease the positive predictive value. The probability of a patient with a negative test result being disease-free or not showing the trait is the *negative predictive value*. False negatives decrease the negative predictive value. The prevalence or base rate of a trait changes the predictive value of tests, but not sensitivity or specificity. It can be demonstrated that predictive value decreases markedly when the prevalence in a new sample is either significantly greater or lower than the validation sample.

In clinical practice, sensitivity and specificity are rarely 100 percent. There will always be a certain degree of false positives and false negatives over time. The consumer of tests must independently decide which type of error is more tolerable, given the application of test results. For example, a high degree of sensitivity, sacrificing specificity may be appropriate for medical tests used to diagnose life-threatening disease, while greater specificity and lower sensitivity may be more acceptable in establishing a psychiatric diagnosis (Diamond & Forrester, 1979; Galen & Gambino, 1975). Presently, many soft sign measures typically demonstrate high sensitivity with low specificity.

We can also view our prior discussion of pathognomonic signs in this light. Pathognomonic signs can be considered one-time tests with reliability and validity coefficients of .99, having sensitivity and specificity estimates of 100 percent. This is the situation for discrete disease states. Yet, soft signs do not appear to represent a discrete, homogeneous entity. For this reason, the search for "the soft sign" may be fruitless.

Norms and Interpretations of Tests

Raw scores from any soft sign test or battery, in the absence of additional data, are quantitatively meaningless. Scores must be interpreted in relation to norms, collected from a representative standardization sample. Raw scores should be converted to derived scores in order to: (1) determine the subject's relative standing among a general or selected population and (2) permit comparisons between tests for the same subject.

The most common derived score is a standard score or *z-score*. These scores are computed by dividing the difference between the raw score and the mean of the normative group by the standard deviation (SD) of the normative sample. Raw scores that are equal to the mean have a z-score of zero. Because z-scores often produce numbers that are awkward to interpret (e.g., negative or positive decimals), a number of *linear transformations* for z-scores are commonly used. Deviation IQs on the Wechsler Scales are one example where IQ = 100 + 15(z). Hence, an IQ of 85 is equivalent to a z-score of -1.0. The T-Score is another transformation defined as: 50 + 10(z).

The use of test scores in a clinical setting best demonstrates the importance of standard scores.

During a case conference at a rehabilitation hospital, a health care professional reported that a 5-year-old boy achieved an "average" score of 90 percent correct on a certain neurodevelopmental test. A second team member disagreed with this finding, noting that the child performed deficiently on a similar test, only in the 20th percentile. A heated debate followed these presentations. Percentiles are another example of a z-score transformation, while percent correct scores are raw scores. Percentiles allow comparison to age peers and comparison between test performances; percent correct scores do not. Percentiles and percent correct scores are therefore not equivalent.

In many cases, consumers of tests also wish to know how "good" is the reliability or validity of a given measure. Reliability estimates of .80 - .95 are considered acceptable. In general, the validity coefficient does not usually exceed the square of the reliability coefficient; reliability sets the upper limit upon validity. For example, if test A has a test-retest reliability of .90, it is unlikely that the validity coefficient will exceed .81. If we wish to use test B, with a test-retest reliability of .80, we may expect a validity coefficient of .64, under the best circumstances. Apparently small differences in reliability coefficients may significantly alter the predictive validity of any test. Alternate methods for empirically determining reliability and validity include the *standard error of measure* and the *standard error of estimate*. These are used to construct confidence intervals (depending upon the desired alpha level) in order to assess the significance of intertest score differences and degree of possible error in predicted criterion scores.

Finally, we wish to emphasize that no one test may be "better" than another in the assessment of neurobehavioral deficits. Certain measures are more valid or reliable for certain applications. Given the heterogeneity of soft signs, multiple measures are likely necessary to achieve reliable and valid assessments (Taylor, 1983). Adherence to the guidelines discussed above provide most prerequisites necessary for a taxonomic study of subtle neurobehavioral deficits, as suggested by Adams (1985).

QUALITATIVE ASSESSMENT

In terms of measurement, Russell (1986) and Rourke and Brown (1986) consider the difference between qualitative and quantitative measurement to be spurious since quality and quantity are very closely related. In fact, since "everything that exists, exists in some quantity" (Russell, 1986), a qualitative measurement approach can be translated into a quantitative one when we realize that a number based approach presupposes qualitative classification. From a purely psychometric point of view, a qualitative measurement is based only on nominal scales rather than the usual interval or ratio scales required for quantitative measurement.

Clinically, however, qualitative examination has been described elegantly by Luria (1980) for adults, although many of his interpretations are based upon clear pathognomonic signs. Qualitative examination may be useful in determining *how* a client approaches a more complex psychological problem (a "process-oriented" approach) but loses its empirical basis when applied to measurement of soft neurological signs. We would argue that qualitative observations are important in evaluating subtle neurobehavioral deficit, but that more focused, well-validated measures are the method of choice both clinically and in research investigating soft sign correlates of neurologic dysfunction.

Once qualitative data is collected, it should be integrated with other quantitative information in some standard fashion. A number of studies have consistently demonstrated that the most efficient and accurate conclusions from behavioral assessments results from integrating both clinical and objective data in a standard fashion (Sawyer, 1966).

One of the methods by which clinical observations can be completed in a standardized fashion is the structured interview. Observations from structured interviews may also be recorded in a consistent manner through the use of a variety of symptom rating scales or behavior checklists. We believe rating scales are best utilized in this capacity; as adjuncts to quantitative data.

Although symptom checklists do not rely upon structured interviews in all cases, they too may provide additional, useful information. This type of information may be frequently ignored, or dismissed as unrelated to the issue of soft sign assessment. However, there is ample evidence to suggest that neurological soft signs are associated with behavioral and cognitive disturbance (Hertzig, 1983; Shaffer, O'Connor, Shafer, et al, 1983; Shaffer, Schonfeld, O'Conner, et al, 1985).

We consider the assessment of personality an important adjunct to any soft sign battery as a measure of behavior tendencies and not necessarily as a pure neurological sign. As an example, a well standardized, multidimensional personality scale for children is the *Personality Inventory for Children-Revised* (PIC) (Lachar, 1982). This instrument is a parental report or rating of observed childhood behaviors designed for caretakers with a sixth grade reading level. This inventory requires true-false responses to 600 questions (abbreviated versions are available). An important consideration in rating personality, as with soft signs, is the heterogeneity and diversity of behavior. This scale is particularly well suited for clinical and research applications for the following reasons: (1) it is a criterion-referenced test, with 12 homogeneous scales, (2) it provides standard scores for within and between child comparisons, (3) it allows multidimensional profile analyses, (4) it demonstrates high internal consistencies *within* each homogeneous scale, and (5) it has high predictive validity to external criteria (Gdowski, Lachar, & Kline, 1985). This tool permits standard evaluation of what many might consider purely qualitative and clinical information. The PIC represents an excellent example of measurement theory applied to problems in obtaining useful "clinical" data. Thus, it is a useful qualitative assessment tool when attempting to measure neurobehavioral deficit.

In cases where soft signs must be assessed by less standardized and clinical methods, we suggest the approach presented by Rutter, Graham, and Yule (1970). This study presents a step by step manual for the assessment of soft signs, including an abbreviated version of the Oseretsky Test of Motor Proficiency. As is the case with most rating scales, however, there are no standard scores reported by Rutter et al. The absence of standard scores makes individual decisions regarding the significance of findings difficult at best. The descriptions provided in their manual do, however, facilitate comparisons of findings in individual cases.

CONCEPTUAL INTEGRATION

Quantitative and qualitative data can provide essential information for the study and treatment of subtle neurobehavioral deficit. However, a persistent problem regarding these data (especially "soft signs") concerns the appropriate means of data interpretation. The heterogeneity and multidetermined nature of soft signs suggest the need for *multivariate* statistical approaches (see also, Tupper & Rosenblood, 1984). In the past, this has also been referred to as a *configural approach* (Meehl, 1954). Specific statistical analytic techniques included under this heading are factor analysis, cluster analysis, canonical correlation, and multiple regression. The basis for these techniques involves discovering relationships between clusters or sets of independent variables and how they can *collectively* predict to an especially multidetermined criteria such as "soft signs." This methodology relies upon sets of independent measures assessing specific behavioral domains; reducing or eliminating the need to speak of soft signs as a general category of behavior. Rather than stating that: "soft signs predict cognitive and psychiatric difficulties," we might say "fine motor incoordination, motor perseveration and tactile sensory impairments" are associated with certain types of psychiatric disorders for children at certain ages with certain family backgrounds. Attempts at defining these more specific relationships might significantly improve the specificity of test findings related to what we now call "soft signs."

The neuropsychological approach conforms to configural or multivariate data analysis, including a variety of reliable measurement tools assessing heterogeneous behavioral and cognitive domains (see Voeller's Extended Neurological Examination in Appendix D). Yet, according to Chadwick and Rutter (1983), the utility of this methodology remains to be demonstrated in the study of soft neurological signs. One consideration neglected by these and other authors involves the possibility that cognitive, neuropsychological and soft sign deficits covary together. In other words, stating that soft signs "predict" certain behavioral problems may not be accurate if research indicates that certain patterns of behavioral, neuropsychological, and soft signs consistently occur together. While current methodology permits such analyses (e.g., by Q-factor analysis and clustering techniques), they have not been applied to the study of soft signs. Issues concerning the construct validity of soft signs may also be resolved with the application of such an approach. Similar diagnostic and classification problems were encountered in recent studies of "dyslexic" and learning impaired children.

Fletcher and Satz (1985) reviewed a series of studies from the Florida Longitudinal Project, which attempted to classify disabled learners into homogeneous groups. A major difficulty encountered in completing these studies involved findings that indicated that children diagnosed as MBD or dyslexic could not be differentiated from other disabled learners with low intelligence, low SES, and other problems. The terms *MBD* and *dyslexia*, similar to soft signs or subtle neurobehavioral deficit, should be considered hypothetical constructs (Rutter, 1974). The great heterogeneity of findings in the Florida Longitudinal Project prevented pure definitions of learning disability. The investigators were forced to derive empirically defined clusters of deficits (based on within subject pattern analysis) and relate common clusters of deficits to specific learning and behavioral problems. The net result of these studies was the description of five separate subtypes of learning impaired children. The subtypes of neuropsychological deficits predicted longitudinal course, showed high internal consistency, and differentially predicted external criteria such as teacher ratings and academic achievement.

Our prior discussions indicated that statistical analysis of both clinical and empirical data significantly improve prediction. We believe data collection methods presented here with multivariate analytic techniques provide exciting alternatives to the study of soft signs. However, rather than discussing soft signs, we suggest measurement, description, and analysis of specific behavioral deficits assessed by reliable and valid instruments. At this time, soft sign measures of subtle neurobehavioral deficit appear to represent a hypothetical construct in need of more specific validation. Intervening variables associated with hypothetical constructs are what we actually measure. A taxonomy of soft signs may best be served by multivariate analyses of intervening variables (Taylor, 1983). Such a taxonomic approach has been applied to the study of learning disabilities, with significant advances in defining subtypes, predicting outcome, and planning remedial programs (Rourke, 1985; Rourke, Bakker, Fisk, et al, 1983). These studies emphasize the use of empirical measures, whether collecting qualitative or quantitative data. In addition, neuropsychological methods in these studies are usually complemented with emotional or personality measures. We believe the same methodology applied to the study of soft signs and other subtle neurobehavioral deficits may produce similar advances.

REFERENCES

Adams KM. Theoretical, methodological and statistical issues. In Rourke B (Ed.). Neuropsychology of Learning Disabilities. New York: Guilford, 1985

American Psychiatric Association. Diagnostic and Statistical Manual of Mental Disorders (3rd ed.). Washington: American Psychiatric Association, 1980

Anastasi A. Psychological Testing. New York: MacMillan, 1982

Buchsbaum MS, & Haier RJ. Psychopathology: biological approaches. Annual Review of Psychology, 1983, 34, 401-430

Campbell DT, & Fiske DW. Convergent and dicriminant validation by the multitrait-multimethod matrix. Psychological Bulletin, 1959, 56, 81-105

Chadwick O, & Rutter M. Neuropsychological assessment. In Rutter M (Ed.). Developmental Neuropsychiatry. New York: Guilford, 1983

Clements SD. Minimal brain dysfunction in children, Monograph No. 3, Bethesda, MD: U.S. National Institute of Neurological Disease and Blindness, 1966

Cohen J. A coefficient of agreement for nominal scales. Educational and Psychological Measurement, 1968, 20, 37-46

Cohen J. Weighted kappa: Nominal scale agreement with provisions for scaled disagreement or partial credit. Psychological Bulletin, 1968, 70, 213-220

Cronbach LJ. Essentials of Psychological Testing (3rd ed.). New York: Harper International Editions, 1970

Cronbach LJ, Gleser G, Nanda H, & Rajaratnam N. The Dependability of Behavioral Measurements: Theory of Generalizability for Scores and Profits. New York: Wiley, 1972

Diamond GA, & Forester JS. Analysis of probability as an aid in the clinical diagnosis of coronary-artery disease. New England Journal of Medicine, 1979, 300, 1350-1358

Ebel RL. Measuring Educational Achievement. Englewood Cliffs, NJ: Prentice Hall, 1965

Fleiss JL. Statistical Methods for Rates and Proportions (2nd ed.). New York: Wiley, 1981

Fletcher JM, & Satz P. Cluster analysis and the search for learning disability subtypes. In Rourke B (Ed.). Neuropsychology of Learning Disabilities. New York: Guilford, 1985

Galen RS, & Gamino SR. Beyond Normality: The Predictive Value and Efficiency of Medical Diagnosis. New York: Wiley, 1975

Gdowski CL, Lachar D, & Kline RB. A PIC profile typology of children and adolescents: 1. Empirically derived alternative to traditional diagnosis. Journal of Abnormal Psychology, 1985, 94, 346-361

Hertzig ME. Temperament and neurological status. In Rutter M (Ed.). Developmental Neuropsychiatry. New York: Guilford, 1983

Lachar D. PersonalityInventory for Children (PIC); Revised Format Manual Supplement. Los Angeles: Western Psychological Services, 1982

Lahey MA, Downey RG, & Saal FE. Intraclass correlations: There's more there than meets the eye. Psychological Bulletin, 1982, 93, 586-595

Landy FJ, & Farr JH. Performance rating. Psychological Bulletin, 1980, 87, 72-107

Luria AR. Higher Cortical Functions in Man (2nd Ed.). New York: Basic

Books, 1980

MacCorquodale K, & Meehl PE. On a distinction between hypothetical constructs and intervening variables. Psychological Review, 1948, 55, 95-107

McMahon SA, & Greenberg LM. Serial neurologic examination of hyperactive children. Pediatrics, 1977, 59, 584-587

Meehl P. Clinical versus Statistical Prediction. Minneapolis: University of Minnesota Press, 1954

Meehl PE. Psychodiagnosis: Selected Papers. Minneapolis, MN: University of Minnesota Press, 1973

Meehl P, & Rosen A. Antecedent probability and the effficiency of psychometric signs, patterns or cutting scores. Psychological Bulletin, 1955, 52, 194-216

Nichols PL, & Chen TC. Minimal Brain Dysfunction: A Prospective Study. Hillsdale, NJ: Erlbaum, 1981

Nunnally JC. Psychometric Theory. New York: McGraw Hill, 1978

Quitkin F, Rifkin A, & Klein DF. Neurologic soft signs in schizophrenia and character disorder. Archives of General Psychiatry, 1976, 33, 845-853

Rie ED, Rie HE, Stewart S, & Rettemnier SC. An analysis of neurological soft signs in children with learning problems. Brain and Language, 1978, 6, 32-46

Rourke BP (Ed.). Neuropsychology of Learning Disabilities: Essentials of Subtype Analysis. New York: Guilford, 1985

Rourke BP, Bakker, DJ, Fisk JL, & Strang JD. (Eds.). Child Neuropsychology: An Introduction to Theory, Research and Clinical Practice. New York: Guilford, 1983

Rourke BP, & Brown GG. Clinical neuropsychology and behavioral neurology: Similarities and differences. In Filskov SB, & Boll TJ (Eds.). Handbook of Clinical Neuropsychology (Vol. 2). New York: Wiley-Interscience, 1986, pp. 3-10

Russell EW. The psychometric foundation of clinical neuropsychology. In Filskov SB, & Boll TJ (Eds.). Handbook of Clinical Neuropsychology (Vol. 2). New York: Wiley-Interscience, 1986, pp. 45-80

Rutter M. Emotional disorder and educational under-achievement. Archives of Diseases in Childhood, 1974, 49, 249-256

Rutter M, Graham P, & Yule W. A Neuropsychiatric Study in Childhood. Clinics in Developmental Medicine, Vol. 35-36. London: Spastics International Medical Publications, 1970

Sawyer J. Measurement and prediction, clinical and statistical. Psychological Bulletin, 1966, 66, 178-200

Shafer SQ, Shaffer D, O'Connor PA, & Stokman CJ. Hard thoughts on neurological "soft signs." In Rutter M (Ed.). Developmental Neuropsychiatry. New York: Guilford, 1983

Shaffer D, O'Connor PA, Shafer SQ, & Prupis S. Neurological "soft signs:" Their origins and significance for behavior. In Rutter M (Ed.). Developmental Neuropsychiatry. New York: Guilford, 1983

Shaffer D, Schonfeld I, O'Connor PA, et al. Neurological soft signs: Their relationship to psychiatric disorder and intelligence in childhood and adolescence. Archives of General Psychiatry, 1985, 42, 342-351

Skinner HA. Toward the integration of classification theory and methods. Journal of Abnormal Psychology, 1981, 90, 68-87

Taylor E. Measurement issues and approaches. In Rutter M (Ed.). Developmental Neuropsychiatry. New York: Guilford, 1983

Tupper DE, & Rosenblood LK. Methodological considerations in the use of attribute variables in neuropsychological research. Journal of Clinical Neuropsychology, 1984, 6, 441-453

Wiggins JS. Personality and Prediciton: Principles of Personality Assessment. Reading, MA: Addison-Wesley, 1980

Margaret E. Hertzig
Theodore Shapiro

4

The Assessment of Nonfocal Neurological Signs in School-Aged Children

There are two views concerning the significance of nonfocal neurological signs (NFNS). The first view seeks to establish regular association between specific and varied disorders of behavior and NFNS. The second view considers the persistent NFNS to be a nonspecific indicator of delayed maturation. The first vantage will be referred to as the *specificity hypothesis*, and the second as the *nonspecific developmental view*. What follows seeks to examine the reasons for these views in the poor uniformity of existing systems of assessment of NFNS. Although it is clear that in general such signs can be readily recognized and reliably elicited in the course of the clinical examination of an individual patient (Quitkin, Rifkin, & Klein, 1976; Rutter, Graham, & Yule, 1970a; Shapiro, Burke, Petti, & Ranz, 1978; Werry, Minde, & Gusman, 1972) both the origin and significance of anatomically nonspecific deviations in motor, sensory, and neuro-integrative functions remains obscure (Rutter, 1982; Rutter et al, 1970a; Shaffer, 1978).

Some investigators have suggested that nonfocal signs represent a direct measure of central nervous system dysfunction, and argue that increased frequency of occurrence of abnormalities of this type in behaviorally disturbed and/or cognitively impaired children is evidence for an "organic" substrate for their disorders (Birch, Richardson, & Baird, 1970; Hertzig & Birch, 1966; Kennard, 1960; Strauss & Lehtinen, 1947). Bender (1947) interpreted the developmental irregularities in the organization of motor functions found in some psychotic children as but another manifestation of the "diffuse encephalopathy affecting every area of patterning in the central

SOFT NEUROLOGICAL SIGNS
ISBN 0-8089-1841-9

nervous system," which, in her view, determined the emergence of symptoms of schizophrenia during childhood. Fish (1977), following the Bender tradition, has argued that nonfocal signs may represent a genetic marker for schizophrenia in a population at risk. Such views, however, are always tempered by consideration of normal maturation of perception and motor development. There is some agreement that one can expect that by age 7 that NFNS elicited earlier will disappear (Shapiro & Perry, 1976). A number of different investigators also have consistently demonstrated a greater frequency of occurrence of nonfocal signs among children with lower IQ (Adams, Kocsis, & Estes, 1974; Bortner, Hertzig, & Birch, 1972; Hertzig, 1982; Rutter et al, 1970a; Stine, Saratsiotis, & Mosser, 1975). In addition, nonfocal signs have been observed to occur (albeit with decreased frequency) in many otherwise normally developing children (Adams et al, 1974; Peters, Romine, & Dykman, 1975; Rutter et al, 1970a; Wolff & Hurwitz, 1966). Rutter (1970a; 1977; 1982) has interpreted this pattern of findings as indicating that nonfocal signs are but another nonspecific manifestation of generalized developmental delay and therefore an unsatisfactory guide to the presence of brain damage.

Reconciliation between these opposing views has been difficult because, to date, *there is no generally accepted wide-range system of pediatric neurological examination* (Werry, 1972; Werry & Aman, 1976). Some investigators and clinicians have restricted assessment to only those functions for which interexaminer reliability is relatively high such as speech, motor coordination, or adventitious motor overflow. Others have expanded consideration to include minor asymetries of tone, muscle strength, or reflex organization that are much more difficult to detect (Rutter et al, 1970a). Rutter (1970a; 1977; 1982), has indicated that the pooling of signs that represent deficits of function characteristic of younger children (right-left discrimination and clumsiness) together with those that may be due to either neurological or nonneurological causes (strabismus and nystagmus) as well as those that are difficult to reliably assess (asymmetries and equivocal Babinski responses) can only lead to confusion. The confusion introduced by lack of uniformity in the selection of what is to be examined is further augmented by the fact that different investigators and clinicians utilize different techniques of examination.

Despite this generally pessimistic picture, a good deal is known about the neurological assessment of the school-aged child. Child neurologists, psychiatrists, and pediatricians, as well as psychometricians and educators have all addressed the problem from their respective clinical and research perspectives. In the subsequent sections of this chapter we shall review representative examples of approaches to assessment. Our discussion will include a consideration of purpose, theoretical principles underlying the selection of particular items, procedures for examination and scoring, as well as issues of reliability and validity, in order to finally define the requirements of an effective clinical and research tool.

Although some neurologists have categorically dismissed concern over the clinical significance of nonfocal signs as indicative only of "soft thinking" (Ingram, 1973) on the part of "soft neurologists" (Barlow, 1974), others (Kennard, 1960) have puzzled over their utility in diagnosis ever since the turn of the century when routine neurological examination was first established. The standard neurological assessment requires that the examiner systemically evaluates the following areas of function: mental status and orientation, speech and language organization, intactness of cranial nerves, sensory organization, reflexes, directed and voluntary movement, muscle strength and tone, and motor coordination. The criteria for designating abnormality are those developed by each clinician in the course of his or her education and experience. In addition, individual clinicians also have developed idiosyncratic lists of deviations from normal expectations that, if present, cause them to suspect neuropathology.

For example Strauss (Strauss & Lehtinen, 1947) offers the following list of "Valuable Neurologic Signs for the Diagnosis of a Lesion in the Central Nervous System" (p. 110).

Solitary Signs
- Babinski sign pure (dorsal-extension of great toe with plantar flexion of the other toes)
- Paralysis of cranial nerves III, IV, VI, VII, XII.

Combined signs (valuable only when two or more are noted)
- Pupils: light reflex sluggish or absent
- Nystagmus, especially when unilateral
- Adiadochokinesis
- Mayer's and Leri's signs absent unilaterally
- Oppenheim's sign
- Babinski sign, modified (dorsal-extension of the great toe with reflex or fan reflex alone)
- Increase or decrease of deep or cutaneous reflexes especially when unilateral.

By contrast, Kennard (1960) directed attention to the following list of nonfocal abnormalities: visual acuity, extraocular muscle dysfunction, tremor, left sided dominance, left-right confusion, auditory impairment, intention tremor, reflex asymmetry, athetoid movements, speech deficit, hyperkinesis, adiadochokinesis, graphesthesia, equivocal Babinski sign, nystagmus, tics or grimacing, pupiliary responses, and whirling.

Although some items appear on both lists (i.e., extraocular muscle dysfunction, Babinski signs, adiadochokinesis, pupillary responses, and reflex asymmetry), it is remarkable that two workers, utilizing essentially the same instrument, i.e., the clinical neurological examination, could direct attention to such widely different indicators of abnormality or deviance. Yet all of the items listed by Strauss and all but one listed by Kennard (the whirling response, which was initially described by Lauretta Bender) are a routine part of clinical neurological assessment.

Paine and Oppe (1966) directly address the problem of selection in their discussion of the clinical neurological examination of children. These workers have provided a conceptual framework within which the observations of individual clinicians may be organized. They have developed an examination designed for use by pediatric neurologists, who may be required to evaluate children with gross impairments of motor function as well as intellectual retardation, learning problems, and behavioral disorder. Paine and Oppe (1966) point out that the purpose of the neurological examination is to test cerebral function, and that the testable facets of cerebral function include motor activity, mental ability (thought and learning), cortical blindness or deafness, and epilepsy respectively. They also admit to subclinical abnormalities in each area: i.e., general awkwardness; borderline or noncertifiable mental retardation or irregularities in the ability to learn; perceptual abnormalities; and EEG abnormalities without actual seizures. Clinical and subclinical abnormalities in the different spheres of cerebral function potentially exist in any combination, the number of permutations running into the hundreds. As a consequence each affected child will be in some way different from every other.

Thus, these clinicians outline a neurological examination that provides for the identification of subclinical abnormalities in motor, mental, and sensory functions. Coordination is tested along with the presence of adventitious and associated movements; and higher cerebral functions such as short-term memory and recall, various linguistic functions, perception of design, gnosis, praxis, concept of body image, concept of extracorporeal space, directional orientation, right-left orientation, abstraction, and cerebral inhibition also are described. Guidelines for interpreting the findings against chronologic and mental age are found throughout their presentation. These clinicians believe that testing higher cerebral functions in some depth will often be diagnostically useful, "although a directly treatable cerebral lesion is seldom found ... and the diagnosis is usually left as 'chronic brain syndrome' due to whatever cause is presumed and manifested by a listing of disproportionate deficits as compared with overall intellectual ablility as measured by IQ." (Paine & Oppe, 1966, pp. 66-67). "In making the diagnosis of chronic brain syndrome, the physician depends on the association of a number of minimal abnormal findings with (commonly) a history of past insult to the cerebrum" (p. 84).

Thus, in this clinical approach to neurological assessment, diagnosis is not restricted to findings on physical examination alone, but is the result of the clinician's integration of data deriving from both history and clinical examination.

As clinicians, Paine and Oppe (1966) did not focus on the reliability of their proposed examination schedule, nor were they very concerned with the problem of the validity, except as the requirement of consistency between history and physical findings may be considered to reflect an aspect of validation. The proposed system is a clinical examination for use by clinicians in the diagnosis and management of individual cases. Nevertheless, thay have advanced a number of principles against which both the proposed intent of a neurological appraisal and the interpretation of findings can be assessed.

1. Item selection must be broad-based and insure the identification of possible abnormality or dysfunction.
2. The designation of performance on any given item as abnormal must occur within a developmental context.
3. The designation of neurological impairment requires a number of abnormal findings. Single deviations should be interpreted conservatively.
4. As abnormalities in the different spheres of cerebral function (motor, sensory, mental/cognitive) may potentially occur in any combination it is to be expected that children designated as neurologically abnormal will exhibit widely different patterns of deviancy.

Following on this more general examination several different groups of investigators (Birch, Richardson, Baird, et al, 1970; Bortner et al, 1972; Hertzig, 1982; Hertzig & Birch, 1966; Hertzig et al, 1969; Rutter et al, 1970a; Rutter, Tizard, & Whitmore, 1970b), have all adapted aspects of the clinical neurological examination to particular research situtions.

Rutter, Graham, and Yule (1970a) have described an examination to be used in a psychiatric clinic to detect those children requiring further neurological study. However, it was specifically developed as an epidemiologic instrument to study the associations between education, health, and behavior conducted on the Isle of Wight (Rutter et al, 1970b). These workers directed their primary attention to the development of a reliable procedure for neurological assessment. The schedule followed the standard format of a clinical examination and provided for the assessment of cranial signs, coordination, power and tone of limbs, and reflex organization as well as laterality, constructional ability, limb dyspraxia, and speech and mirror movements (Table 4-1).

Test-retest reliability (Rutter et al, 1970a) was conceptualized as reflecting both of the following: (1) comparability between different examiners with respect to administration and scoring and (2) stability in the performance of subjects over time. Two examiners jointly evaluated a series of children to insure correspondence between methods of eliciting signs and application of scoring criteria. Children were then reexamined at intervals ranging from 1 day to 1 month. The results with respect to individual items are presented in Table 4-1. If 90 percent is accepted as a satisfactory level of test-retest agreement, this level was achieved over all scale points for only the following items: nystagmus, side-to-side movements of the tongue, power of both upper and lower limbs, and foot laterality. However, if agreement is defined as including any discrepancies that did not exceed 2 scale points, only finger to nose, and speech syntax failed to meet the 90 percent level.

These data leave little doubt that the individual items of the clinical neurological examination can be reliably assessed, although, as is the case with respect to other assessments, test-retest reliability is better at the extremes of established scales. The data do not permit minor disagreements that arise as a consequence of examiner variability or subject instability to be distinguished.

Item reliability however, is only a first step in the interpretation of findings on clinical examination. Rutter provides additional information with respect to the reliability of overall neurological judgment. On a 4-point scale the level of agreement was: normal — 85 percent; dubious — 62 percent; slight — 79 percent; and marked — 92 percent. These findings are difficult to interpret, however, because the criteria utilized for assignment to each category are not specified. As a consequence it is not possible to determine if children in the slight or dubious categories have evidence of neurological disease that is symptomatically mild or have an aggregate of abnormalities that do not conform to a recognizable clinical pattern. Nonetheless, only 1 percent of disagreements with respect to global neurological status exceed 2 scale points.

Table 4-1
Test–Retest Reliability of Findings on Clinical Neurologic Examination of 10–11-year-old Children*

Sign	N	% Overall Agreement	Number of Points on Scale	% Agreement within 2 Scale Points
Cranial Signs				
Nystagmus	88	92	3	98
Strabismus	88	89	3	93
Facial Power	26	81	—	—
Facial Assymetry	27	85	—	—
Tongue—Licking Lip	87	85	3	98
Tongue—Side to Side	87	91	3	100
Skull Asymmetry	89	78	3	100
Coordination				
Threading Beads	27	85	3	100
Holding Pencil	27	70	3	100
Touching Fingers with Thimb	26	54	3	96
Finger to Nose	27	70	3	89
Kicking Ball of Paper	26	81	3	100
Throwing Ball of Paper	26	58	3	96
Hopping on One Foot	26	85	3	100
Walking and Turning	26	88	3	100
Tremor	27	85	3	93
Power of Limbs				
Upper Limbs	81	95	3	100
Lower Limbs	82	94	3	100
Tone of Limbs				
Upper Limbs	87	86	5	100
Lower Limbs	87	86	5	100
Reflexes				
Supinator	88	54	5	99
Biceps	88	65	5	100
Triceps	88	60	5	98
Knee	88	76	5	99
Ankle	88	63	5	99
Plantar	84	74	5	97
Laterality				
Hand	88	80	4	95
Foot	81	98	3	99
Age	85	87	4	94
Developmental Abnormalities				
Constructional Difficulties	87	76	4	100
†Limb "dyspraxia"	86	77	3	99
Articulation Defect	89	78	3	98
Speech Syntax	88	58	5	89
Speech Complexity	88	82	4	100
Adequacy of Description	88	76	3	100
Mirror Movements	83	63	3	93

*Data from Rutter et al, 1970a.

†This item is a composite of performance on the following tasks: threading beads, holding pencil, touching fingers with thumb, finger-to-nose test, kicking ball of paper, throwing ball of paper, hopping on one foot, walking and turning.

What then, does the presence or absence of positive findings on clinical neurological examination mean? Rutter has chosen to examine discriminant validity, i.e., the ability of the examination to distinguish between normal children and defined clinical groups. The clinical groups selected for study included intellectually retarded and reading retarded children who were without overt neurological disorder, and children with known neurological disorder conventionally diagnosed on the basis of information derived from history, physical examination, and ancillary tests, i.e., EEG.

The latter group was further subdivided into those with uncomplicated epilepsy and those with neurological disorder without epilepsy. The discriminant validity of each sign was examined, both individually and in combination.

Poor right-left discrimination, constructional difficulties, limb dyspraxia, articulation defects, speech complexity, and mirror-movements were likely to occur with greater frequency among all of the clinically defined contrast groups. Rutter advances two principle reasons for hesitating to attach significance to these findings. First he views the presence of such abnormalities in school-aged children as reflecting delays in the development of normal functions rather than as signs of abnormality. Thus, he argues that the attribution of neurological abnormality must take *chronologic age* into account, and that there is a great need for the establishment of age-specific norms for all items included in an assessment schedule.

Rutter cites the high frequency of occurence of so-called developmental signs among children with low IQ who are without overt evidence of neurological disease as a second reason for believing that no necessary neurologic significance attaches to abnormal nonfocal signs. In his view, such findings may merely be another manifestation of intellectual immaturity. However, it should be noted that not all mentally retarded children exhibit nonfocal abnormalities. Birch et al (1970) using a somewhat different assessment schedule (to be described in a later section of this chapter) demonstrated that only ¼ of 101 mentally retarded children between the ages of 8 and 10 years exhibited 2 or more nonfocal signs. Moreover, psychiatric disturbance occurred significantly more frequently among neurologically impaired mentally retarded children than among those whose neurological examinations were considered normal. In yet another study Bortner et al (1972) showed that although the correlation between IQ and number of nonfocal signs among children in special educational placement is significant ($r = -.578$, $N = 129$) this negative association accounts for only one third of the variance.

Thus, the overlap between abnormalities detected in the course of clinical neurological examination and standardized intellectual assessment is not complete. The two approaches are also divergent in tapping different aspects of the function of the central nervous system. To require that any given neurological sign be fully independent of IQ is unreasonable given the current state of knowledge with respect to brain-damage as one of the possible etiologies of mental retardation (Birch et al, 1970). However, it does seem reasonable to suggest that the clinical neurological examination not duplicate the assessment of aspects of higher cortical functions that are systemically evaluated during the course of standardized IQ testing.

Rutter has also addressed the problem of utilizing aggregate scores as a way of determining the presence or absence of neurological abnormality. However, his procedure for the calculation of a "Total Composite Neurologic Score" fails to distinguish between signs that may be neurological or nonneurological in nature (i.e., nystagmus), and those that may be only slight or difficult to detect (i.e., slight deviations in muscle tone or reflexes) or those that in his views reflect developmental delays (i.e., coordination). No consideration is given to either the type or severity of abnormal findings, or whether they occurred in the presence or absence of diagnosable neurological disease. Thus, Rutter's conclusion that Total Composite Neurologic Score is not a useful way of distinguishing between normals and various diagnostic groups is impossible to evaluate, and his verdict on the validity of aggregate scores, must, on the basis of this body of data, be considered "not proven."

In summary, Rutter and his colleagues have devised a clinical neurological schedule that has content validity when measured against the standards suggested by Paine and Oppe (1966). The individual items of the instrument are demonstrably reliable, particularly at the extremes of the established measurement scales. The reasons advanced for eliminating abnormalities such as nystagmus, which cannot be uniformally considered to reflect CNS dysfunction, or those that are doubtfully present are sound. However, the distinction between "delay" in the development of normal functions and the emergence of abnormal neurological organizations is less clear. Moreover, there is a lack of discriminant validity of aggregates or combinations of signs.

Hertzig and Birch (Birch et al, 1970; Bortner et al, 1972; Hertzig, 1974; 1981; 1982; Hertzig & Birch, 1966; 1968; Hertzig et al, 1969) utilized a modification of the schedule proposed by Paine and Oppe (1966) to examine the neurological status of psychiatrically disturbed and learning disabled adolescents, as well as low birthweight, mentally retarded, learning disabled, and normally developing school-aged children. While clinically based, the procedure was specifically developed for research use. The entire schedule required from between 20 and 30 minutes to administer and all responses were recorded on a specially designed protocol during the course of the examination (see Appendix B). The procedures for the administration and scoring of individual items are well described (Hertzig, 1981; 1982). A child was judged to be neurologically abnormal if (1) any localizing signs of central nervous system abnormality were present or if (2) two or more nonlocalizing signs were found.

Localizing signs included such standard indicators of central nervous system dysfunction as abnormalities in cranial nerves, lateralized dysfunctions, and the presence of pathologic reflexes when those were noted to occur in a pattern consistent with conventional neurological diagnosis.

Assessment of the presence or absence of NFNS was more complex. Individual tasks were grouped to permit the development of judgments about the integrity of broader areas of central nervous sytem function: (1) speech, (2) balance, (3) coordination, (4) double simultaneous stimulation (DSS), (5) gait, (6) sequential finger-thumb opposition, (7) muscle tone, (8) graphesthesia, (9) asterognosis, and (10) choreiform movements. Mild or questionable abnormalities were not scored and in addition, much information obtained in the course of the examination (i.e., hand, eye, and foot dominance and right-left awareness) was ignored in designating a given child as neurologically abnormal for research purposes.

While these workers present no data on the reliability of the instrument, Quitkin et al (1976) have examined both the reliability and short-term persistence of many of the individual items of this instrument. Difficulties in establishing the reliability of observing infrequently occurring events led Quitkin and his colleagues to confine consideration only to those items that were found to occur in at least 2 percent of 298 drug-free young adult psychiatric patients. Reliability (i.e., agreement between examiners) was distinguished from persistence (i.e., consistency of subject performance over time). Reliability was determined in joint examination of 25 subjects by 2 examiners who made independent ratings of their findings. The Pearson correlation coefficient for total number of signs was 0.94 ($p < .001$). There was a statistically significant level of agreement between the two examiners with respect to the presence or absence of the following items: speech, coordination, finger-thumb opposition (right and left hands), pronation-supination, foot taps, dominance, right/left errors, DSS, graphesthesia (right and left hands), and tandem walking.

In addition, persistence was assessed on 16 subjects examined 24-48 hours apart. There was little variation for the total number of signs ($r = .96$,

$p < 0.001$) but consistency of performance on individual signs was more variable. Speech, finger-thumb opposition, dominance, and graphesthesia were significantly persistent, while foot-tapping behavior, pronation-supination as well as response to double simultaneous stimulation were not.

A similar pattern of persistence of subject performance over the longer interval of 4 years has been described by Hertzig (1982) in 53 children and adolescents. (First exam mean age: 10 years 6 months ± 15.06 months; second exam mean age 14 years ± 21.31 months). While the number of subjects who exhibited 2 or more nonfocal signs on both examinations did not differ significantly, the likelihood that findings of the first examination were replicated on the second varied from sign to sign. Overall consistency was highest for responses to DSS (75 percent); and then astereognosis (74 percent); speech, choreiform movements, and finger-thumb opposition (72 percent); balance (68 percent); gait (58 percent); graphesthesia (57 percent); coordination (55 percent); and tone (47 percent).

Normally developing children between the ages of 8 and 12 years show less than a 5 percent rate of 2 or more nonfocal signs (Hertzig & Birch, 1968; Bortner et al, 1972). Samples of mentally retarded (Birch et al, 1970), psychiatrically disturbed (Hertzig & Birch, 1966; 1968; Quitkin et al, 1976), and low birthweight (Hertzig, 1981), children and adolescents as well as those in special educational placements (Hertzig et al, 1968; Bortner et al, 1972; Hertzig, 1982), all have been shown to have a significantly higher frequency of occurrence of two or more nonfocal signs. Thus, the examination schedule *adequately discriminates* between normally developing and clinically defined groups of children. Further evidence of the discriminant validity of the instrument is provided by the fact that within samples of mentally retarded (Birch et al, 1970) and low birthweight (Hertzig 1981; 1983) children, those with and without nonfocal signs exhibit significant differences with respect to antecedent perinatal risk conditions as well as concurrent patterns of behavioral organization.

In summary, Hertzig and Birch utilize data derived in the course of clinical neurological examination to arrive at judgments with respect to the presence or absence of both localized central nervous system abnormality and nonfocal neurological signs. The examination schedule indicates a range of items that, in accordance with traditional neurological practice, permit the systematic assessment of motor, sensory, and higher cortical functions. Ten nonfocal signs are abstracted from the array of items and scoring criteria are well specified. Minor variation in muscle tone or reflex organization, nystagmus, or lateralized abnormalities (i.e., those observed to affect only one side of the body) are not considered as nonfocal signs.

The instrument discriminates between normally developing children above 8 years of age and a variety of clinically defined groups including psychiatrically disturbed, mentally retarded, and low birthweight children as well as those in special educational placement. The ability of the instrument as designed to differentiate between clinically defined groups of younger children has not been systematically examined. Available data suggest that although normally developing children between 3 and 5 ½ years are able to perform the finger-thumb opposition task with an overall accuracy rate of 87 percent (Lefford, 1971), it is not until 8 years that correct responses to double simultaneous stimulation exceed chance levels (Bender, Fink, & Green, 1951). Despite the fact that total number of nonfocal signs decreases significantly with increasing age, children who exhibited 2 or more signs when they were between 8 and 12 years of age continue to do so when reexamined 4 years later. Moreover, only abnormalities in graphesthesia and coordination occur significantly less often among older as opposed to younger children (Hertzig, 1982). These findings suggest that the presence or absence of nonfocal signs is only minimally affected by increasing age in older children and adolescents.

Touwen (1979) has approached the problem of design of an instrument for the examination of the child with minor neurological dysfunction from a somewhat different vantage point. He proposes techniques and procedures to be used by pediatricians and neurologists in clinical settings. In his view, systematic attention to the recognition and description of minor deviations is required (1) when the history suggests the possibility of neurological disease in its early stages; (2) as a basis for the adequate planning of treatment for the child with an obvious neurological disorder; and (3) for the full assessment of children who present with behavioral and/or learning difficulties. The neurological examination of the child with behavioral and learning problems is a necessary part of the diagnostic process according to Touwen (1979). He cautions, however, that the neurological examination is limited and can assess only those behaviors that fall within its scope.

What then is to be included as a routine part of the clinical neurological assessment of children? Touwen (1979) believes

> ... it is impossible to design a series of 'crucial' neurologic tests that will indicate whether the brain is functioning normally or abnormally. A plea for a short form of neurologic screening for this purpose, though understandable, ignores essential properties of the central nervous system. A test of a single part of the neurologic repertoire, for example grasping or walking, may

give information about that particular function but will not evaluate the neurologic mechanisms on which the function is based ... the examination of a single aspect of the nervous system — coordination for example — does not give sufficient information about other aspects such as muscle power or reflexes (p. 3).

Nevertheless, choices must be made. Touwen (1979) offers the following rationale for his selection. First, the neurologic examination is concerned with the quality of performance within a developmental context and is to be distinguished from a developmental assessment that is viewed as a means of determining if performance is consistent with an established maturational timetable. The examination described is considered suitable for children between 3 and 12 years of age. The examination procedures include modifications of administration and scoring appropriate for differences in age based upon clinical experience with large numbers of normally developing and deviant children. Touwen (1979) questions the value of population norms and urges that each clinician utilize a standardized method to determine his or her own norms for a particular population.

Second, Touwen (1979) has chosen to eliminate items in which the reasons for poor performance are multidetermined. Thus, his schedule does not include graphesthesia, astereognosis, and constructional abilities because the influence of attention, learning, verbal ability, social factors, intelligence, and motivation cannot be assessed unequivocally.

In Touwen's (1979) view, the least problematic aspects of the neurological examination lie in the assessment of a large number of motor and sensory functions. Individual tasks are grouped into 10 areas: (1) sensory-motor apparatus (13 items); (2) posture (8 items); (3) balance of trunk (5 items); (4) coordination of extremities (5 items); (5) fine manipulative ability (3 items); (6) dyskinesia (4 items); (7) gross motor functions (7 items); (8) quality of motility (6 items); (9) associated movements (5 items); and (10) visual system (7 items).

Touwen does not consider that the presence of a single nonoptimal sign has any clinical significance, and suggests that a neurological profile be drawn in order to show the distribution of optimal signs over the subsystems of the nervous system. Touwen suggests that further insight into the pattern of deficit may be obtained by determining the discrepancy between the total number of items in each subsector and the number of items a particular child performs adquately. The resulting array of discrepancy scores enables the examiner to describe findings that cannot be arranged in traditional diagnostic patterns as well as to easily recognize multiple areas of deficit. In addition, the profile provides an opportunity for distinguishing groups of children with various kinds of nontraditional neurological dysfunction.

In summary, Touwen has proposed a clinical neurological examination for use in clinical settings, which focuses on the detailed study of a large number of motor and sensory functions. Although the schedule is constructed in accordance with developmental principles it is clearly distinguished from a developmental assessment, the design of items and their scoring emphasizing qualitative aspects of performance. Little systematic information is available with respect to either examiner reliability or consistency of findings over time. Nor have issues of validity been systematically addressed. The length of the examination, while clinically appropriate, limits its usefulness for research purposes. However, the principles underlying its construction are clearly applicable to research settings.

Several other investigators have reported on the use of an expanded clinical neurological examination for the assessment of children with school problems (Lucas, Rodin, & Simson, 1965) and academic underachievement (Stine et al, 1975), as well as those at genetic risk for schizophrenia (Marcus, 1974; Rieder & Nichols, 1979), and hyperactivity (Lerer & Lerer, 1975; McMahon & Greenberg, 1977). Although conducted within the context of a standard traditional neurological assessment, these workers variously included a miscellany of additional items ranging from those designed to assess aspects of motor functions to those that tapped higher cortical functions. Little information is provided with respect to either administration or scoring. While some investigators (Hart, Rennick, Klinge, & Schwartz,1978) have utilized findings with respect to NFNS to make judgments about the presence or absence of neurological abnormality or dysfunction, the criteria for arriving at these judgments are poorly specified. In the absence of adequate description, neither the reliability or validity of these examination schedules can be further assessed.

The principle approaches to the assessment of nonfocal signs (Hertzig 1981; 1982; Paine & Oppe, 1966; Rutter et al, 1970a; Touwen, 1979) have all utilized information obtained during clinical examination to formulate a neurological diagnosis in a traditional sense as well as to describe and categorize diagnostically nonspecific deviations in motor, sensory, and higher cortical integrative functions. While each schedule differs somewhat with respect to content, administration, scoring, and interpretation, all permit (either actually or potentially) a distinction to be made between nonspecific deviations occurring in the absence of localizing disease and disturbances (i.e., in gait, balance, coordination, etc.), which occur as a consequence of or in association with a defined neurological entity (e.g., hemiplegia). The logical impossibility of specifying any particular deviation as nonfocal, in the absence of at least clinical certainty with respect to the absence of localizing abnormality is apparent. Nevertheless, numerous investigators have attempted to construct an examination schedule limited to the assessment of only nonfocal signs (Adams et al, 1974; Close, 1973; Peters et al, 1975; Shapiro et al, 1978; Stine et al, 1975; Werry et al, 1972).

Werry (Werry et al, 1972) reports that a review of the literature has revealed a total of 140 signs that have been utilized in the neurological examination of children, including individual items relevant to the examination of the head (51 items), motor system (22 items), coordination (26 items), reflexes (15 items), sensory examination (15 items), and speech (11 items). Different investigators have selected items from this array in the construction of schedules for the examination of nonfocal neurological signs. By far the most comprehensive effort in this regard is the *PANESS, a 43 item scale*, constructed by Close (1973) (see Appendix A). The scale contains items designed to assess gross motor coordination (1-8), fine motor coordination (37-42), balance (21-26), persistence (31-36), optokinetic responses (43), cortical sensitivity (27-29), graphesthesia (9-16), and stereognosis (17-20). Thus, the scale has some degree of face validity in that the items allow for the assessment of aspects of motor, sensory, and higher cortical functions. Werry (Werry & Aman, 1976) has examined the reliability of individual items in 21 children (6 normal, 10 hyperactive, and 5 neurologically impaired), who ranged in age from 61 to 146 months. Two different examiners assessed the children with an interval between examinations from 1 to 110 days. Thus, the procedure makes it impossible to separate examiner reliability from persistence. Werry and Aman (1976) raise concerns about the adequacy of the instrument because of the infrequency with which many of the items occurred. Despite the fact that 75 percent of the study sample was composed of children who might be expected to exhibit abnormality, only 12 percent of the signs occurred in as many as 50 percent of the children, making the assessment of reliability difficult. Moreover, it suggests that a large number of items are probably noncontributory. Moreover, of 7 items that occurred in over 50 percent of the subjects, 5 were present in more than 80 percent. Thus, although these items (40A, 41C, 42A, 39A, 41A) are reliable, they most probably do not clearly distinguish between clinical groups.

Bialer (Camp, Bialer, Sverd, & Winsberg, 1978) has examined the diagnostic validity of the PANESS. The mean PANESS scores of hyperactive and normal children ranging in age from 5 to 11 years were compared and contrasted. The 43 item scale yields a total of 56 scores as some items are scored in more than one dimension. Each score receives a numerical weight ranging in some way or another over a 4 point scale from "no impairment" through "severe impairment." The performance of both hyperactive and normal children was found to improve with age. However, the only significant difference between the groups was at the 9 year level, where the hyperactive children showed superior performance. Both Bialer (Camp et al, 1978) and Werry and Aman (1976) caution against the routine acceptance of the PANESS as a definitive examination for NFNS in view of inadequate information about the reliability, diagnostic power, and predictive qualities of both individual items and the examination as a whole.

Similar concerns can be raised about other examination batteries, the content of which overlaps with that of the clinical neurologic examination. One such instrument is the Lincoln-Oseretsky Motor Development Scale. While the original version of the scale is described as unduly long and cumbersome to administer (Sloan, 1955) shortened forms are available (Rutter et al 1970; Bialer et al, 1974). Bialer (Bialer et al, 1974) has provided age-specific normative data. Rutter has examined the test-retest reliability of the short modification used in the Isle of Wight Studies in 10-11-year-old children. Despite the fact that scores tended to increase when children were reexamined between 1 and 29 days after the first assessment (presumably as a consequence of "practice effects") the reliability was considered adequate (r = 0.69, N = 74). Rutter (Rutter et al, 1970) has also reported that scores obtained on the modified scale correlate well with the limb dyspraxia sign of the clinical neurological assessment employed in these studies. However, the Lincoln-Oseretsky Scale does not allow for differentiation between types of incoordination, i.e., paresis, a central deficit in motor control, or that due to tremor. Moreover, as Touwen (1979) has indicated, the scale assesses only a single dimension of neurological organization, and the presence or absence of findings cannot be readily generalized. While the instrument certainly has a place in the clarification of functional motor organization for the purposes of planning strategies of intervention, its restricted scope limits its diagnostic utility.

A consideration of strategies for the assessment of NFNS would be incomplete without reference to neuropsychological approaches to the problem. Clinical neuropsychology is concerned with the exploration of human brain behavior relations as applied to clinical situations. For the most part, neuropsychologists have tried to develop instruments to examine the impact of cerebral injury on intellectual, sensory, motor, adaptive, and personality organization. Perhaps the most sophisticated of the approaches is that of Reitan (Reitan & Davison, 1974), who has both developed testing procedures and assembled items from existing instruments to assess (1) motor functions, (2) tactile perceptual functions, (3) academic ability, (4) intelligence, (5) verbal abilities, (6) visual-spatial and sequential abilities, (7) immediate alertness, (8) incidental memory, and (9) concept formation and reasoning ability. Thus, the battery although extremely useful as an approach to the elucidation of the possible mechanisms underlying behavioral organization in both normally functioning and brain injured children is both more inclusive and more restrictive than the clinical neurological examinations. Tests of motor functioning test aspects of motor strength and motor coordination that fall within the province of clinical neurological assessment as well as motor speed and motor problem solving, which are most often beyond the scope. While the instrument is a valuable research tool and has clinical ramifications (i.e., in the monitoring of neurologically impaired patients over time) it is in no sense a substitute for clinical neurological assessment.

Conclusions

In conclusion, no wholly satisfactory method for the assessment of nonfocal neurological signs in the school-aged child is currently available for use in either clinical or research settings. Nevertheless, this review provides a basis for the development of guidelines for the construction of such an instrument.

1. The assessment of nonfocal neurological signs must occur within the context of a clinical neurological examination, sufficiently comprehensive in scope to permit the identification of localizing neurological abnormality. This is necessary because disturbances in many areas of function often considered as nonfocal signs may occur in conjunction with localizing neurological disease. Abnormalities in such areas of function as gait, balance, coordination as well as astereognosis and graphesthesia can only be designated as nonfocal signs if there is reasonable clinical certainty localizing abnormalities are absent.

2. "Nonfocal signs" are best defined as aggregate abnormalities in areas of CNS function, rather than discrete deviations from the norm in response to individual tasks. This approach reduces the overlap between normally developing and clinically defined groups of children augmenting the discriminant validity of the instrument. In addition, the frequency of occurrence of abnormalities defined as aggregates is higher than for discrete items in populations of "at risk children" facilitating the assessment of reliability.

3. How should areas of CNS functions be defined and described? The problem of the organization of discrete tasks into functional areas involves decisions with respect to what should be excluded as well as what should be included.

   A. *Exclusion criteria*

      1. *Items deriving from standard intelligence tests* (or other well standardized psychometric instruments) or closely resembling such items should not be included. Examples include such tasks as copying geometric forms, or tests of constructional abilities (Touwen, 1979).
      2. Items such as *nystagmus should be excluded* as abnormalities. These may be of either neurological or nonneurological origin. (Rutter et al, 1970a).
      3. Items that studies have shown to be *clearly inadequate* as indicators of CNS dysfunction or abnormality, i.e. *laterality and dominance* (Touwen, 1979).
      4. Minor *examples of classical neurological signs* that are *difficult to detect or unreliably assess* should be eliminated. Examples include slight asymmetries of tone or reflexes, just perceptible hemiparesis, minimal athetosis, or mild asymmetry of skull or limbs (Rutter et al, 1970a).

   B. *Inclusion criteria*

      1. Functional areas should encompass a range of motor, sensory, and cortical integrative functions.
      2. Items selected should be able to be performed without evidence of marked deviation (c.f. Touwen, 1979) by 90 percent of school-aged children (8 years and older).

3. A suggested list is that of Hertzig (1982, 1983) (see Appendix B).
4. Additional tasks to assess associated or mirror movements might be considered for inclusions.
5. Tasks subsumed by Hertzig (1982), under the headings of balance, gait, and coordination, might be arranged to reflect global judgments, with respect to balance of trunk, coordination of extremities, fine manipulative ability, and gross motor functions (Touwen, 1979). The discriminant validity of various groupings of individual items is an empirical issue that requires further study.

4. Scoring procedures must be developed for both individual items and functional areas. While it is possible to develop a scoring system that permits a numerical weight to be assigned to no findings, mild or questionable abnormality and marked or severe abnormality, in our judgment, only marked deviations from expected performance should be considered in developing judgments about the functional integrity of the central nervous system. Thus, we do not advocate the computation of a total neurological score per se, but rather either a listing of the number or type of markedly impaired functional areas or a graphic depiction of the pattern of functional organization of the nervous system (Touwen, 1979).

5. Studies of reliability must clearly distinguish between examiner and subject characteristics as they may contribute to the replicability of findings on reexamination. As studies of both short-term (Quitkin et al, 1976; Shapiro, 1978) and long-term (Hertzig, 1982) persistence of nonfocal signs strongly suggest that inconsistency of performance per se may well be a characteristic of a disordered nervous system, examiner reliability can only be assessed when two examiners independently record findings elicited during joint examination.

6. The ability of the instrument to discriminate between normally developing children above the age of 8 years and defined clinical groups must be adequately assessed before any instrument is widely adopted for either clinical or research purposes. If discriminant validity is established, the association between clinical neurological findings and either chronologic or mental age should not preclude its use. Further validation awaits the application of nonclinically based

technologies such as the CT scan or NMR for the assessment of the integrity of the central nervous system.

REFERENCES

Adams RM, Kocsis J, & Estes RE. Soft neurologic signs in learning disabled children and controls. American Journal of Diseases of Children, 1974, 128, 614-618

Barlow CF. Soft signs in children with learning disorders. American Journal of Diseases of Children, 1974, 128, 605-606

Bender L. Clinical study of 100 schizophrenic children. American Journal of Orthopsychiatry, 1947, 17, 40-46

Bender M, Fink M, & Green M. Patterns in perception on simultaneous tests of face and hand. Archives of Neurology and Psychiatry, 1951, 66, 350-362

Bialer I, Doll L, & Winsberg BG. A modified Lincoln-Oseretsky motor development scale: Provisional standardization. Perceptual and Motor Skills, 1974, 38, 599-614

Birch HG, Richardson SA, Baird D, et al. Mental Subnormality in the Community. A Clinical and Epidemiologic Study. Baltimore: Williams & Wilkins, 1970

Bortner M, Hertzig ME, & Birch HG. Neurologic signs and intelligence in brain-damaged children. Journal of Special Educucation, 1972, 6, 325-333

Camp JA, Bialer I, Sverd J, & Winsberg B. Clinical usefulness of the NIMH physical and neurological examination for soft signs. American Journal of Psychiatry, 1978, 135, 362-364

Close J. Scored neurological examination in pharmacotherapy of children. Psychopharmacology Bulletin Special Issue — Pharmacotherapy of Children, 1973, 142-148

Fish B. Neurobiologic antecedents of schizophrenia in children. Archives of General Psychiatry, 1977, 34, 1297-1313

Hart L, Rennick PM, Klinge V, & Schwartz ML. A pediatric neurologist's contribution to evaluation of school underachievers. American Journal of Diseases of Children, 1978, 128, 319-323

Hertzig ME. Neurologic findings in prematurely born children at school age. In Rolf M, & Thomas A (Eds.). Proceedings of the Fifth Conference the Society for Life History Research. Minneapois, MN: University of Minnesota Press, 1974

Hertzig ME. Neurologic "soft" signs in low birthweight children. Developmental Medicine and Child Neurology, 1981, 21, 778-791

Hertzig ME. Stability and change in nonfocal neurologic signs. Journal of the American Academy of Child Psychiatry, 1982, 21, 231-236

Hertzig ME. Temperament and neurologic status. In Rutter M (Ed.). Developmental Neuropsychiatary. New York: Guilford, 1983

Hertzig ME, & Birch HG. Neurologic organization in psychiatrically disturbed adolescent girls. Archives of General Psychiatry, 1966, 15, 590-598

Hertzig ME, & Birch HG. Neurologic organization in psychiatrically disturbed adolescents. A comparative consideration of sex differences. Archives of General Psychiatry, 1968, 19, 528-537

Hertzig ME, Bortner M, & Birch HG. Neurologic findings in children educationally designated as "brain-damaged." American Journal of Orthopsychiatry, 1969, 39, 437-446

Ingram TTS. Soft signs. Developmental Medicine and Child Neurology, 1973, 15, 527-529

Kennard M. Value of equivocal signs in neurologic diagnosis. Neurology, 1960, 10, 753-764

Lefford A. Sensory, perceptual and cognitive factors in the development of voluntary action. In Connolly K (Ed.). The Mechanisms of Motor Skill Development. New York: Academic Press, 1971, pp. 207-224

Lerer RJ, & Lerer MD. The effects of methylphenidate on the soft neurologic signs of hyperactive children. Pediatrics, 1976, 57, 521-525

Lucas AR, Rodin EA, & Simson CB. Neurologic assessment of children with early school problems. Developmental Medicine and Child Neurology, 1965, 7, 145-156

Marcus J. Cerebral functioning in offspring of schizophrenics. A possible genetic factor. International Journal of Mental Health, 1974, 3, 57-75

McMahon SA, Greenberg LM. Serial neurologic examination of hyperactive children. Pediatrics 1977, 59, 584-587

Paine RS, Oppe TS. Neurological Examination of Children. Clinics in Developmental Medicine No 20/21. London: Heinemann Medical Books, 1966

Peters JE, Romine JS, & Dykman RA. A special neurological examinationof children with learning disabilities. Developmental Medicine and Child Neurology, 1975, 17, 63-78

Quitkin R, Rifkin A, & Klein D. Neurologic 'soft' signs in schizophrenia and character disorders. Archives of General Psychiatry, 1976, 33, 845-853

Rieder HO, & Nichols PL. Offspring of schizophrenics III. Hyperactivity and neurologic soft signs. Archives of General Psychiatry, 1979, 36, 665-674

Reitan RM, & Davison LA (Eds.). Clinical Neuropsychology: Current Status and Applications. New York: Halsted Press, 1974

Rutter M. Brain damage syndromes in childhood: Concepts and findings. Journal of Child Psychology and Psychiatry, 1977, 18, 1-21

Rutter M. Syndromes attributed to “minimal brain dysfunction” in childhood. American Journal of Psychiatry, 1982, 139, 21-33

Rutter M, Graham P, & Yule W. A Neuropsychiatric Study in Childhood. Clinicis in Developmental Medicine, No. 35/36. London: Heinemann Medical Books, 1970a

Rutter M, Tizard J, & Whitmore K (Eds.). Education, Health and Behavior. London: Longmans, 1970b

Shaffer D. Soft neurologic signs and later psychiatric disorder — a review. Journal of Child Psychology and Psychiatry, 1978, 19, 63-65

Shapiro T, Burkes L, Petti T, & Ranz J. Consistency of “non-focal” neurologic signs. Journal of American Academy of Child Psychiatry, 1978, 19, 63-65

Shapiro T, & Perry R. Latency revisited. The Psychoanalytic Study of the Child, 1976, 31, 79-105

Sloan W. The Lincoln-Oseretsky motor development scale. Genetic Psychology Monographs, 1955, 51, 183-252

Stine OC, Saratsiotis JB, & Mosser RS. Relationships between neurologic findings and classroom behavior. American Journal of Diseases of Children, 1975, 129, 1036-1040

Strauss A, & Lehtinen L. Psychopathology and Education of the Brain-injured Child. New York: Grune & Sratton, 1947

Touwen BCL. Examination of the Child with Minor Neurological Dysfunction, 2nd ed. Clinics in Developmental Medicine, No, 71, London: Spastics International Publishers, 1979

Werry JS. Organic factors. In Quay HC, & Werry JS (Eds.). Psycho-

pathological Disorders of Childhood. New York: Wiley, 1972
Werry JS, & Aman MG. The reliability and diagnostic validity of the physical and neurological examination for soft signs (PANESS). Journal of Autism and Child Schizophrenia, 1976, 6, 253-262
Werry JS, Minde K, Gusman A, et al. Studies on the hyperactive child. American Journal of Orthopsychiatry, 1972, 42, 441-450
Wolff PH, & Hurwitz J. The choreiform syndrome. Developmental Medicine and Child Neurology, 1966, 8, 160-165

Ruthmary K. Deuel
Dora Jean Robinson

5

Developmental Motor Signs

In 1925, in reporting his series of dyslexic children, Samuel Orton spoke of "that mild motor incoordinate type in whom many exact motor acts are acquired slowly and with difficulty" (Orton, 1925). In so doing, Orton opened a discussion of motor abnormalities in children who demonstrate the neuropsychiatric syndromes of childhood. While these syndromes have been extensively investigated in the 60 years that have passed, the significance of such motor abnormalities in children of normal intelligence, but poor academic and social performance, is still unknown. It has become clear that many of the pertinent motor abnormalities are developmentally determined in that they are found in all young children, and only persist to a later chronological age in a small percentage of children, in whom they then may be considered abnormal.

Several generalizations arise from our review of a modest proportion of the literature that followed Orton. First, concepts of childhood neuropsychological disorders have undergone an evolution. Initially, motor soft signs were thought to validate the origin of childhood neuropsychiatric syndromes in mild brain damage (Bender, 1970; Benton, 1956; Clements, 1966; Hertzig, Bortner, & Birch, 1969; Kennard, 1960; Orton, 1925; Paine, Werry, & Quay, 1968; Strauss & Lehtinen, 1947). Gomez (1967) pointed out the circular nature of this proposition in his article *Minimal cerebral dysfunction (maximal neurologic confusion)*. Brain damage must be present to create signs, thus soft signs mean brain damage. Other authors also countered the claim that motor soft signs were inevitable indicators of brain damage (Barlow, 1974; Gomez, 1967; Touwen & Sporrel, 1979), although pointing out that they did occur along with localizing signs in cases of cerebral palsy (Hertzig et al, 1969; Reitan, 1971). Later, soft signs were

SOFT NEUROLOGICAL SIGNS
ISBN 0-8089-1841-9

attributed to "developmental lag," an entity that could be genetically determined (Bakwin, 1968; Kinsbourne, 1973) or caused by an acquired condition, such as prematurity (Gillberg & Rasmussen, 1978; Gomez, 1967). Examination for soft signs in dyslexic, otherwise learning disabled, hyperkinetic, and conduct disordered children is clinically assiduously pursued to the present day (Adams 1973; Aram & Horwitz, 1973; Bishop, 1980; DSM III, 1980; Gillberg & Rosmussen, 1982; Johnston, Stark, Mellits, & Tallal, 1981; Kornse, Manni, & Rubenstein, 1981; Lucas, Rodin, & Simson, 1965; Peters, Rumine, & Dykman, 1975; Rie, Rie, Stewart, et al, 1978; Rutter, 1977; Seidel, Chadwick, & Rutter, 1975). Examinations are conducted in part because there is a clearly documented high incidence of developmental motor soft signs in cohorts of children with neuropsychiatric syndromes even if the significance of this association is unclear; and in part because developmental motor disorders sometimes form a handicapping condition in and of themselves (Baker, 1981; Dare & Gordon, 1970; David & Ferry, 1981; Dawdy, 1981; Gubbay, 1975, 1978; McKinley, 1978; Rutter, 1977).

The motor findings we shall address as "developmentally determined motor soft signs," are those readily assessed on physical exam, and that have been shown to be frequent (normal) in toddlers and preschool children, but to be of low incidence (abnormal) at a later age. It is important to note that the term *developmental* does not mean that the child *will* "grow out" of the motor traits, only that in the course of *normal* development they usually disappear. The complex matter of the age at which each sign becomes abnormal and the quality of the evidence in the literature that supports this judgment is discussed in later sections. We will not cover signs generally recognized as clear indicators of location of pathology in the nervous sytem (e.g., Babinski signs) nor any recognized as indicating specific etiology.

The most commonly reported motor soft signs include (1) clumsiness (maladroitness), (2) dyspraxia (poor motor planning), (3) synkinesis (movement overflow), (4) choreiform movements, and (5) reversed or incomplete manual dominance. While called soft signs, these are not specific signs in the classic sense. Instead they are inferential categories that classify aspects of various motor performances (Wolff, 1981). Evidence for these categories is derived from neurologic examination and sometimes from more highly standardized tests that have been elaborated from items of the neurologic exam. We will review selected papers that provide data on normal populations, and discuss the incidence and significance of soft signs in various abnormal populations. Finally, vis a vis the handicap that the developmental motor soft signs can cause in and of themselves, we will review the clinical syndrome and the means that have been used for remediation.

STUDIES OF NORMAL MOTOR DEVELOPMENT

The normal mean and range of ability development in a sense define developmental motor abnormalities. Studies of this development fall into two general categories. One surveys large numbers of motor behaviors including complex coordinated voluntary movements such as walking and writing, and comes up with some sort of general rating in relation to normal for age. The other evaluates one or a limited number of simple acts such as finger tapping. This latter type of study generally uses carefully controlled interval measurements. We reviewed numerous articles reporting both categories of study, and discuss a few in detail. Table 5-1 lists some of the first variety, while Table 5-2 lists the second.

The theoretical approach to motor development taken by early 20th century authorities provides the underpinning of the current concepts of normal development and thus developmental motor soft signs. Such theories are succintly articulated by Bobath (1966), Peiper (1963), Paine (1964), and others (Doman, Delacato, & Doman, 1960; Gesell & Amatruda, 1947; McCarthy, 1972; McGraw , 1968). In general, early infant mass synergistic reflex actions are said to be superceded by variously described patterns of discrete unilateral voluntary motions. For instance, Peiper says unilateral thumb-finger apposition evolves from a "clumsy and explosive" (Peiper, 1963, p. 255) synkinetic activity of both hands. He mentions choreiform movements as characteristic of infancy, and cites the study of Gesell and Ames (1947) on the point that handedness is fully established by about 4 years of age. Bobath (1966) describes two sets of processes that characterize normal motor development. The first process facilitates the development of mass movements and postural tone. These reflex regulated mass movements allow for the maintenance of body and limb position against gravity and form the postural background for voluntary sitting, standing, and walking. For example, "if one leg is extended at the knee and hip, the other will be flexed at the same time and visa-versa" (Peiper, 1963, p. 253). The second process involves inhibition of the mass responses so that "performance of selective movement ..., especially the perfection of manipulative skill" is allowed (Bobath, 1966, p. 1). That movements have goals in

Table 5-1
Test Batteries for Soft Neurological Signs in Children

Authors Year (Reference)	Number of Subjects	Ages	Reliability Precautions	Total No. Tests for Soft Signs	Specific Motor Items	Developmental Motor Soft Signs Addressed
Kennard 1960	nl = 65 abnl = 123	13–16 yrs	Subject selection	18	1. Resting and intention tremor 2. Left as marked dominant 3. Dysdiadochokinesis 4. Athetoid movements	Clumsiness, chorea, incomplete dominance, adventitious movements (substantial overlap of findings between controls and patients)
Gubbay 1965	nl = 10 abnl = 21		Subject selection	12	1. Skipping 2. Dribble ball 3. Thread beads 4. Pierce holes in paper 5. Form board	Incomplete dominance, apraxia, adventitious movements, (minimal overlap of findings between controls and abnormals)
Roach & Kepart 1966	nl = 200	6–10 yrs	Test–retest test intercorrelations. Teacher rating to test validity.	30	1. Imitation of movements 2. Rythmic writing	Apraxia, adventitious movements
Spreen & Gaddes 1969	nl = 129	6–15 yrs	Subject selection	15	1. Finger tapping test 2. Grip strength 3. Reaction times 4. Three-dimensional construction praxis	Clumsiness, constructional apraxia
Adams, Kocsis, & Estes 1974	nl = 130 LD = 139	9y 3mo 11y 8mo	Subject selection	8	1. Suppination–pronation of wrist 2. Extend arms in space, abduct fingers with eyes open while seated 3. Hopping 4. Writing	Clumsiness, chorea, manual preference, dysgraphia, (substantial overlap between normal and abnormals)
Hart, Rennick, Klinge, & Schwartz 1974	nl = 30 LD = 129	6–11 yrs	Subject selection by referring source I.Q. (full-scale WISC 80 or above)	16	1. Imitation of hand movements 2. Finger-tapping 3. Foot-tapping 4. Wrist pronation-suppination 5. Heel-walking 6. Standing with feet together, eyes closed, tongue and arms extended, fingers abducted	Apraxia, clumsiness, chorea, synkinesis

Authors Year (Reference)	Number of Subjects	Ages	Reliability Precautions	Total No. Tests for Soft Signs	Specific Motor Items	Developmental Motor Soft Signs Addressed
Gubbay 1975	982 total school population	8–12 yrs	External validation of tests on history and other types of tests	8	1. Form board 2. Whistle 3. Skip 4. Dribble ball 5. Throw ball and clap 6. Tie shoelaces 7. Thread beads 8. Piece holes in paper	Clumsiness, apraxia
Peters, Romine, & Dykman 1975	nl = 45 abnl = 82	8–11 yrs	Subject selection	80	1. Writing 2. Copy finger movements 3. Hopping 4. Tandem walk 5. Foot-tapping 6. Facial movements 7. Finger–nose test 8. Suppination–pronation 9. Finger-tapping 10. Papers and clip 11. Associated movements, asymmetrical 12. Associated movements, symmetrical	Choreaform movements, clumsiness, apraxia, synkinesis, tremor, manual preference, dysgraphia (material-specific apraxia), (substantial overlap of findings between controls and abnormals)

The batteries are listed in chronological order by year of publication.
Abbreviations: mo = months, y = year, nl = normal, abnl = abnormal

Table 5-2
Specific Motor Tests: Normative Data at Specific Ages

Authors Year (Reference)	Number of Subjects	Ages	Reliabilty	Tests and Results	Pertinent SSss
Goodenough, 1935	240	3.5–5.5 yrs	Subject selection sample size	Key tapping with index finger 3½ yrs 18.9 taps in 10 sec R males 14.9 taps in 10 sec L males 4½ yrs 28.7 taps in 10 sec R males 23.2 taps in 10 sec L males 5½ yrs 32.0 taps in 10 sec R males 23.7 taps in 10 sec L males	Manual clumsiness
Costa, 1964 Rapin, 1966	183	6 y	3 subject reselection	Cut-off scores chosen to allow correct classification of subjects, classified 75% of "abnl"	Manual clumsiness
Spreen & Gaddes, 1969	Specified per test (e.g., 222 for key tapping)	6–15 yrs	4 subject selection sample size per age	Key tapping with index finger 6y 30 in 10 sec 8y 38 in 10 sec 12y 47 in 10 sec	
				Preference test some with change with age. Increase in strength of grip. Reaction time steadily decrease with age. Three-dimensional constructional praxis—time to complete steadily declines with age.	Incomplete lateral dominance Not specific constructional apraxia
Boll, 1972	35	10–14 yrs	Subject selection	Index finger-tapping, dominant hand 38 in 10 sec, nondominant hand 34 in 10 sec	Clumsiness, lateral dominance

Authors Year (Reference)	Number of Subjects	Ages	Reliabilty	Tests and Results	Pertinent SSss
Denckla, 1973	237 (normal + right handed)	5–7 yrs	Subject pool test–retest reliability tests	Index finger taps on thumb 5y male R hand 7.30 sec/20 taps (27/10 sec) L hand 7.95/20 taps (25/10 sec) Successive finger tap on thumb 5 y male R hand 16.70 L hand 16.86	Manual clumsiness
Denckla, 1974	168 (normal + right Handed)	5–10 yrs	Subject pool test–retest reliability tests	10 y male R hand 5.55 sec/20 repetitive finger tap (36 taps in 10 sec) 10 y male R hand 7.09 sec/20 turns arm supination–pronation (28 turns in 10 sec) L hand 7.41 sec/20 taps (26.9 in 10 secs) Comparison of L and R hand perform in all tasks. Hands become more similar at older ages. Other hand and some foot tasks increasing speed with increasing age.	Manual clumsiness, pedal clumsiness, incomplete lateral dominance
Adams, 1974	130 nl	9y 3mo to 11y 8mo	Subject selection, then statistical determination of "abnormal": cut off set at 1.5 SD from mean	S pronation Dominant hand 30.35 turns in 10 sec Nondominant 26.73 turns in 10 sec	Manual clumsiness
Annet, 1975 1970	73 nl	11–45 yrs	Test–retest	Peg-moving test consistent difference between hands. Both hands improve with practice.	Incomplete lateral dominance

Table 5-2 *continued*
Specific Motor Tests: Normative Data at Specific Ages

Authors Year (Reference)	Number of Subjects	Ages	Reliabilty	Tests and Results	Pertinent SSss
Kornse D, 1981	18 nl	3y 8mo to 7y 6mo	Subject selection	Peg insertion 5.22 pegs in 30 sec RH male Removal 9.78 pegs/30 sec RH male Sequencing 4.52 pegs/30 sec RH male	Manual apraxia and clumsiness
Hulme C, 1982	16 nl	9y 5mo to 11y 3mo	Subject selection	Pedal ball manipulation about matchbox scored elaborately mean 30.6 pnts Tennis ball throwing scored 10.13 Posting box 15.25 scored Skipping 91.25 scored (gubbay battery)	Clumsiness and apraxia
Wolff, Gunnoe & Cohen, 1983	100 nl (R handed)	5–7 yrs	Subject selection	Associated movements of hands and arms with Fog test. Decrease over 12 mo (rating scales). Mirror movements to finger displacements. Decrease over 12 mo (rating scales). Mirror movements to repetitive–sequential hand and finger tapping. Decrease— particularly in finger tapping over 12 mo.	Synkinesis (mirror and heterotopic)
Rudel, Healey & Denckla, 1984	96 (normal + left handed)	5–10 yrs	Subject selection	10 y male R hand (nondominant) manual clumsiness 5.46 sec/20 finger taps (= 36.3 taps in 10 sec) L hand (dominant) 4.74 sec/20 taps (= 42 taps in 10 sec)	Manual clumsiness

time as well as space is considered (McGuinness, 1981). "In order for ... a motor system to act the time course of a movement trajectory must be reproducible" (Shaffer, 1982). Mature efficient movement requires rapid, orderly temporal and spatial sequences. Failure of the theorized developmental processes would lead to the motor soft signs we are considering.

While we found considerable information on normal motor development, the documentation varies in reliability. A number of older studies (Gesell & Amatruda, 1947; Illingworth, 1966, 1968) and the Denver Developmental Screening Test (Frankenberg, 1983; Frankenberg & Dodds, 1967; 1971) clearly show that the range of normal development is great (the clear-cut "walks alone" milestone occurs over a 6 month range in normal children). When it comes to applications of this knowledge to developmental motor soft signs, the *range* of "normal" to be expected is often poorly defined, or even forgotten in favor of a single milestone. The problem of normal milestones is in part related to the multiplicity of facets of "normal" motor development (Clinton & Boyce, 1975). Strength, tone, coordination (Kelso, Suthard, & Goodman, 1979; Tupper, 1983a; Werry & Aman, 1976; Wolff & Cohen, 1980), sensation (Roland, 1979; Skubic & Anderson, 1970), primitive reflexes (Paine, 1964), equilibrium responses (Shapiro, Burkes, Petti, & Ranz, 1978), manual dominance (Annett, 1970; Kimura & Vanderwolf, 1970), related cognitive processes (Capute, Shapiro, Accardo, et al, 1982; Skubic & Anderson, 1970) and practice opportunity (Foster, Margolin, Alexander, et al, 1978) are some of them.

The best known pioneer in measuring complex voluntary motor development in children was Oseretsky. His tests, published in Russian in 1923 (Oseretsky, 1931) are still being used today. His method comprised organized observation of motions as well as carefully defined measurements of specific performance tests: "static coordination of the hands," "dynamic coordination of the hands," "general dynamic coordination," "motor speed," "simultaneous voluntary movements" and "asynkinesia" (he defined the latter as the ability to perform without synkinesis) (Costa & Fosa, 1946). His tasks were constructed with increasing difficulty for increasing ages, providing, for complex movements, a standard of normal development that was similar in quality to that provided by the Binet intelligence test in the 1930s. He does not give his sources of information concerning the age appropriateness of his items, but when the Oseretsky scales were adapted for use with American school children in 1948 (Sloan, 1948), they were standardized on a group of 730 children from 6 to 14 years of age and do yield a general motor developmental measure that correlates well with age and grade (Espenschade, 1978). Although Oseretsky carefully took specific elemental characteristics of motor activity (such as speed or force), as well as the complex interplay of innervations during serial voluntary motor behaviors (as can be subsumed under the heading of praxis) into account when constructing his tasks, his test does not isolate or overtly measure any one of these characteristics.

Before embarking on our detailed discussion of other developmental motor scales, we should point out that the reliability (defined as reproducibility, in the same individual, of a given motor trait discovered by the same and/or other examiners) was generally not established in earlier studies (see also Table 5-1). Other design problems that occur in studies directed at abnormal populations are further discussed at the end of this section and in a later section (Satz & Morris, 1981). Among papers that do address such issues, Foster's (Foster, Margolin, Alexander, et al, 1978) study assesses the reliability of five items: successive finger movements, tandem walking, closing one eye and then the other, moving the eyes to one side or the other conjugately, and the Babinski response. Physicians repeatedly examine 10 pediatric psychiatric patients in 6-12 sessions. On the successive finger movements task, the performance of all subjects, independent of age and sex, improved. Tandem walking also significantly improved. The highest score achieved on the successive finger approximations was achieved by a child who played the piano, suggesting that practice and exposure may alter the index motor traits. It casts new light on such studies as that of Lerer and Lerer (1976) and McMahon and Greenberg (1977) that draw conclusions concerning the disappearance of soft signs in relation to treatments. Among the factors that must be considered in differentiating between "normal" and "abnormal," is the state of the patient's sleep satiation. While sleep deprivation may not seem a likely source of developmental motor signs, children with attention deficit disorder (ADD) frequently exhibit chronic sleep deprivation, that could, if Sassin's study (1970) is correct, contribute to an increased incidence of soft neurological signs. In the 1950s and 1960s, as part of a large collaborative project, neurological exams were carried out on thousands of children seen at 14 centers around the United States, and the results related to neuropsychiatric syndromes were recently reported by Nichols and Chen (1981). Among other points, this excellent review of "minimal cerebral dysfunction" makes its tabulation of the incidence of soft signs reported from the different collaborating institutions. There was a marked variability in the incidence of certain developmental motor soft signs from institution to institution. Such studies and others (Adams, Kocsis, & Este, 1974; Annett, 1970) certainly serve to highlight the tentative reproducibility of motor soft sign findings. The crux

Table 5-3
Some Tests for Chorea

Authors/Year (Reference)	Tests for Chorea
Prechtl & Stemmer, 1962	Test not specified. Chorea described as slight jerky movements occurring irregularly and arrhythmically in different muscles.
Lucas, Rodin, & Simpson, 1965	Hold arms extended.
Wolff & Hurwitz, 1966	Extend both arms in space at shoulder level, hands pronated, fingers abducted, while standing, for 30 secs.
Barlow, 1974	Extend arms in space, hands suppinated.
Hart, Rennick, Klinge, & Schwartz, 1974	Extend arms in space, finger abducted, eyes closed, tongue protruded, standing with feet together, for 40 secs.
Adams, Kocsis, & Estes, 1974	Extend arms in space six inches above table, abduct fingers, eyes open, sitting, for 30 secs.
Ayers, 1977	Arms outstretched, abduct fingers, eyes closed, standing with feet together, count aloud to 20.

of the issue is lack of uniformly accepted test items and developmental normal ranges (see Tables 5-1 to 5-3).

Frankenberg's Denver Developmental Screening Test (Frankenberg & Dodds, 1967; 1971) uses a gross and a fine motor category. Not only are the standard data derived from a large population, over 1000 normal children of varied socioeconomic status, but the ages at which a given percent of normal children pass an item is given. Thus, 25 percent of children walk by 11.3 months of age and 90 percent walk by 14.2 months of age. This method of reporting results is far more useful than reporting 12 months (the point at which 50 percent of children are walking) as the normal walking milestone. While a screening test is designed to point out areas of concern, rather than to make specific diagnoses, the Frankenberg approach to normative values seems desirable even for more exacting measures, giving, in a manner of speaking, confidence limits for the appearance of certain motor activites in normal SES and racially mixed groups.

The McCarthy Scales of Children's Abilities (McCarthy, 1972) consists of 18 tests, 5 of which directly address motor performance, that are scored on 6 separate scales. The motor items, although not specifically structured to analyze for soft signs, would clearly be impaired by clumsiness and apraxia. This test battery was also carefully standardized. Interestingly, careful selection of normal subjects fulfilling specifically defined socio-economic, sex, and age statuses from preselected United States urban and rural geographic areas was used. Such a standardizing population is quite statistically satisfying. Following collection of scores, reliability was tested primarily by statistical means, and validity by using other tests of cognitive ability, with which there was high correlation, although the motor items were not well correlated. This standardization, reliability, and validity testing (Satz & Morris, 1981) is discussed to point out some of the methods that can be employed to ensure that data are reproducible enough to use with (cautious) confidence to determine probability of abnormality at a given age. The McCarthy Test, like the Denver and Oseretsky is an indicator of developmental level, and does not purpose to provide information as the cause of deviance from its norms. To validate the Purdue Perceptual Motor Survey, Roach and Kephart (1966) did test-retest evaluations of their 200 normal subjects who were from 6 to 10 years. They did test intercorrelations and teacher rating scales to test the test score correlations, thus, further validating their method. A number of surveys derive directly from the neurological exam. These, unlike the standard clinical neurological exam, use specified scoring systems, but the derivation of their normal limits is not always clear. The Physical and Neurological Examination for Soft Signs (PANESS) (Camp, Bailey, & Press, 1977; Camp, Bailer, & Sverd, 1978; Werry & Aman, 1976) is a 43 item examination of a number of motor and sensory items, specifically to evaluate soft signs for drug studies (Close, 1973). While styled after the clinical neurological exam it has an administration and scoring manual, thus helping to standardize the administration, and provides a basis for uniform judgment of normalcy. A revalidation of the PANESS yielded quite acceptable test-retest reliability for the entire battery, but not for many individual items (Holden, Tarnowski, & Prinz, 1982). Touwen and Prechtl's (1970) The Neurological Examination of the Child With Nervous Dysfunction is likewise a carefully directed neurological exam. Peters, Romine, and Dykman (1975) tested 45 normal children, ages 8-11, against their disabled school classmates on tests for choreoathetosis, copying finger movements, hopping, tandem walk, foot tapping, paper clipping, associated movements, facial movements, and writing. They, like Kennard (1960), found considerable overlap between their 45 normal subjects and their index patients. Clearly, the development of general normal values for any of the types of motor survey was not a simple matter.

Selective studies that determine developmental norms for one specific motor item (Denckla, 1973; 1974; Denckla & Rudel, 1978; Kinsbourne, 1973; Spreen & Gaddes, 1969; Tupper, 1983a; 1983b) appear more satisfying, at least at first glance, for such studies generally yield quantitative data (rates of tapping for instance) rather than overall motor developmental ratings. On closer scrutiny, such studies may conflict with each other in important details, so that normative data is only valid for that exact version of the test and cannot be used as a standard for a population or individual that is tested in a somewhat different way. For instance, the most frequently studied activity is finger tapping, done according to sex, respective age group, and often, hand preference. In Table 5-2 it can be seen that when the data of Spreen and Gaddes (1969) for right-handed 8-year-old boys is compared with that of Denkla (1973) for 10-year-old boys for the dominant hand, Denckla obtained a figure of 36 taps in 10 seconds and Spreen 38 taps in 10 seconds. Some of this discrepancy may be related to the methods used. Denckla's subjects tapped on the thumb whereas Spreen's subjects were tapping a key. Goodenough (1935) used a key tapping test in very young children and her 5 ½-year-old males could tap 32 times in 10 seconds compared to Denckla's 5-year-olds (Denckla, 1973) who tapped 27 times in 10 seconds. Perhaps discrepancies in the mode of testing account for the discrepancies in rates of tapping. Denckla and Rudels' (Denckla, 1973, 1974; Denckla & Rudel, 1978; Rudel, Healey, & Denckla, 1984) studies evaluate motor activities for both feet and hands between the ages of 5 and 10. In addition to finger tapping, they tested subjects on successive movements of the fingers upon the thumb, repetitive hand patting, alternating hand pronation and supination (for dysdiadochokinesis), alternating hand flexion and extension, and repetitive tapping on the foot. Subjects were retested, for reliability, and finger successive movements were found the most reliable, followed by the finger tapping test. Practice tended to equalize right and left performances. Further, while a relative plateau in speed of motor performance appeared for ages 8-10, there was also a marked increase in speed of tapping between ages 5 and 7. The distal tasks such as finger tapping, hand flexion and extension, repetitive tapping of the toes, and the heel and the toe were significantly asymmetrical with better scores uniformly produced by the dominant side, but improvement in both, as also noted by Spreen and Gaddes (1969).

Tupper's (1983a, 1983b) studies evaluated manual activities in younger children. Tupper assessed a group of 219 3–8-year-olds on the Purdue Peg Board, lateral preference, bilateral alternating finger tapping, and the Oseretsky Test for reciprocal coordination. Tupper reported that lateral preference did not change dramatically from ages 3-8 while unilateral motor performance skill increased linearly for both hands. While improvement of reciprocal coordination and bilateral alternating activities were found, Tupper's study also showed that synkinesis declined steadily with increasing age, particularly in what he calls "contralateral associated movements" (mirror movements). He concluded, however, that bimanual coordinated movements did not improve as rapidly as mirror movements disappeared, suggesting dissociation of the two developmental trends, even though they may both be related to an "inhibition" system, consistent with the developmental notions of Bobath (1966), Kinsbourne (1973), and Peiper (1963).

Overall, quantitative studies substantiate the notion that adroitness normally evolves rapidly between the ages of 3 and 8, and then, more slowly, evolves to an asymptote in early adulthood, and serve to highlight the problem of presenting norms for motor tasks used to test for soft signs. Differences in theoretical construct, methodology, and task selection obviously affect performance outcomes: each study has a somewhat different outcome related to these factors. A major factor is the definition of normal. Motor soft signs are defined as developmental on the basis of being present in most members of a young population but infrequent in members of an older population. Given that understanding of "developmental," the age at which the slowness of finger tapping or the overflow of movements or the difficulty in producing a sequence of voluntary acts becomes abnormal is a matter of definition (Rapin, Tourke, & Costa, 1960). One may define a phenomenon as deviant, for instance, if it appears in 10 percent of an age cohort (as the Denver Developmental Screening Test does), or one might rather define it as abnormal if it appears only in 2 percent of a cohort.

DEFINITIONS OF SOME DEVELOPMENTAL MOTOR SOFT SIGNS AND TESTS FOR SOFT SIGNS

There is no definite consensus as to what constitutes the motor soft signs and still less the optimal way to test for them. Nonetheless, in most articles reviewed at least one, and often several, of the motor traits we will define below were investigated. We will concentrate this discussion on measures of dexterity, praxis, measures of what might be called orthokinesis (as the opposite of synkinesis), tremor and chorea, and measures of manual preference. Although we have alluded to clumsiness, apraxia, synkinesis, chorea and tremor, and incomplete manual dominance as soft signs, they are in fact inferential categories. In this section, in addition to defining each soft sign category, we will discuss the individual test items that are used to evaluate the category.

The term clumsiness in common parlance means inability to manipulate objects well, and says nothing about why the objects are not manipulated well. The most commonly used test for dexterity (the opposite of clumsiness) is index finger tapping on the thumb. The second most often used test is successive fingers tapping on the thumb. Some authors very clearly separate these two tests (Denckla, 1973), while in the work of others it is difficult to determine which finger tapping test was used. Some testers require that both hands be suspended in the air while the index finger taps on the thumb (in order to simultaneously evaluate for associated movements), while others do not specify hand position (Hertzig, 1981). Finger tapping on a key may also be used (Holden et al, 1982). Table 5-2 lists several studies where this test has been used and their specific findings (Boll & Reitan, 1972; Denckla, 1973; 1974; Goodenough, 1935; Spreen & Gaddes, 1969). Peg placing, often as part of the Purdue Pegboard Test (Costa, Scarda, & Rapin, 1964; Rapin, Tourke, & Costa, 1960), or peg moving aside from that used in formalized tests (Annett, 1970; Deuel & Moran, 1980), is often used. Alternating supination and pronation of the wrist is frequently used as a measure of dexterity. A number of other items are occasionally used (e.g., bead stringing, hand clapping) and others rarely or only in a single study. Deficits in individual tests, of course, can be due to a number of totally disparate factors; for instance, weakness, spasticity, or cerebellar tremor. Thus, one must be able to say that weakness or spasticity are not present before inferring the observed clumsiness is not due to a localizing lesion of the nervous system, or other factors.

In neurologic terms, clumsiness implies a lower order deficit; that is, a deficit in alteration of joint angles by effector structures according to the speed and direction specified by the cerebral innervation. But the inability of the cerebral apparatus to judge distance and directions for movement trajectories will also lead to clumsiness in that the incorrect specifications will be transmitted to the effector structures. Such difficulty with judgment of distance and direction (a problem that may be termed perceptual) (Bender, 1970; Denckla & Rudel, 1978), could also occur for reasons of poor eyesight or visual acuity, i.e., a sensory deficit. Thus sensory deficits must be ruled out before labeling as clumsiness. In summary, neurologic clumsiness is of two varieties, poor execution because joint angles will not alter fast and accurately enough, and poor execution due to transmission of improper spatial information (a type of agnosia), as discussed by Walton,-Ellis, and Court (1965). The former, according to Oseretsky, is a variety of apraxia first delineated by Liepmann, who called it limb kinetic apraxia (Liepmann, 1908). In adults with strokes, this entity is so difficult to dissociate from mild paresis that it has been abandoned as a category of apraxia (Botez, 1961). In the developmental variety of clumsiness, in contradistinction to mild paresis due to focal cerebral lesions, clumsiness is not unilateral. One of its hallmarks is that it does not change much with the task at hand; it is as bad when buttoning a Barbie doll's dress or when writing. The muscle groups and joints should all be surveyed, as clumsiness may affect only distal joints, only proximal and axial joints, or both.

Apraxia of the ideomotor or ideational variety (DeRenzi, Pieczoro, & Vignolo, 1968; Haaland, Porch, & Delaney, 1980; Heilman, Schwartz, & Geschwind, 1975; Kelso & Tupper, 1981), as opposed to clumsiness or limb kinetic apraxia, is manifest as the inability of the subject, despite preserved sensation, strength, coordination, dexterity, and volition, to make a sequence of voluntary movements that are appropriately directed and effective. An apraxic (some prefer to use "dyspraxic" for the developmental variety) disability may be manifest particularly in acts to verbal command (with or without the use of actual objects), or on the imitation of movements. As sequences of voluntary movement are affected, the dyspraxic difficulty is often spoken of as a difficulty in motor planning. Of course, conscious planning of a motor act is not necessarily affected, but the order of the elemental motions is improper and the entire act may not produce the finished effect desired by the subject. If the command has been attended to and the child understands and wishes to attempt the act and the correct action is not forthcoming despite observed attempts to perform, requiring the child to point to a picture of the requested action may differentiate failure of understanding from failure of actual ability to produce the movement sequences. Tests that are most often used for praxis include pantomiming on command, following serial commands, manipulating complex objects, and imitating hand and finger postures produced by the examiner. In children the differentiation of the two major varieties of dyspraxia, ideomotor and ideational (DeRenzi et al, 1968), has seldom been attempted. In a small study of matched normal and LD subjects (Deuel, Feely, & Bonskowski, 1984), and in the study of Gubbay and coauthors (Gubbay, Ellis, & Walton, 1965), both types were present concomitantly.

Synkinesis is a term referring to a specific type of involuntary movement that occurs when a voluntary movement is intended and carried out. The synkinetic movement occurs involuntarily in muscle groups that are not required for the intended action, for example, with an *intended* tapping of the *nondominant* thumb, an involuntary tapping of the dominant thumb occurs. Naturally, the hands must be held in a position where this can be noted. As voluntary motor acts become more difficult or require more muscle groups, mirror synkinesis may occur in any subject, even in a normal young adult. Mirror synkinesis may be defined as that movement appearing in muscle groups that are innervated by the same segmental levels as the intended movement, but on the opposite side of the body. Heterotopic synkineses occur at the same time as intended movements, but in heterotopic muscle groups. A common heterotopic synkinesis occurs when a child is asked to open his eyes as wide as possible, and the mouth opens involuntarily. The Fog test, that requires the child to walk on the sides of his feet, often brings out heterotopic synkinesis in the hands and mouth (Fog & Fog, 1963). The mechanism of abnormal synkinesis is not known but it is hypothesized that insufficient "inhibitory" influence is being exterted (Wolff & Cohen, 1980; Wolff, Gunnoe, & Cohen, 1983) via the corpus callosuum and other intracortical pathways (Preilowski, 1972; Roland, 1979).

Chorea and tremor are both involuntary adventitious movements. Chorea consists of irregular, rather sudden movements of whole muscle groups (Prechtl & Stemmer, 1962), but does not invariably involve muscle groups on ongoing intended movement and so is quite different from synkinesis. The maneuver most commonly used to bring out chorea, particularly of the hands, is to have the patient extend the pronated arms in front of him, close his eyes, abduct his fingers, and maintain the position for at least 10 seconds (Rutter, Graham, & Birch, 1966; Wolff & Hurwitz, 1966). Table 5-3 documents some of the many variations on this test for chorea. Prior vigorous exercise may lead to markedly increased choreiform movements (Rutter et al, 1966). Chorea may also be observed pari passu while the child is walking or running. Chorea may sometimes be appreciated in the patient's grip, when different fingers exert different forces at different times. Extending the hands over the head may bring out a posture of pronation that is commonly associated with chorea. Hypotonia may be associated particularly with severe chorea. Tremor may be of several varieties, and all may be seen in children with neuropsychiatric disorders. Intention tremor is tested by finger-nose-finger test. The finger-nose-finger test, as with items we have discussed earlier, is performed differently by different examiners.

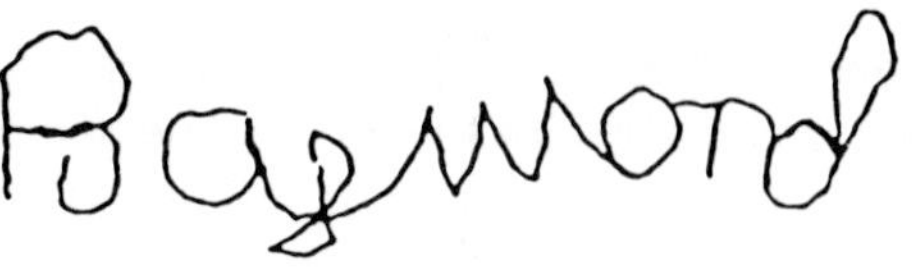

Cursive writing of a 10y 2mo male with normal intelligence (I.Q. 96), CT scan, but marked tremor, chorea and clumsiness.

Figure 5-1. A 10-year-old boy with tremor, hypotonia, chorea, and clumsiness writes his name (Raymond). The oscillations of his hand during writing are apparent in the lines he draws.

One version is to have the child seated or standing, touch his nose with his forefinger, touch the examiner's forefinger with his forefinger, return his finger to his nose. Another version has the child close his eyes, extend his arms to the side and bring each forefinger to his own nose. This version excludes vision and forces use of kinesthetic sensation. Action tremor may be seen during movements of a pencil or pen and writing is frequently used, or drawing, to observe for action tremor. Figure 5-1 shows the writing of a child referred for clumsiness and learning problems. His tremor is evident in his writing.

The last developmental motor sign we will discuss is mixed dominance and/or incomplete manual dominance. Manual dominance, of course, is a full topic in its own right, and what constitutes an abnormality of manual dominance (too much ambidexterity or left handedness) is not clear (Annett 1970; Annett, Hudson, & Turner, 1974; Bishop, 1980; Hicks & Dusek, 1980). Approximately 10 percent of the normal population in all countries, and all eras of human civilization have been left handed (Deuel & Dunlop, 1980). The age at which manual dominance should be manifest is a matter of controversy (Deuel & Moran, 1980; Gesell and Ames, 1947). So called mixed dominance is when the manual preference and ocular and/or pedal preference are different. Of course ocular preference may be dependent upon local interocular factors, not cerebral organization. All of these lateralities are generally tested by the preference method (which eye is preferred for sighting through a telescope, which foot for kicking a ball). Manual dominance is tested generally in two fashions, by questionaire, which appears to be highly accurate (Annett et al, 1974; Deuel & Moran, 1980) or by actual performance tests (Annett, 1970). Tests of hand preference allow the subject to choose the hand he or she prefers. Tests of performance actually pit the measured abilities of one hand against the other. It has been found that the dominant hand is more dexterous than the nondominant hand (Annett, 1970; Annett et al, 1974; Denckla, 1973; Spreen & Gades, 1969). One notion behind the search for mixed cerebral dominance in children is that "brain damage" will lead to mixed or even shifted dominance (Bishop, 1980). This is due to the presence of documented "pathological left handers" in the left-handed population. However, that subliminal brain damage always creates left handedness or ambidexterity, or that left handedness is often due to brain damage is not substantiated. For instance, a recent study demonstrates a higher proportion of left handers in the intellectually gifted (where there is an underrepresentation of individuals with the neuropsychological syndromes of childhood) than the average population (Hicks & Dusek, 1980).

INCIDENCE OF MOTOR SOFT SIGNS

This section will present the reported incidence of the five motor soft signs in groups with learning disabilities (LD), conduct and emotional disorders, the clumsy child syndrome, hyperactivity-attention deficit disorder (HA), and minimal brain dysfunction (MBD) (see Table 5-4). A synopsis of the conceptual issues and problems that are apparent in the reports that use neurologic soft signs as evidence of (assumed) etiology or as evidence for specific neuropsychiatric syndromes will also be made.

As repeatedly demonstrated (Abbie, Douglas, & Ross, 1978; Gubbay, 1975; 1978; Gubbay et al, 1965; Henderson & Hall, 1982; Hulme, Biggerstaff, & Morgan, 1982), motor abilities can statistically discriminate groups of normal from groups of children with neuropsychiatric syndromes. Authors consistently find that the "abnormal group" takes longer to complete tasks and fails more items than normal groups (Henderson & Hall, 1982; Hulme et al, 1982), although many report a considerable incidence of the soft signs of interest in the "normal" group as well (Adams et al, 1974; Kennard, 1960; Peters et al, 1975). Thus, with respect to the discriminatory function of these motor tests, they seem to facilitate post facto group categorical differentiations only. The evidence we have reviewed does not indicate that they shed any light on causal relationships (Beggs & Breslaw, 1982; Berger & Marqulies, 1978; Corey, 1980; Foster et al, 1978; Touwen & Sporrel, 1979), nor do they appear to facilitate clini-

Table 5-4
The Percent of Abnormal Subjects, as Designated by the Authors, Reported to Demonstrate the Given Soft Sign

Authors Year (Reference)	Index Syndrome	Sample Characteristics	Clumsiness	Apraxia	Chorea	Synkinesis	Altered Dominance
Kennard, 1960	Behavior Disorders	135 abnl, nl IQ 65 nl 13–16 y	17% (15% nl)	NR	21% (5%)	NR	28% (12% nl)
Prechtl & Stemmer, 1962	Learning Disability	157 LD males 876 nl males	prsent	NR	45% (20% nl)	NR	NR
Walton, Ellis & Court, 1962	Clumsiness	5 clumsy 9–14yr nl IQ (verbal 87–137, perf 44–97)	100%	60%	NR	NR	80%
Gubbay, Ellis, Walton & Court, 1965	Clumsiness	21 clumsy 9y 5mo to 17y 4mo Verbal IQ >80 nl 10	100%	100% (20% nl)	23%	NR	33%
Belmont & Birch, 1965	Reading Disability	50 disabled readers, 9y 4mo to 10y 4mo	NR	NR	NR	NR	31%
Wolff & Hurwitz, 1966	MBD	210 abnls 9–15y delinquent and neurotic males 1772 nl males	NR	NR	43% (11.7% nl)	NR	NR

Authors Year (Reference)	Index Syndrome	Sample Characteristics	Clumsiness	Apraxia	Chorea	Synkinesis	Altered Dominance
Paine, Werry & Quay, 1968	MBD	83 referrals for MBD mean age 84y SD 2.6y mean IQ 96.3	43%	NR	present	NR	NR
Hertzig, Bartmer & Birch, 1969	MBD	59 educationally designated brain damaged children 10–12y	57.6%	33.9%	42.4%	NR	NR
Adams, Kocis & Estes, 1974	Learning Disabilities (LD)	368 school children 9y 3mo to 11y 8mo designated as nl, borderline or LD on basis of achievement and IQ testing	37% (9% nl)	NR	36% (35%nl)	NR	43% (46% nl)
Peters, Romaine & Dykman, 1975	Learning Disabilities (LD)	82 LD-BD males 8–11y, IQ >90 45 nls	46% (9% nl)	29% (14% nl)	57% (29% nl)	42% (16% nl)	46% (27% nl)

Table 5-4 *continued*
The Percent of Abnormal Subjects, as Designated by the Authors, Reported to Demonstrate the Given Soft Sign

Authors Year (Reference)	Index Syndrome	Sample Characteristics	Clumsiness	Apraxia	Chorea	Synkinesis	Altered Dominance
Denckla & Rudel, 1978	Hyperactivity (HA)	43 HA males 5–11y, right handed IQ >90, 50 nls	present	NR	NR	present	NR
Lerer & Lerer, 1976	Hyperactivity (HA)	40 HA 7.3y to 11.3y IQ 87–120	77%	NR	10%	18%	NR
McMahon & Greenberg, 1977	Hyperactivity	102 HA 6.5y to 11y IQ >70	75%	NR	0%	82%	NR
Deuel, 1981	MBD	40 MBD referrals 18–12y IQ 85–125	42%	NR	NR	NR	NR
Gilberg & Rasmussen, 1982	MBD	42 MBD on clinical designations	NR	NR	NR	NR	33%
Henderson & Hall, 1982	Clumsiness	16 teacher-designated as clumsy, mean age 6.6y IQ 102.7 mean	present	present	NR	NR	NR

For the sake of uniformity and simplicity, when multiple categories were reported by a given author (e.g., right-handed versus left-handed males versus males), this table uses the category with the highest incidence of a given soft sign. We suggest referring to the original articles for the details of each study. We will not discuss the controversies surrounding the terms and titles of these syndromes; rather, articles will be reviewed under the syndrome name used by their authors. NR = not reported.

cal management of individuals apart from remediation of motor abnormalities (Critchley, 1970; Deuel, 1981; Hart, Rennick, & Klinge, 1974; Hertzig et al, 1969; Kenney, Clemmens, Cicci et al, 1972; Shapiro et al, 1978). Signs may change in the face of maturation and repeated examination (Foster et al, 1978; Ingram, 1973; Lerer & Lerer, 1976; Sassin, 1970), which certainly must add to their lack of reliability in diagnosis. For example, although Peters (Peters et al, 1975) reported that 57 percent of 82 boys with learning disabilities exhibited choreiform movements, the sign did not discriminate older members of this group from older normal children. In a recent study, intended to reappraise the motor performances of previously diagnosed clumsy and normal children, Knuckey and Gubbay (1983) found that 13 children who originally had evidenced mild to moderate degrees of clumsiness, improved to normal, while 7 children who originally had severe clumsiness still differed significantly from their normal counterparts, suggesting a favorable prognosis for children who initially evidence a mild to moderate impairment. Although evaluating a different population, Hertzig's (1981) longitudinal study on low birth weight children found similar interactions of development with severity of deficit. As evidenced by Hart, Rennick, and Klinge's study, in which the poor motor performances of young children were interpreted as abnormal when in fact they could be within the range of normal (Hart et al, 1974), developmental range norms are a critical issue.

At times, results are based on test items that are dissimilar among studies. Barlow's (Barlow, 1974) test of chorea is with the supinated outstretched forearm. Wolff (Wolff & Cohen, 1980), on the other hand, wants subjects to pronate the forearm. Signs generally are used to either substantiate etiology (Bishop, 1980; Geshwind & Behan, 1982) or to discern significant differences between groups of normal and disordered children (Adams et al 1974; Peters et al, 1975). As can be noted in Table 5-4, different studies report different incidences of soft signs among children wth the same syndrome. For example, Adams (Adams et al, 1974) reports an incidence of reversed or mixed dominance of 36.1 percent in LD males and 43 percent for LD females, while Belmont and Birch (1965) report 31 percent for both and Peters (Peters et al, 1975) reports 46 percent mixed laterality in LD males. In some instances, however, dominance findings did not significantly differentiate between normal and disordered groups (Adams et al, 1974) let alone provide clinically useful data on individual children. Fagan-Dubin's (1974) two phase study that surveyed 667 kindergarden boys and 590 girls, reported that 12.3 percent of the boys and 10.3 percent of the girls were left handed. In a second phase of this study, the authors also found no significant differences in the verbal and performance abilities of the left from the right-handed children. Others that examined the relationship between left handedness or eye-hand preference among children with reading (dyslexia) and behavior problems also failed to find significant results (Belmont & Birch, 1965). Although Stine (Stine, Saratsiotis, & Mosser, 1975) found significant associations between mixed dominance and hyperactivity (69 out of 283 children) and variable day to day performance (69 out of 272 children = 24 percent), their commentary about the sources of unreliability in their own study is noteworthy; (1) differences in interpretation of terms, i.e., hyperactivity versus aggressiveness can lead to misdiagnosis, (2) test failures can involve factors that are uncontrolled, making it difficult to discern the exact cause, (3) the relatively common occurrence of a sign in their study (mixed dominance) among normal children makes the clinical interpretation of the sign difficult.

In a study that examined left handers (Bishop, 1980), one of the inherent concerns of studies that examine dominance is evident. Bishop hypothesizes that a certain percentage of children evidence "extended pathologic left handedness" (EPLH, natural right handers that shifted hand preference). Using a square tracing test he devised to assess handedness, Bishop evaluated 170 children (ages 8-9) and did a further analysis of the performance of 33 children (target group) who were selected from the original sample on the basis of inferior performance with their nonpreferred as opposed to preferred hand. Bishop (1980) found a higher incidence of left-handed subjects among the target group and concluded: "... left handedness represents a mild unilateral brain abnormality which renders the contralateral hand clumsy and depresses cognitive ability" (p. 577). Studying this same point, Hicks and Dusek (1980) hypothesized that if left handedness is caused by brain damage, the frequency of left-handers among normal and gifted children should be less. They evaluated 578 intellectually gifted and 31 average children, with the gifted group demonstrating more left-handedness than their normal counterparts. The authors conclude that handedness is not a reliable indicator in the assessment of individual brain dysfunction, nor is handedness a viable discriminator between groups of gifted and nongifted children. All together, the studies we reviewed suggest that if a child is left handed he or she is just as likely to be gifted as brain damaged or (according to Geschwind & Behan, 1982) learning disabled with a disposition to immune disease or migraine.

As can be seen in Table 5-4 studies not only report widely differing incidence rates of mixed or altered dominance, but also synkinesis, apraxia, clumsiness, and choreiform movements (0 percent to 57 percent in abnormals). For example, Wolff and Hurwitz's MBD study (Wolff & Hurwitz, 1966) reported that chorea was more frequent among delinquents, learning disabled, and emotionally disabled children, although present in approximately 12 percent of the normal population. Hertzig et al's (1969) study of 59 designated brain damaged children reported a high incidence of chorea, 42.1 percent, while Lerer and Lerer (1976), who evaluated 40 hyperactive children, found an incidence of 10 percent. Prechtl and Stemmer's (1962) investigation of 50 children with behavior problems, reported an incidence of 100 percent, however, subject selection was predicated upon the observed presence of the sign. McMahon and Greenberg (1977), on the other hand, reported that none of their hyperactive sample of 102 children evidenced chorea. Such radical differences in incidence are likely due to: (1) differences in subject selection criteria; (2) differences in methods of testing (shown in Table 5-3 for chorea); and (3) differences in scoring interpretation. To summarize, it is the dissimilarity among these factors, particularly the subjective interpretation of soft sign absence or presence, that makes study comparisons in each category of disorder difficult and indicates a need to temper acceptance of incidence reports and claims of cause and effect relationships.

MOTOR SOFT SIGNS WITH HANDICAPPING SIGNIFICANCE

Clumsiness in the sense discussed above, apraxia in the sense discussed above, tremor (see Fig. 5-1), and adventitious movements as discussed by Tupper (Tupper, 1983a, 1983b) are all potentially handicapping conditions. The motor soft sign most commonly found to be handicapping is clumsiness of unknown etiology (Ford, 1960; Orton, 1925; Walton et al, 1965). A child with this disturbance, the classical "klutz," suffers from poor self-esteem from the very first time he can't tie a shoe or button a button. At times this motor disability is the primary cause of school failure even without cognitive deficits, as secondary low self-esteem mediates the continued failure. It must be recalled that the clumsy child's problem, unlike the dyslexic's, has often created difficulties and tensions at home, years before he ever gets to school.

The first cornerstone of management, advocated early on, was a common sense diminishing of motor demands (don't make him write the word 50 times if he can spell it correctly after the first 10). Beyond that, several disciplines can help in the management of the clumsy child (Gordon &

McKinley, 1980). Clumsiness may improve with the practice of a specific sequence of movements. For instance, after practicing buckling a given belt, the child may do it fairly well. However, a new belt with a new type of buckle will be a new challenge, and will have to be practiced all over again before reasonable facility is achieved. Furthermore, stress usually makes the situation more difficult and will bring back the slowness of movement. Frustration or fear of failing the first attempt evokes worse performance and further frustration and failure. Before planning a remedial program detailed testing is useful to determine the extent and type of motor handicap (David et al, 1981) and associated cognitive and motivational problems (Paulsen & O'Donnell, 1979; Quitkin, Rifkin, & Klein, 1976; Rutter, 1981; Shaffer, 1978). Occupational therapy can provide activities to enhance coordination in such necessary activities as use of everyday tools such as scissors, writing (Towle, 1978), and self care activities. Some of the more arcane therapies, touted as promoting "sensorimotor integration" are not of proven value (Weeks & Zona, 1979). Physical therapy and physical education (adaptive PE) will provide exercises to promote gross motor improvement. Psychologists, psychiatric and speech therapists should be deployed as required. Parental knowledge of the ramifications of the problem, and their continued efforts to promote social comptence appear of paramount importance (Abbie et al, 1978).

CONCLUSION

Our review has highlighted several needs in this area. One is to establish a consensus on the tests to be used to evaluate the signs, another is to establish the age range of normal disappearance of the developmental motor soft signs. To accomplish the latter, it would be optimal to make a longitudinal study (that is, would follow the same individuals throughout development) of a large representative population of children not designated as normal or abnormal. Such a study might well show that some children change slowly but smoothly from one stage of the development of an ability to the next and in those children the apparent "abnormality" (looked at from the point of view of inclusion in the lowest 10 percent or 5 percent of an age bracket) would be part of an individual "normal" pattern of development, much in the way that head circumference, height, and weight follow growth curves. A third need is to establish the functional significance of these motor soft signs. A comprehensive study of handicap that can be attributed to soft signs, considered in conjunction with pertinent congnitive and emotional factors (Deuel, 1981; Quitkin et al, 1976; Rutter, 1981; 1982) is much needed. When motor traits are clearly handicapping, appropriate remediation should be attempted. Despite the views of many purists such as Ford (1960) and Gomez (1967) and the evidence that eventual disappearance of soft signs as the subject matures may occur (Knuckey, Apsimon, & Gubbay, 1983), children with severe soft signs may retain difficulty in performance at least until late teenage (Knuckey et al, 1983). Not only may the motor signs persist, but several authorities are of the opinion that early motor handicap may cause later psychiatric problems whether or not the signs persist (Quitkin et al, 1976; Shaffer, 1978). It is our belief that the handicapping potential of each soft sign should be considered separately and with full realization that many soft signs may be without functional significance, as far as can be determined from our review of the literature. Why some children with motor soft signs have no trouble coping with school and life while others with no worse signs have dire problems seems to be related to a complex interplay between physical, psychological, and environmental factors that may produce the actual functional achievement of the child. These factors all have to be evaluated to find the answer to this question for each individual patient (David et al, 1981; Touwen & Sporrel, 1979).

REFERENCES

Abbie M, Douglas H, & Ross K. The clumsy child syndrome: Observation in cases referred to the gymnasium of the Adelaide Children's Hospital over a three-year period. Medical Journal of Australia, 1978, 1, 65-69

Adams J. Clinical neuropsychological study of learning disorders. Pediatric Clinics of North America, 1973, 29, 587-598

Adams R, Kocsis J, & Estes R. Soft neurological signs in learning disabled children and controls. American Journal of Diseases of Children, 1979, 128, 614-618

Annett M. The growth of manual preference and speed. British Journal of Psychology, 1970, 61, 544-558

Annett M, Hudson P, & Turner A. The reliability of differences between the hands in motor skill. Neuropsychologia, 1974, 12, 527-531

Aram D, & Horwitz S. Sequential and non-speech praxic abilities in developmental verbal apraxia. Developmental Medicine and Child Neurology, 1983, 25, 197-206

Ayers J. Effect of sensory integrative therapy on the coordination of children with choreaoathetoid movements. American Journal of Occupational Therapy, 1983, 31, 291-293

Baker J. A psychomotor approach to the assessment and treatment of clumsy children. Physiotherapy, 1981, 67, 356-365

Bakwin H. Symposium on developmental disorders of motility and language. Pediatric Clinics of North America, 1968, 15, 565-567

Barlow C. "Soft signs" in children with learning disorders. American Journal of Diseases of Children, 1974, 128, 605-606

Beggs W, & Breslaw P. Reading, clumsiness and the deaf child. American Annals of the Deaf, 1982, 127, 32-37

Belmont L, & Birch H. Lateral dominance, lateral awareness, and reading disabilities. Child Development, 1965, 36, 57-71

Bender L. Psychopathology of Children with Organic Brain Disorders. Springfield, Ill: Charles C. Thomas, 1970

Bennett F, & Sherman R. Management of childhood "hyperactivity" by Primary Care Physicians. Developmental and Behavioral Pediatrics, 1983, 4, 88-93

Benton A. Right-left discrimination and finger localization in defective children. Archives of Neurology and Psychiatry, 1956, 74, 583-589

Berger E, & Marqulies J. Frequency of minor nervous dysfinction in school children. Journal of Neurology, 1978, 219, 205-212

Bishop D. Handedness, clumsiness and cognitive ability. Developmental Medicine and Child Neurology, 1980, 22, 569-579

Bobath C. The motor deficit in patients with cerebral palsy. Clinics in Developmental Medicine, 23, London: Spastics Society and William Heinemann, 1966

Boll T, & Reitan R. Motor and tactile perceptual deficits in brain-damaged children. Perceptual and Motor Skills, 1972, 34, 343-350

Botez M. Mild forms of aphasia, apraxia and agnosia. Acta Neurologica Scandinavica, 1961, 37, 111-128

Camp J, Bialer I, & Sverd J. Clinical usefulness of the NIMH physical and neurological examination for soft signs. American Journal of Psychiatry, 1978, 135, 362-364

Camp J, Bialer I, & Press M. The PANESS: norms and comparisons between normal and deviant boys. Psychopharmacology Bulletin, 1977, 13, 39-41

Capute A, Shapiro B, Accardo, P, et al. Motor functions: associated primative reflex profiles. Developmental Medicine and Child Neurology, 1982, 24, 662-669

Clements S. Minimal brain dysfunction in children. (USPHS Publication #141). Washington, DC: U.S.Government Printing Office, 1966

Clinton L, & Boyce K. Acquisition of simple motor imitative behavior in mentally retarded and nonretarded children. American Journal of Mental Deficiency, 1975, 79, 695-700

Close J. Scored neurological examination. Psychopharmacology Bulletin: Special Issue, Psychopharmacology of Children, 1973, 9, 142-148

Corey WB. Minimal brain dysfunction and hyperkinesis. American Journal of Diseases of Children, 1980, 134, 926-930

Costa M, & Fosa E. The Oseretsky Tests of Motor Proficiency: A Translation for the Portugese Adaptation. In Doll E (Ed.). Philadelphia Educational Test Bureau Educational Publishers, 1946

Costa L, Scarda L, & Rapin L. Purdue Peg Board Scores for normal grammar school children. Perceptual and Motor Skills, 1964, 18, 748

Critchley M. The Dyslexic Child. Springfield, Ill: Charles C. Thomas, 1970

Dare M, & Gordon N. Clumsy children: A disorder of perception and motor organizaton. Developmental Medicine and Child Neurology, 1970, 12, 178-185

David R, Deuel D, & Ferry P. Proposed nosology of disorders of higher cerebral function in children. Task Force on Nosology of Disorders of Higher Cerebral Function in Children. Child Neurology Society, 1981

Dawdy S. Pediatric neuropsychology: Caring for the developmental dyspraxic child. Clinical Neuropsychology, 1981, 3, 30-37

Denckla M. Development of speed in repetitive and successive finger movements in normal children. Developmental Medicine and Child Neurology, 1973, 15, 635-645

Denckla M. Development of motor co-ordination in normal children. Developmental Medicine and Child Neurology, 1974, 16, 729-741

Denckla M, & Rudel R. Anomalies of motor development in hyperactive boys. Annals of Neurology, 1978, 3, 231-233

DeRenzi E, Pieczoro A, & Vignolo L. Ideational apraxia: A quantitative study. Neuropsychologia, 1968, 6, 41-52

Deuel R. Minimal brain dysfunction, hyperkinesis, learning disabilities, attention deficit disorder. Journal of Pediatrics, 1981, 98, 912-915

Deuel R, & Dunlop N. Hand preferences in the rhesus monkey: Implications for the study of cerebral dominance. Archives of Neurology, 1980, 37, 217-221

Deuel R, Feely C, & Bonskowski C. Manual apraxia in learning disabled children (Abstract). Annals of Neurology, 1984, 16, 388

Deuel R, & Moran C. Cerebral dominance and cerebral asymmetries on computed tomogram in childhood. Neurology, 1980, 30, 934-938

Doman G, Delacato C, & Doman R. The Doman-Delacato developmental mobility scale. The Rehabilitation Center at Philadelphia, Philadelphia: The Rehabilitation Center at Philadelphia, 1960

DSM III. Diagnostic and Statistical Manual of Mental Disorders. Disorders usually evident in infancy, childhood, and adolescence (Chapter 2). Washington, DC: American Psychiatric Association, 1980

Espenschade A. In Buros O (Ed.). 5th Mental Measurement Yearbook. Highland Park, NJ: Buros Institute, 1978, p. 768

Fagan-Dubin L. Lateral dominance and development of cerebral specialization. Cortex, 1974, 10, 69-74

Fog E, & Fog M. Cerebral inhibition examined by associated movements. In MacKeith R, & Bax M (Eds.). Minimal Cerebral Dysfunction. Clinics in Developmental Medicine (#10). London: Spastics Society and Heinemann Medical, 1963

Ford F. Diseases of the Nervous System in Infancy, Childhood and Adolescence. (2nd ed.), Springfield, Ill: Charles C. Thomas, 1960, p. 197

Foster R, Margolin L, Alexander O, et al. Equivocal neurological signs, child development and learned behavior. Child Psychiatry and Human Development, 1978, 90, 728-32

Frankenberg W. Infant and preschool developmental screening. In Levine M, Carey W, & Crocken A (Eds.). Developmental-Behavioral Pediatrics (Chap. 45A). Philadelphia: W.B. Saunders, 1983

Frankenberg W, & Dodds J. The Denver Developmental Screening Test. Journal of Pediatrics, 1967, 71, 181-191

Frankenberg W, & Dodds J. Validation of the Revised Denver Development Screening Test. Journal of Pediatrics, 1971, 79, 988-995

Geschwind N, & Behan P. Lcft handedness associated with immuno disease, migraine and development disorder. Proceedings of the National Academy of Science, 1982, 79, 5097-5100

Gesell A, & Amatruda C. Developmental Diagnosis. New York: Hoeber, 1947

Gesell A, & Ames L. The development of handedness. Journal of Genetic Psychology, 1947, 70, 155-176

Gillberg C, & Rasmussen P. Perceptual, motor and attentional deficits in seven-year-old children: Background factors. Developmental Medicine and Child Neurology, 1982, 24, 752-770

Gomez M. Minimal cerebral dysfunction (maximal neurologic confusion). Clinical Pediatrics, 1967, 6, 589-591

Goodenough F. A further study of speed of tapping in early childhood. Journal of Applied Psychology, 1935, 19, 309-315

Gordon N, & McKinley I. Helping Clumsy Children. New York: Churchill Livingstone, 1980

Gubbay S. The Clumsy Child: A Study of Developmental Apraxic and Agnostic Ataxia. London: Saunders, 1975

Gubbay S. The management of developmental apraxia. Developmental Medicine and Child Neurology, 1978, 20, 643-646

Gubbay S, Ellis E, & Walton J. Clumsy children: a study of apraxic and agnosic defects in children. Brain, 1965, 88, 295-312

Haaland K, Porch E, & Delaney D. Limb apraxia and motor performance. Brain and Language, 1980, 9, 315-323

Hart Z, Rennick P, & Klinge U. A pediatric neurologists contribution to evaluations of school underachievers. American Journal of Diseases of Children, 1974, 128, 319-323

Heilman K, Schwartz H, & Geschwind N. Defective motor learning in ideomotor apraxia. Neurology, 1975, 25, 1018-1020

Henderson E, & Hall D. Concomitants of clumsiness in young school children. Developmental Medicine and Child Neurology, 1982, 24, 448-460

Hertzig M. Neurological soft signs in low-birth weight children. Developmental Medicine and Child Neurology, 1981, 23, 778-791

Hertzig M, Bortner M, & Birch H. Neurologic findings in children educationally designated as "brain-damaged." American Journal of Orthopsychiatry, 1969, 39, 437-446

Hicks R, & Dusek C. The handedness distributions of gifted and nongifted children. Cortex, 1980, 16, 479-481

Holden W, Tarnowski K, & Prinz R. Reliability of neurological soft signs in children: Reevaluation of the PANESS. Journal of Abnormal Child Psychology, 1982, 10, 163-172

Hulme C, Biggerstaff A, & Morgan G. Visual, kinaesthetic and cross-modal judgements of length by normal and clumsy children. Developmental Medicine and Child Neurology, 1982, 24, 461-471

Illingworth R. The Development of the Infant and Young Child (3rd Ed.). Baltimore: Williams and Wilkins, 1966

Illingworth R. Delayed motor development. Pediatric Clinics of North America, 1968, 15, 569-580

Ingram T. Soft signs. Developmental Medicine and Child Neurology, 1973, 15, 527-530

Johnston R, Stark R, Mellitis E, & Tallal P. Neurological status of language impaired and normal children. Annals of Neurology, 1981, 10, 159-165

Kelso J, Southard D, & Goodman D. On the coordination of two-handed movements. Journal of Experimental Psychiatry, 1979, 5, 229-238

Kelso J, & Tupper B. Toward a theory of apractic syndromes. Brain and Language, 1981, 12, 224-245

Kennard M. Value of equivocal signs in neurologic diagnosis. Neurology, 1960, 10, 753-764

Kenney T, Clemmens R, Cicci R, et al. Diagnosis and treatment: The medical evaluation of children with reading problems (dyslexia). Pediatrics, 1972, 49, 438-442

Kimura D, & Vanderwolf C. The relation between hand preference and the performance of individual finger movements by left and right hands. Brain, 1970, 93, 769-774

Kinsbourne M. Minimal brain dysfunction as a neurodevelopmental lag. Annals of the New York Academy of Science, 1973, 265, 268-273

Knuckey N, Apsimon T, & Gubbay S. Computerized axial tomography in clumsy children with developmental apraxia and agnosia. Brain and Development, 1983, 5, 14-19

Knuckey N, & Gubbay S. Clumsy children: A prognostic study. Australian Pediatric Journal, 1983, 19, 9-13

Kornse D, Manni JL, & Robenstein H, et al. Developmental apraxia of speech and manual dexterity. Journal of Communication Disorders, 1981,14, 321-330

Lerer R, & Lerer M. The effects of methylphenidate on the soft neurological signs of hyperactive children. Pediatrics, 1976, 57, 521-525

Liepmann H. Drei afsatze aus dem Apraxiegebiet. B Berlin, Korger, 1980

Lucas AR, Rodin EA, & Simson CB. Neurological assessment of children with early school problems. Developmental Medicine and Child Neurology, 1965, 7, 145-56

McCarthy D. McCarthy Scales of Children's Abilities. New York: The Psychological Corporation, 1972

McGraw MB. The Neuromuscular Maturation of the Human Infant. New York: Hafner, 1968

McGuinness D. Auditory and motor aspects of language development in males and females. In Ansara A, Geschwind N, & Galaburda A (Eds.). Sex Differences in Dyslexia. Towson, Md: The Orton Dyslexia Society, 1981

McKinley I. Strategies for clumsy children. Developmental Medicine and Child Neurology, 1978, 20, 494-496

McMahon S, & Greenberg L. Serial neurological examination of hyperactive children. Pediatrics, 1977, 59, 584-587

Nichols P, & Chen T. Minimal Brain Dysfunction: A Prospective Study. Hillsdale, New Jersey: Earlbaum, 1981

Orton S. "Word-blindness" in school children. Archives of Neurology, 1925, 14, 582-615

Oseretsky N. Methoden der untersuchung der motorile. Heft 57 Beihefte Zur Zeitschrift Fur Angewandte Psychologie, Barth, Leipzig, 1931

Paine R. The evolution of infantile postural reflexes in the presence of chronic brain syndromes. Developmental Medicine and Child Neurology, 1964, 6, 345-361

Paine R, Werry J, & Quay H. A study of minimal cerebral dysfunction. Developmental Medicine and Child Neurology, 1968, 10, 505-520

Paulsen K, & O'Donnell, J. Construct validation of children's behavior problem dimensions: Relationship to activity level, impulsivity, and soft neurological signs. Journal of Psychology, 1979, 101, 273-278

Peiper A. Cerebral Function in Infancy and Childhood. New York: Consultants Bureau, 1963

Peters J, Romine J, & Dykman R. A special neurological examination of children with learning disabilities. Developmental Medicine and Child Neurology, 1975, 17, 63-78

Prechtl H, & Stemmer C. The choreiform syndrome in children. Developmental Medicine and Child Neurology, 1962, 4, 119-127

Preilowski B. Possible contribution of the anterior forebrain commissures to bilateral motor coordination. Neuropsychologia, 1972, 10, 267-277

Quitkin F, Rifkin A, & Klein D. Neurologic soft signs in schizophrenia and character disorders. Archives of General Psychiatry, 1976, 33, 845-853

Rapin J, Tourke K, & Costa L. Evaluation of the Purdue Peg Board as a screening test for brain damage. Developmental Medicine and Child Neurology, 1960, 8, 45-54

Reitan R. Complex motor functions of the preferred and nonpreferred hands in brain damaged and normal children. Perceptual and Motor Skills, 1971, 33, 671-675

Rie E, Rie H, Stewart S, et al. An analysis of neurological soft signs in children with learning problems. Brain and Language, 1978, 6, 32-46

Roach E, & Kephart N. The Purdue Perceptual Motor Survey. Columbus, OH: Charles C. Merrill, 1966

Roland P. Sensory feedback to the cerebral cortex during voluntary movement in man. The Behavioral and Brain Sciences, 1979, 1, 129-171

Rudel R, Healey J, & Denckla M. Development of motor coordination by normal left handed children. Developmental Medicine and Clinical

Neurology, 1984, 26, 104-111

Rutter M. Brain damage syndromes in childhood: concepts and findings. Journal of Child Psychiatry, 1977, 18, 1-21

Rutter M. Psychological sequelae of brain damage in children. American Journal of Psychiatry, 1981, 138, 1533-1544

Rutter M. Symptoms attributed to minimal brain damage in children. American Journal of Psychiatry, 1982, 134, 21-33

Rutter M, Graham P, & Birch H. Interrelationship between the choreiform syndrome, reading disorder in children of 8-11 years. Developmental Medicine and Child Neurology, 1966, 8, 149-159

Sassin J. Neurological findings following short term sleep deprivation. Archives of Neurology, 1970, 22, 54-56

Satz P, & Morris R. Learning disability subtypes: A review. In Pirozollo F, & Wittrock M (Eds.). Neuropsychological and Cognitive Processes in Reading. New York: Academic Press, 1981

Seidel UP, Chadwick O, & Rutter M. Psychological disorders in crippled children. A comparative study of children with and without brain damage. Developmental Medicine and Child Neurology, 1975, 17, 563

Shaffer D. "Soft" neurological signs and later psychiatric disorder — a review. Journal of Child Psychiatry, 1978, 19, 63-65

Shaffer L. Rhythm and timing in skill. Psychological Review, 1982, 89, 109

Shankweiler O. A study of developmental dyslexia. Neuropsychologia, 1963, 1, 267-286

Shapiro T, Burkes L, Petti T, & Ranz J. Consistency of "nonfocal" neurological signs. American Journal of Child Psychiatry, 1978, 17, 70-79

Sharp J. Assessment of normal motor development in the child. Journal of American Psychological Association, 1981, 71, 109-114

Skubic V, & Anderson M. The interrelationship of perceptual motor achievement, academic achievement, and intelligence in fourth grade children. Journal of Learning Disabilities, 1970, 3, 33-40

Sloan W. The Lincoln Adaptation of the Oseretsky Tests: A Measure of Motor Proficiency. Lincoln, Ill: Lincoln State School and Colony, 1948

Spreen O, & Gaddes W. Developmental norms for 15 neuropsychological tests age 6-15. Cortex, 1969, 5, 170-181

Stine O, Saratsiotis J, & Mosser R. Relationships between neurological findings and classroom behavior. American Journal of Diseases of Children, 1975, 129, 1036-1040

Strauss A, & Lehtinen NC. Psychopathology and Education of the Brain Injured Child. New York: Grune & Stratton, 1947

Touwen B, & Prechtl H. The Neurological Examination of the Child with Minor Nervous Dysfunction, Clinics in Developmental Medicine (38). London: Heinemann Medical, 1970

Touwen B, & Sporrell T. Soft signs and MBD. Developmental Medicine and Child Neurology, 1979, 21, 528-530

Towle M. Assessment and remediation of handwriting defects for children with LD. Journal of Learning Disabilities, 1978, 11, 43-50

Tupper D. Development of bimanual and unimanual coordination in children ages 3 to 8: Involvement of one system or two? Paper presented at the 11th annual meeting of the International Neuropsychological Society, Mexico City, 1983a

Tupper D. The pattern of lateral preference and motor dominance in children. Paper presented at the 11th annual meeting of the International Neuropsychological Society, Mexico City, 1983b

Walton J, Ellis E, & Court S. Clumsy children: Developmental apraxia and agnosia. Brain, 1965, 85, 603-612

Weeks, & Zora R. Effects on vestibular stimulation on mentally retarded, emotionally disturbed, and learning disabled individuals. The American Journal of Occupational Therapy, 1979, 3, 450-457

Werry J, & Aman M. The reliability and diagnostic validity of the physical and neurological exam for soft signs (PANESS). Journal of Autism and Childhood Schizophrenia, 1976, 6, 253-262

Wolff PH. Theoretical issues in the development of motor skills. In Lewis M, & Taft L (Eds.). Developmental Disabilities. Jamaica, NY: SP Medical and Scientific Books, 1981

Wolff PH, & Cohen C. Dual task performance during bimanual coordination. Cortex, 1980, 16, 119-133

Wolff PH, Gunnoe C, & Cohen C. Associated movements as a measure of developmental age. Developmental Medicine and Child Neurology, 1983, 25, 417-429

Wolff P, & Hurwitz I. The choreiform syndrome. Developmental Medicine and Child Neurology, 1966, 4, 160-165

John R. Hughes

6

Electroencephalography Soft Signs

The term *soft sign* is used in clinical neurology but not usually in clinical electroencephalography (EEG), and therefore its definition in this latter field must be initially clarified. The term will be used in this chapter to imply both subtlety and nonspecificity; thus, this chapter will deal with subtle, rather than gross EEG findings that are nonspecific, rather than those that are highly suggestive or pathognomonic of a particular kind of disorder.

SPECIFIC EEG PATTERNS WITH NONSPECIFIC SIGNIFICANCE

Premature

The premature baby, by definition, is an infant born prior to full term and the EEG maturity of that infant usually depends upon the conceptional age (CA), i.e., the number of weeks after conception (Ellingson & Peters, 1980a). Abnormalities, both clinical and electrographic, may appear in the form of signs characteristic of a younger CA. Thus, an EEG pattern in a 36-week-old infant that is characteristic of a 28-week-old premature would be considered abnormal and such patterns are often called immature or dysmature (Schulte, Michaels, Nolte, et al, 1969). Occasionally, bioelectric patterns that represent *different* stages of development may be found together in the same baby; this condition has been called heterochronism (Lombroso, 1982), which may qualify as an EEG soft sign.

Decreased Activity, Increased Quiescent Periods (see Fig. 6-1)

In the youngest of prematures (22-24 weeks CA) who can possibly survive, the most characteristic EEG pattern consists of bursts of activity alter-

SOFT NEUROLOGICAL SIGNS
ISBN 0-8089-1841-9

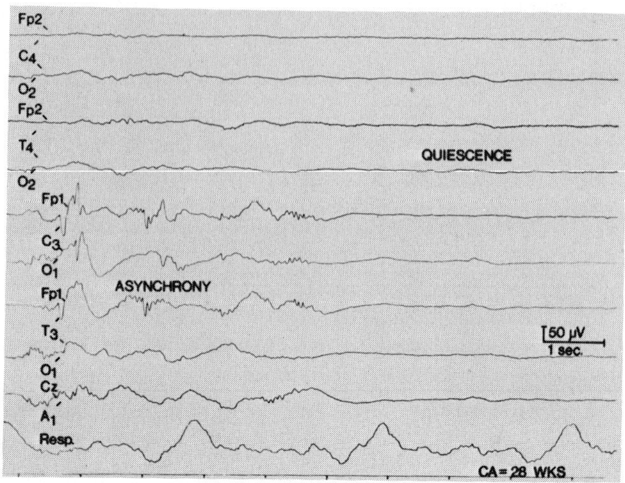

Figure 6-1. Asynchrony (on the left) and quiescence (on the right). Note that high voltage activity is seen on channels 5-8 on the left and not on channels 1-4 on the right. Quiescence appears as an absence of any clear activity. Conceptional age = 28 weeks.

nating with bursts of electrical quiescence (Engel, 1975). With increase in conceptional age, the activity periods increase and the quiescence periods decrease so that by 32 weeks CA only one-half of infants still show quiescence, while the other half demonstrate continuous EEG activity (Hughes, Fino, & Gagnon, 1983a). The percentage of time with clear activity (in nonrapid eye movement sleep) has proven to be of prognostic significance in these infants and may be considered a "soft sign," especially because of its nonspecificity. Data (Hughes et al, 1983a) have shown that infants who later appeared mentally or physically retarded or died had a significantly decreased amount of activity in their EEGs, compared to the group that developed normally or had only mild deficits. Specifically, the amount of activity in a given EEG record increased from 70 to 90 percent from 27 to 38 weeks CA in the near-normal group, significantly increased over the lower values of 50-65 percent from 27 to 38 weeks in the group that either died or later showed definite retardation.

Asynchrony (see Fig. 6-1)

Another characteristic of the very young premature infant is asynchrony of activity, referring to the presence of rhythms from one-half of the brain that are different from those from the other half. Thus, at 22-28 weeks CA only 40-50 percent of the activity on one side of the head also appears on the other side. With increase in CA, the amount of asynchrony gradually diminishes so that at full term the EEG activity in the normal infant should be essentially synchronous between the two sides (Lombroso, 1979; Hughes, 1982). Another example of a dysmature or immature pattern would therefore be the excessive amount of asynchrony that would be characteristic of a significantly younger conceptional age, exemplified by a full-term infant whose activity on the left is also seen on the right only 75 percent of the time, rather than the expected 100 percent.

Late Development of Sleep, Wake Stages (see Fig. 6-2A, B)

As the premature infant matures, the first stage that fully develops is the rapid eye movement (REM) stage, also called active sleep (AS), characterized by irregular respiration, the absence of chin electromyogram (EMG), and EEG activity as a mixture of slow rhythms around 1 c/second and faster rhythms 10-20 c/second (Hughes, 1982). At 32 weeks CA this stage is usually fully developed (Monod & Garma, 1965). The nonrapid eye movement (NREM) stage, also called quiet sleep (QS), consists of

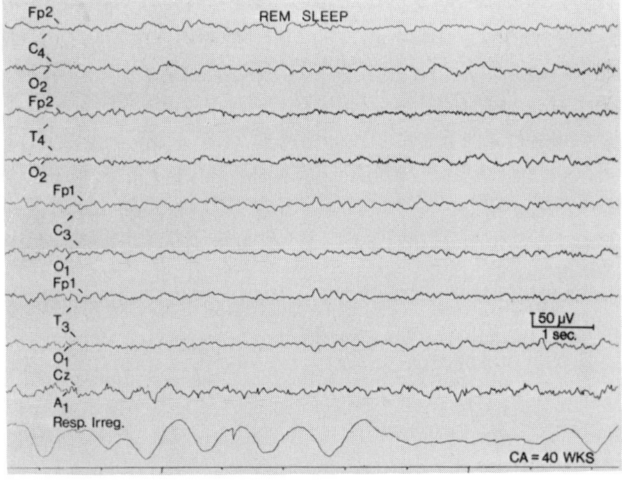

A

Figure 6-2. (A) REM (rapid eye movement) sleep. Note the irregular respiration on the last channel, characteristic of REM sleep. The EEG pattern at this time is low voltage theta (5-6/second) activity.

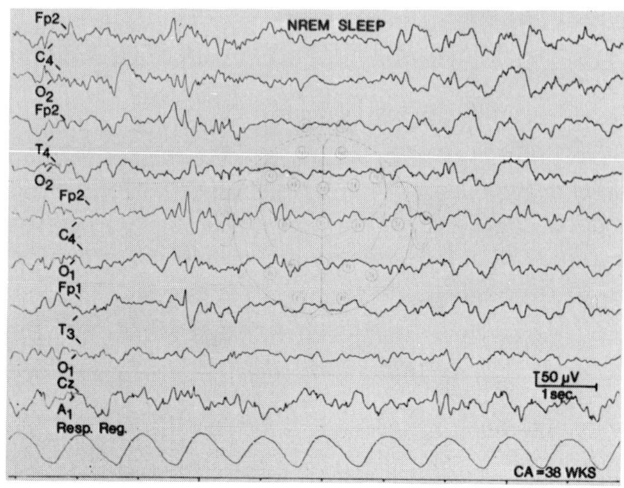

B

Figure 6-2 (Continued). (B) NREM (nonrapid eye movement) sleep. Note the regular respiration on the last channel, characteristic of NREM sleep. The EEG pattern shows alternating high and low voltage patterns.

regular respiration, presence of a chin EMG and an EEG of either high voltage slow activity or a pattern called tracé alternant, i.e., alternation of high and low amplitude activity. At 36 weeks this stage has completely developed (Dreyfus-Brisac,1970). Usually at 37 weeks the waking state has become fully developed (Prechtl, 1974), consisting of irregular respiration, presence of a chin EMG and an EEG of low voltage theta (4-7.5 c/second) rhythms. The soft signs here would include the significant *delay* (by approximately 4 weeks) in the full development of REM or active sleep at 32 weeks, NREM or quiet sleep at 36 weeks, or waking state at 37 weeks.

Infants

A few patterns appear during prematurity and then disappear either at term or shortly thereafter. Soft signs in this age group will include the continuation of those premature patterns beyond the time when they should normally disappear.

Delta Brushes

Delta brushes (Fig. 6-3) refer to activity that consists of very slow delta rhythms (usually at 1 c/second) superimposed onto fast waves, looking like hairs on a brush. This pattern appears in an immature form at 28 weeks, is

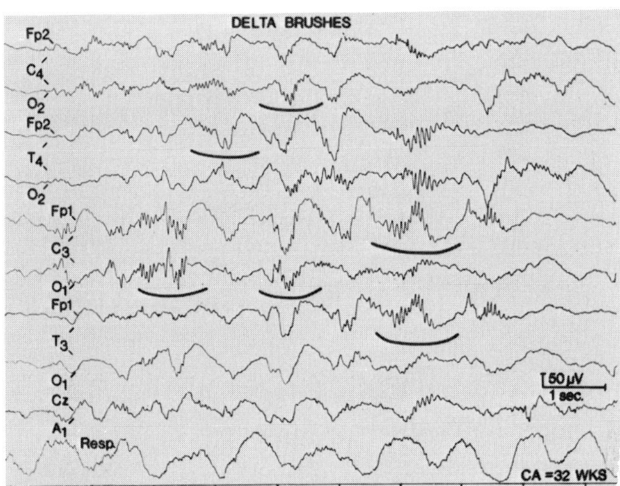

Figure 6-3. Delta brushes. Note very fast activity superimposed on very slow waves (underlined).

prominent at 32 weeks, but disappears at term in the normal infant (Lombroso, 1975). Although some investigators believe that delta brushes may normally extend a few weeks beyond term (Tharp, 1980), the continuation of this pattern into the first few months after 39-40 weeks CA would constitute a maturational lag or an EEG soft sign (Werner, Stockard, & Bickford, 1977). Also, the appearance of unilateral brushes (which are usually seen bilaterally) in quiet sleep beyond 36 weeks also would be a similar sign (Hughes, 1982).

Sporadic Sharp Waves

Sporadic sharp waves (Fig. 6-4) are paroxysmal spike-like events that appear on any and all areas, especially on the central regions, and at frequencies much less than 2/minute on a given region from 30 weeks CA until approximately 2 months post-term (Hughes, Fino, & Gagnon, 1983b). If these sporadic sharp waves extend beyond that 2 month period in the sleep record or appear in the wake or active sleep stage after the first week, they qualify as a soft sign. These paroxysms usually signify a seizure disorder, especially when a given area shows a large number of these events, but a few scattered sporadic sharp waves beyond 2-3 months would likely represent a nonspecific abnormality or soft sign.

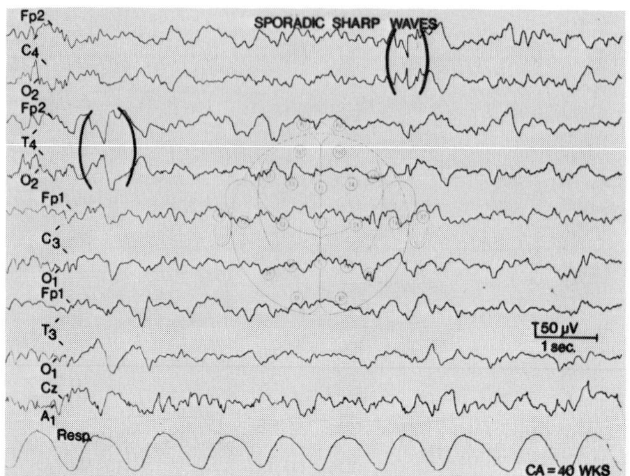

Figure 6-4. Sporadic sharp waves. These sharp events are seen on many different areas, noted here on the T4 (right mid-temporal) electrode (channels 3 and 4) and also on the C4 (right central) electrode (channels 1 and 2).

Frontal Sharp Transient (see Fig. 6- 5)

Sharp transients (Fig. 6-5), which are not as spike-like or paroxysmal as the sporadic sharp wave and are often followed by a wave-like pattern, appear synchronously on the frontal areas in prematures (Kellaway & Crawley, 1964). They are seen first at approximately 26 weeks CA, are prominent with anterior delta patterns at 36 weeks, and usually disappear near term or within 8 weeks after term (Ellingson & Peters, 1980a; Hughes, 1982). Also called "encoches frontales" (Dreyfus-Brisac & Monod, 1975), they may be considered an EEG soft sign if they appear in the waking state at 1 week post-term and also if they continue to be seen in the sleep record after the second month beyond term (Hughes, 1982). Specifically, Ellingson and Peters (1980b) found that these transients disappeared much later (65 days) in Trisomy 21 infants than normal controls (39 days). Finally, these events also qualify as a nonspecific or soft sign if they consistently appear unilaterally (Monod & Dreyfus-Brisac, 1972) or are repetitive in long bursts (Werner et al, 1977). Varner et al (1975) found an excessive number of frontal sharp transients in patients with mild degrees of encephalopathy. Arfel et al (1977) made the same point for patients with "minor pathology" and "stressed babies."

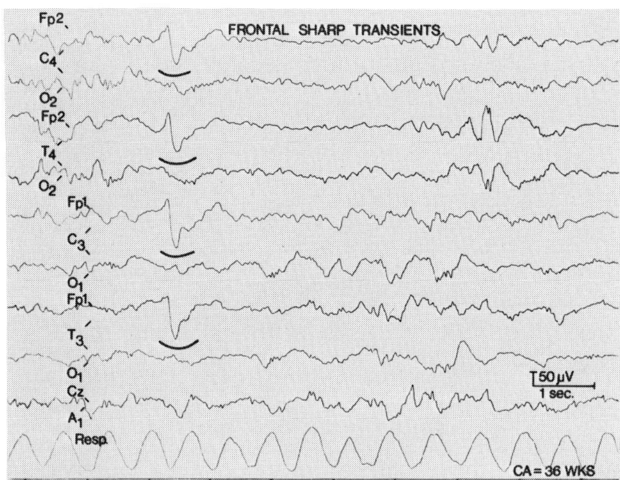

Figure 6-5. Frontal sharp transients. Underlined are these transients that are usually bilaterally synchronous and symmetrical (similar on channels 1 and 3 from the right and channels 5 and 7 from the left).

Wake-Sleep Stages

In premature and newborns, sleep stages can be categorized as active (AS) or quiet sleep (QS) and also indeterminate (IS) when the characteristics are neither AS or QS. In the normal term infant, onset of sleep is usually with AS, then decreasing in incidence to 8 weeks when onset is almost entirely with QS. In Trisomy-21 retardates, AS onset continues to be significantly higher at 5-10 weeks of age than normals as an indication of a developmental delay or soft sign (Ellingson & Peters, 1980b).

The amount of each of these three stages (AS, QS, IS) as a percentage of total sleeptime also is important in assessing maturity. In Trisomy-21 infants the incidence of IS is significantly higher (18 percent) than in controls (11 percent) in the first 3 months and the amount of QS is lower. Also, longer transitional periods between AS and QS have been found in these babies (Goldie, Curtis, Svendsen, & Roberton, 1968), in addition to low percent time AS and paucity of REMs (Petre-Quadens & Jouvet, 1966). Tharp (1981) has reported that IS, also called transitional sleep, increases in infants who are organically "stressed." The amount of AS in normal term infants is 58 percent and the incidence of QS is 39 percent (Dreyfus-Brisac & Monod, 1970), the former decreasing to 29-25 percent at 7-8 weeks after term (Lombroso, 1982) and the latter increasing to 50 percent in time. The failure to decrease the amount of AS and increase QS in time may also be considered an EEG soft sign. Further instances of abnormal amounts of wake-sleep stages include the low incidence (only 4 percent) of the waking stage in hyperbilirubinemic infants who have proportional increases in their AS and QS (Prechtl, Theorell, & Blair, 1973). At times, no sleep cycles may appear at all or sleep may be completely of the indeterminant or transitional type (Lombroso, 1982).

In his 1983 Presidential Address to the American EEG Society, C. Lombroso added that babies at risk show a state variability, compared to normal babies. Data show that the abnormal babies have a decreased coefficient of concordance (0.73 versus 0.99) in the amount of time spent in three different wake and in the two different sleep states (AS and QS) from one day to the next. Also, babies at risk may fail to show any change in the slow delta rhythms on the frontal vertex region in the "alert" stage, different from the changes that usually occur on the central vertex region of similar waves in the normal babies.

Tracé Alternant

This pattern, consisting of bursts of high amplitude rhythms and sharp transients, followed by bursts of low amplitude activity, is a normal waveform, called tracé alternate (TA), so named because these bursts of high and low amplitude activity alternant (Fig. 6-6). This same pattern becomes fully developed at approximately 36 weeks CA and remains until nearly the second month past term (Ellingson & Peters, 1980a). If this activity remains beyond this second month (Lombroso, 1982), its continuation constitutes a soft sign. Specifically, normal controls have lost TA in 33 days (mean), but retardates continue to show this activity until 56 days (Ellingson & Peters 1980b). On the other hand, Goldie et al (1968) found that some retardates never show well-defined TA patterns.

Spindles

Spindles (Fig. 6-7) in the form of short bursts of 14 c/second activity can appear rudimentary in form at 1 week after term, but usually wait for 6 weeks before full expression (Metcalf, 1970; Ellingson & Peters, 1980a,b).

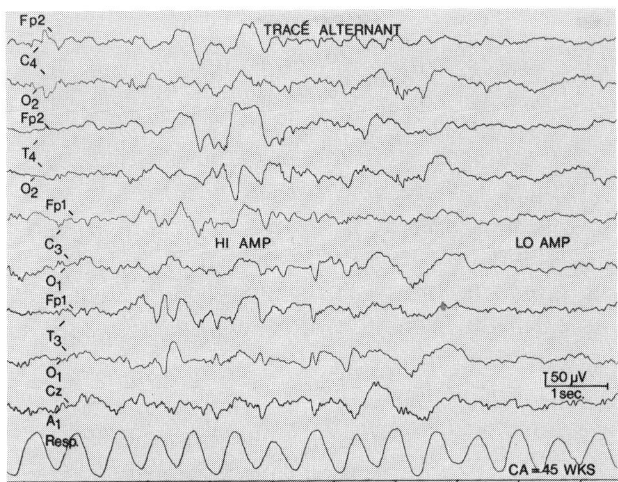

Figure 6-6. Tracé alternant. This pattern consists of high amplitude (voltage) patterns alternating with low amplitude patterns, appearing in NREM sleep (note regular respiration on the last channel).

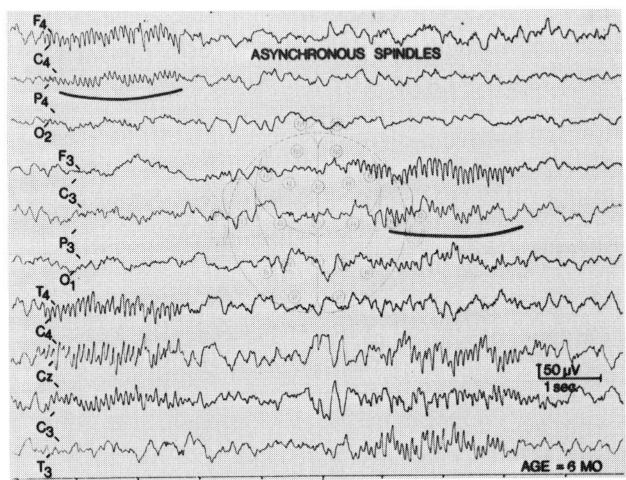

Figure 6-7. Asynchronous spindles. Note (left) the 14/second spindles on channels 1 and 2, also 7-9 only from the right side and (right) similar spindles on channels 4 and 5, also 8-10, only from the left side.

If this activity has not appeared until 2-3 months or later, this delay can be considered an expression of late development or a soft sign, often noted in infants with perinatal asphyxia (Lombroso, 1982) or in Trisomy-21 infants, whose mean onset was 62 days (Ellingson & Peters, 1980b). In the normal infant after a 3-5 month period when the spindles are very long in duration (up to 10 seconds), they then become shortened in duration, take on a sharp monophasic appearance and are seen asynchronously (Hughes, 1982). This asynchrony diminishes at 1 year of age and occurs only occasionally between 1 and 2 years, but completely synchronized spindles should be seen after 2 years. Infants showing a great amount (> 50 percent) of asynchrony between 1 and 2 years or those with clear asynchrony after 2 years (Tharp, 1981), often seen in patients with hydrocephalus (Gibbs & Gibbs, 1964) would demonstrate another example of an EEG soft sign. Also, retardates have shown significantly fewer of their spindles (58 percent) as synchronous and symmetrical at 1 year than normals (70 percent) (Ellingson & Peters, 1980b). The monophasic appearance of spindles lasts until 3 years, but if significantly longer (until 4-5 years), a delayed development or soft sign would again be indicated. Finally, when spindles become very high in amplitude and very long in duration (over 10 seconds) they are called "extreme spindles" (Gibbs & Gibbs, 1962), highly correlating with an organic nonfamilial mental retardation and possibly qualifying as an EEG soft sign. Spindles only slightly longer than usual (3-4 seconds) are often found in deaf children (Hughes, 1971); on the other hand, no spindles at all may be found in some retarded patients (Gibbs & Gibbs, 1964), and also in certain hypothyroid infants (Parmelee & Stern, 1972).

Children

Occipital Alpha (wake) (see Fig. 6-8)

Alpha rhythms at nearly 8 c/second appear on the posterior regions in the resting, wake state as early as 1-2 years of age (Kellaway, 1979). With advances in age the frequency gradually increases so that by 10 years of age the mean frequency is approximately 10 c/second. The 95 percent confidence limit throughout this development is approximately 1.5 c/second (Kellaway, 1979) and at 8 years of age this rhythm should be at least 8 c/second. If this backgound activity is less than 8 c/second at this age or older or if a marked asymmetry (> 50 percent) is seen (Varner et al, 1975; Tharp, 1981), then a soft sign is indicated.

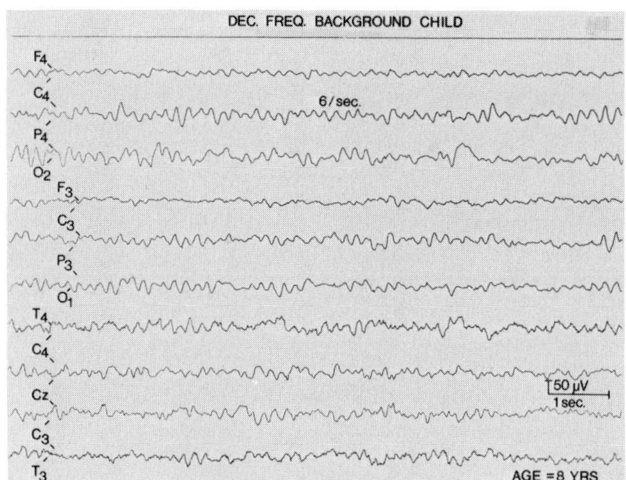

Figure 6-8. Decreased frequency of background rhythm in a child. Note the 6/second activity representing the waking background activity in this 1-year-old.

Fronto-Central Theta (wake) (see Fig. 6-9)

Rhythms of 5-7 c/second maximal on the fronto-central areas become the backgound activity, even in the premature (Dreyfus-Brisac & Monod, 1975), appearing prominent at 3-5 months of age and then tending to diminish in amplitude as the occipital alpha increases in prominence. If these theta waves continue throughout all of childhood as the most dominant rhythm, significantly higher in amplitude than the occipital alpha, they represent a developmental disorder and would therefore qualify as an EEG soft sign.

Occipital Slowing (wake) (see Fig. 6-10)

All children have some slow activity on their occipital areas in the form of slow transients, i.e., pieces of slow waves. They have been called "slow waves found predominantly in youth" by Aird and Gastaut (1959) and polyphasic slow activity by Kellaway (1979). Another normal pattern, described by Petersén and Eeg-Olofsson (1971), is the 2.5-4.5 c/second slow activity seen throughout the posterior regions, appearing in young children, maximal in incidence at 5-7 years of age, and seen up to the age of 15 years. Still a third pattern that is not normal and qualifying as an EEG soft sign is *excessive* occipital slowing, different from the second pattern by its focal localization on the occipital areas, its 4/second frequency, and appearance at all ages. This pattern has been called "slow posterior

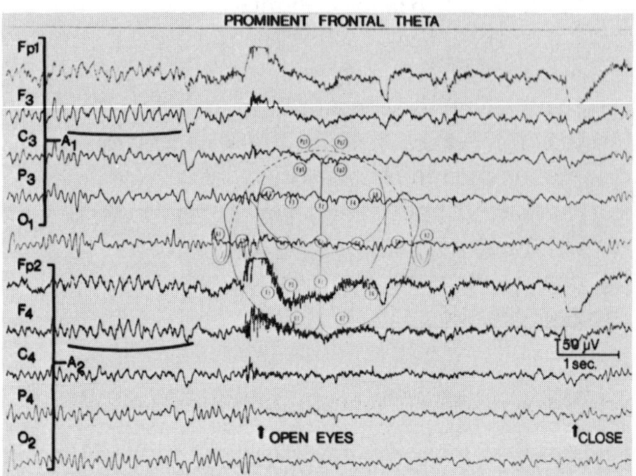

Figure 6-9. Prominent frontal theta. Note on channels 2 (left frontal) and 7 (right frontal) the high voltage 6-7/second theta rhythms that appeared more prominent than the alpha rhythm (10/second) on the occipital areas (channels 5 and 10). Age = 12 years.

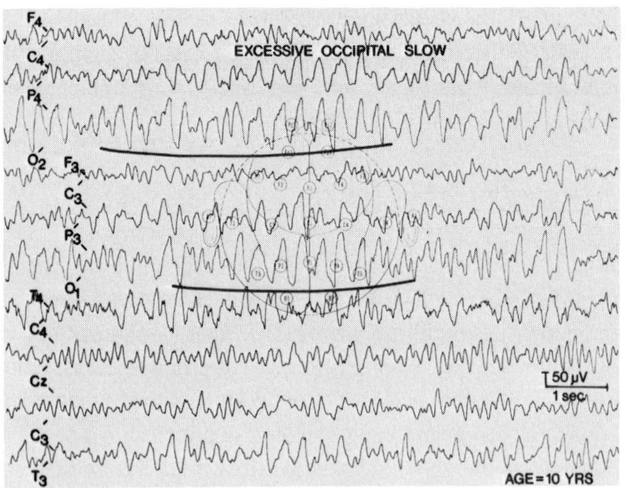

Figure 6-10. Excessive occipital slow. Note the high voltage 3/second rhythms on channels 3 (right) and 6 (left) as an example of rhythmical delta patterns in a child. Age = 14 years.

waves associated with pathology" by Aird and Gastaut (1959) and is found especially in patients with previous head injuries and/or abnormal emotional symptomatology (60 percent). Similar activity can also be seen in patients during the first week after a febrile seizure or head injury (Frantzen, Lennox-Buchthal, & Nygaard, 1968) and only occasionally (7 percent) this type of activity is seen in individuals with a learning disability, dyslexia in particular (Hughes & Park, 1968). Furthermore, excessive occipital slowing can be seen in behavior disorders (Cohn & Nardini, 1958), hyperkinetic syndrome (Knobel, Wolman, & Mason, 1959), and finally visual perceptual disorders (Pavy & Metcalfe, 1965). Occipital accentuation of diffuse delta rhythms has also been described in patients with white matter degenerative disorders (Blume, 1982).

Hypnogogic Hypersynchrony (Drowsy) (see Figs. 6-11A, B)

The term, hypnogogic hypersynchrony, refers to a pattern of high amplitude diffuse slow waves of 2-4 c/seconds seen normally in the drowsiness of children (Kellaway & Fox, 1952). Two forms exist, one continuous and long-lasting and the other paroxysmal in short bursts lasting 2-5 seconds in duration (Gibbs & Gibbs, 1950). Both of these forms disap-

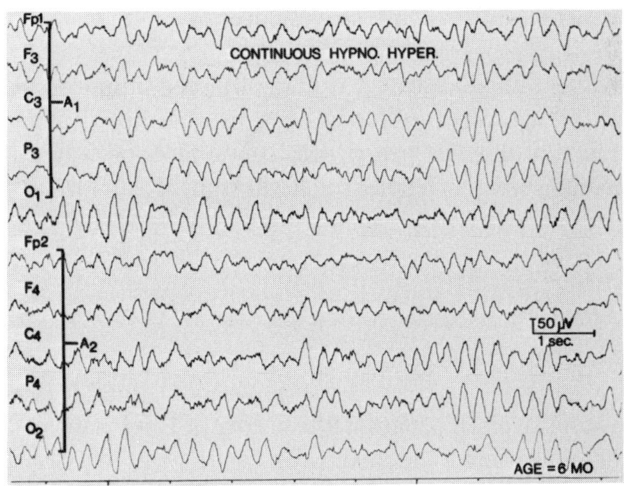

A

Figure 6-11. (A) Continuous hypersynchrony. Note the diffuse 3-4/second rhythms that appear nearly continuously in this drowsy child.

B
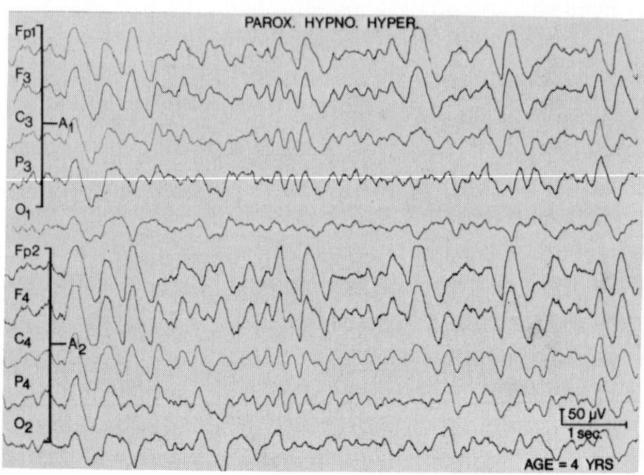

Figure 6-11 ***(Continued).*** (B) Paroxysmal hypnogogic hypersynchrony. Note the bursts of high voltage rhythms at 2-3/second, seen well on the left side of the figure, maximal on the frontal areas (channels 1 and 2 from the left and 6 and 7 from the right).

pear at approximately 9-12 years of age (Hughes, 1982) and the continuation of the pattern beyond that age would qualify as a soft sign.

Fast Rhythms of 20-28 c/second (Drowsy) (see Fig. 6-12)

Fast activity of 20-28 c/second is normally seen in infants and children up to 6 years of age when it becomes rare in incidence (Kellaway, 1979). The appearance of this fast pattern into later childhood would represent a developmental disorder and qualify as a soft sign.

Adolescents

Positive Spikes (see Fig. 6-13)

The most controversial pattern in the history of EEG is the positive spike phenomenon at 6-7 and 14/second. Gibbs and Gibbs first described these spikes in 1951, at first considered by some as an artifact, then becoming the focal point around which every formal EEG organization in the U.S. is duplicated. Hundreds of journal articles support the notion that these spikes

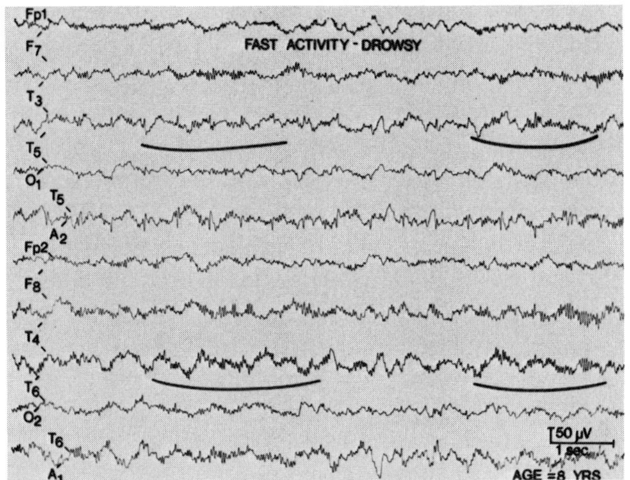

Figure 6-12. Fast activity in a drowsy child (age 2 years). Note the 20-28/second activity seen diffusely on the left side (channels 1-5) and also on the right side (channels 6-10).

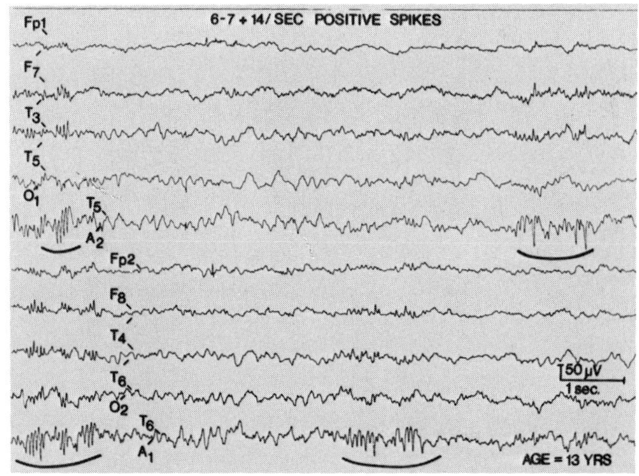

Figure 6-13. Positive spikes at 6-7 and 14/second. Note channels 5 (from the left posterior temporal area) and 10 (from the right posterior temporal area). The positive spikes appear in bursts at either 14/second (left and middle of figure) or 6-7/second (right of figure) and the positivity is seen as sharp downward deflections.

may be significantly related to neurovegetative and/or behavioral disorders, as indicated in the reviews by Hughes (1965, 1983) and Henry (1963). Yet, other studies have reached negative conclusions. One article by Lombroso and his colleagues (1966) reported such a high incidence (58 percent) in "normal" adolescents that many EEGers have determined that this pattern is perfectly normal. On the other hand, evidence continues to be published that indicates the pattern is significantly associated with abnormal signs and symptoms (Hughes, 1983). As an example, after carefully screening nearly 1000 children as a *normal* group, Boseaus and Sellden (1979) selected 200 for further detailed study, especially investigated by pediatric psychiatrists, and found positive spikes significantly related to behavior and neurovegetative disorders. Evidence of the latter type would argue for the possibility that positive spikes may therefore qualify as an EEG soft sign, rather than a completely normal pattern.

Temporal Slow Waves (see Fig. 6-14)

Although slow waves on the temporal areas are more often seen in the elderly (Obrist, 1976), they can also be seen in the adolescent. In a study on adolescents with a learning disability (Hughes, 1971), slow waves (22 percent) represented the major difference between the normal controls with

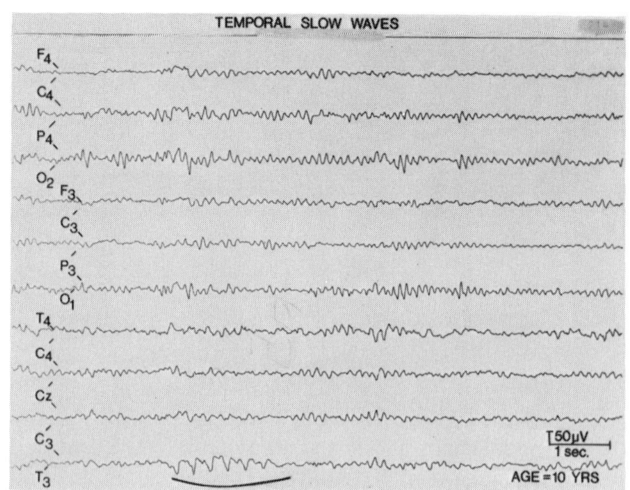

Figure 6-14. Temporal slow waves. Note on the last channel from the T3 electrode (left temporal area) the 3-4/second slow waves.

expected scholastic achievement and the learning disability group with achievement less than expected, based on their IQ level. Among the slow waves, those on the temporal represented the only statistically significant difference between the two groups. This temporal slowing should probably not be considered a specific EEG finding, but instead be considered a soft sign.

Adults and Elderly

Occipital Alpha (see Fig. 6-15)

Especially with the finding that the mean alpha frequency in healthy centenarians is over 8 c/second (Hubbard, Sunde, & Goldensohn, 1976), all elderly individuals should have alpha frequencies (over 8 c/second) as their background rhythm. A decrease below the alpha range is often seen in the elderly (Obrist, 1976) and also in retardates (Gibbs & Gibbs, 1964), but this decrease cannot be considered normal; instead, it may be considered a soft sign that may be either the only abnormality in the tracing or related to other more specific (slow wave) abnormalities. Generally, the background

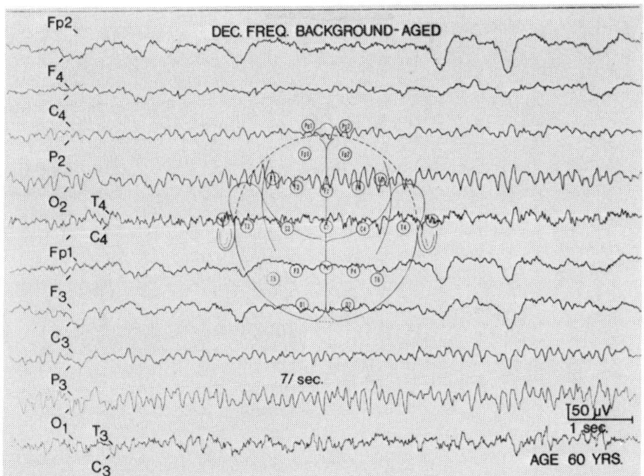

Figure 6-15. Decreased frequency of background rhythm in the aged (70-years-old). Note the 7/second rhythms (channels 4 and 9) as the background waking activity.

rhythm in the theta range (4-7.5 c/second) represents a depressed excitability cycle of neurons incapable of producing rhythms fast enough to qualify as normal.

Temporal Theta (see Fig. 6-16)

Rhythms on the temporal areas in the theta range (and slow transients) are not uncommon in the adult, especially in the elderly (Obrist 1976). They are so common that some EEGers call them normal. However, Drachman and Hughes (1974) separated a group of elderly "normal" hospital volunteers into those *with* and those *without* these slow waves. The presence of this temporal lobe activity reflecting "mildly depressed neuronal function" (Gibbs & Gibbs, 1964) significantly correlated with a nonspecific organic index, based on the difference (> 20 points) between the verbal and performance scores of the Wechsler Adult Intelligence Scale (WAIS). Thus, this slow wave activity on the temporal areas did correlate with abnormal scores on a highly respected IQ test.

A distinctive pattern becomes evident when the unitemporal theta activity is seen in clear bursts, especially in the drowsy record. These patterns

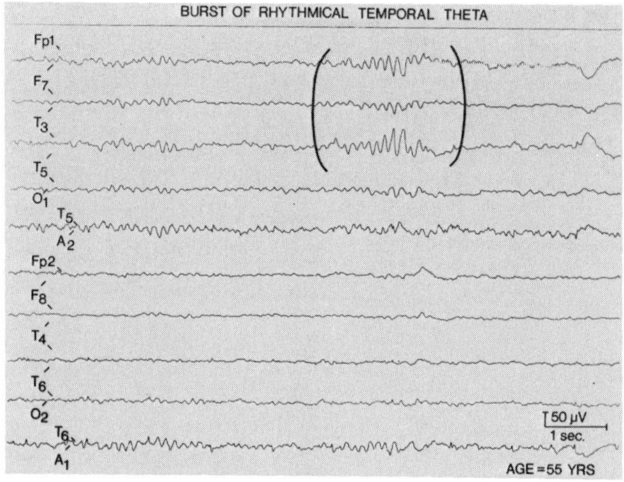

Figure 6-16. Bursts of rhythmical temporal theta (BORTT). Note on channels 1-3 the burst of rhythmical 6-7.5/second rhythms from the left temporal area.

have recently been called BORTT, i.e., bursts of rhythmical temporal theta (Maynard & Hughes, 1984). Their incidence in a hospital group was significantly different from a control group without evidence of organic cerebral disease. Vascular disease, in general, was found in nearly half of the these BORTT patients and evidence of *CNS* vascular disease or previous head injury was also found in half of these same patients. Their major complaints included many symptoms likely related to vascular disease, viz., numbness, paresthesias, and fleeting symptoms of many types. This BORTT pattern may be the forerunner of another electrographic entity that is much sharper in configuration to the point that spikes are evident and therefore the pattern has been called wicket temporal spikes (Reiher & Lebel, 1977). Patients with this waveform are usually in the older age groups, and have symptoms like syncope (33 percent), headaches, and vertigo. Neurovegtative symptoms of the latter type were found in 70 percent of patients with these wicket temporal spikes (Hughes & Olson, 1981). Although BORTT and its possible relative, wicket temporal spikes, have some degree of specificity, especially with regard to a cerebrovascular etiology, there is sufficient polyetiology and the majority of the associated symptoms seem nonspecific; thus, these latter two patterns may qualify as EEG soft signs.

Frontal Delta (see Fig. 6-17)

Frontal intermittent repetitive delta activity (FIRDA) is a nonspecific finding, seen in patients with any type of disturbance of the anterior brainstem and its projection to the frontal areas, associated with metabolic, vascular, infectious or degenerative disorders (Gloor, 1976). As an EEG soft sign, this pattern qualifies especially well by its nonspecificity, but possibly not with regard to its subtlety, since patients with the pattern usually show clear cerebral symptoms and the pattern itself often is high in amplitude.

SUMMARY

EEG soft signs refer to subtle patterns that are nonspecific, as opposed to gross findings that are highly suggestive of a particular type of pathology. Many of the patterns that qualify as EEG soft signs represent developmental delays or manifestations of neurophysiologic immaturity. Examples in

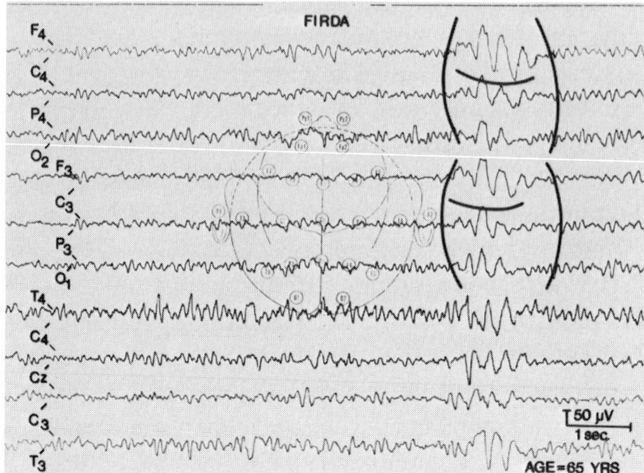

Figure 6-17. FIRDA — Frontal intermittent rhythmic delta activity. Note the burst of rhythmical 3/second activity seen maximal on channels 1 (right frontal) and 4 (left frontal).

the premature infant include decreased activity and increased quiescence, increased asynchrony between the two sides of the head, and the late development of active or quiet sleep or even the waking state.

In infants, examples of EEG soft signs include delta brushes continuing a few months after term and sporadic sharp waves or frontal sharp transients also seen at that time. Other instances are increased amounts of active sleep (AS) for sleep onset, increased incidence of indeterminate sleep, or failure to show decreased amounts of AS or increased amounts of quiet sleep. Furthermore, a low incidence of waking state or the absence of sleep cycles also qualify, as does an increased variability of state from one time to another. The continuation of tracé alternant beyond the second month, late development of spindles or their failure to synchronize by 2 years or to develop a biphasic configuration by 4-5 years are other examples. Finally, extreme spindles or no spindles at all may be further representative of EEG soft signs.

In children, background activity under 8 c/second by 8 years of age, increased frontal-central theta, excessive occipital slow waves, continuing hypnogogic hypersynchrony into the early teens or fast beta rhythms of drowsiness beyond 6 years of age all qualify as EEG soft signs.

In adolescents, positive spikes and temporal slow waves may be considered soft signs. In adults, background activity in the theta rather than alpha frequencies, in addition to bursts of temporal theta rhythms or frontal intermittent repetitive delta patterns, also likely qualify as patterns that are nonspecific in EEG.

REFERENCES

Aird RB, & Gastaut Y. Occipital and posterior electroencephalographic rhythms. Electroencephalography and Clinical Neurophysiology, 1959, 11, 637-656

Arfel G, Leonard N, & Moussalli F. Densié et dynamique des encoches pointues frontales dans le sommeil du nouveau-né et du nourrisson. Revue D Electroencephalographie et de Neurophysiologie Clinique, 1977, 7, 351-360

Blume WT. Atlas of Pediatric Electroencephalography. New York: Raven, 1982, p. 336

Boseaus E, & Sellden U. Psychiatric assessment of healthy children with various EEG patterns. Acta Psychiatrica Scandinavica, 1979, 59, 180-210

Cohn R, & Nardini J. The correlation of bilateral occipital slow activity in the human EEG with certain disorders of behavior. American Journal of Psychiatry, 1958, 115, 44-54

Drachman DA, & Hughes JR. Memory and the hippocampal complexes. III. Aging and temporal EEG abnormalities. Neurology, 1979, 21, 1-14

Dreyfus-Brisac C. Ontogenesis of sleep in human prematures after 32 weeks of conceptual age. Developmental Psychobiology, 1970, 3, 91-121

Dreyfus-Brisac C, & Monod N. Sleeping behavior in abnormal newborn infants. Neuropediatrics, 1970, 1, 354-366

Dreyfus-Brisac C, & Monod N. The electroencephalogram of full term new-born and premature infants. In Lairy GG (Ed.). Handbook of Electroencephalography and Clinical Neurophysiology Vol 6L. Amsterdam: Elsevier, 1975, pp 6-24

Ellingson RJ, & Peters JF. Development of EEG and daytime sleep patterns in low risk premature infants during the first year of life: Longitudinal observations. Electroencephalography and Clinical Neurophysiology, 1980a, 50, 165-171

Ellingson RJ, & Peters JF. Development of EEG and daytime sleep patterns in Trisomy-21 infants during the first year of life: Longitudinal observations. Electroencephalography and Clinical Neurophysiology, 1980b, 50, 457-466

Engel RCH. Abnormal Electroencephalogram in the Neonatal Period. Springfield, IL: Charles C. Thomas, 1975

Frantzen E, Lennox-Buchthal M, & Nygaard A. Longitudinal EEG and clinical study of children with febrile convulsions. Electroencephalography and Clinical Neurophysiology, 1968, 24, 197-212

Gibbs EL, & Gibbs FA. Electroencephalographic evidence of thalamic and hypothalamic epilepsy. Neurology, 1951, 1, 136-144

Gibbs EL, & Gibbs FA. Extreme spindles. Correlation of electroencephalographic sleep patterns with mental retardation. Science, 1962, 138, 1106-1107

Gibbs FA, & Gibbs EL. Atlas of Electroencephalography. Reading, MA: Addison-Wesley, 1950

Gibbs FA, & Gibbs EL. Atlas of Electroencephalography Vol. III. Reading, MA: Addison-Wesley, 1964

Gloor P. Generalized and widespread bilateral paroxysmal activities. Handbook of Electroencephalography and Clinical Neurophysiology, 1976, 11B, 52-87

Goldie L, Curtis JAH, Svendsen U, & Roberton NRC. Abnormal sleep rhythms in mongol babies. Lancet, 1968, 1, 229-230

Henry CE. Positive spike discharges in the EEG and behavior abnormality. In Glaser GH (Ed.). EEG and Behavior. New York: Basic Books, 1963, pp 315-344

Hubbard O, Sunde D, & Goldensohn ES. The EEG in centenarians. Electroencephalography and Clinical Neurophysiology, 1976, 40, 407-417

Hughes JR. A review of the positive spike phenomenon, In Wilson W (Ed.). Applications of Electroencephalography in Psychiatry. Durham: Duke University Press, 1965, pp 54-101

Hughes JR. Electroencephalography and learning disabilities, In Myklebust HR (Ed.). Progress in Learning Disabilities Vol 2. New York: Grune & Stratton, 1971, pp 18-55

Hughes JR. EEG in Clinical Practice. Boston and London: Butterworths, 1982

Hughes JR. A review of the positive spike phenomenon. Recent studies. In Hughes JR, Wilson WE (Eds.). EEG and Evoked Potentials in Psychiatry and Behavioral Neurology. Boston and London: Butterworths, 1983, pp 295-324

Hughes JR, Fino J, & Gagnon L. Period of activity and quiescence in the premature EEG. Neuropediatrics, 1983a, 14, 66-72

Hughes JR, Fino J, & Gagnon L. The use of the electroencephalogram in the confirmation of seizures in premature and neonatal infant. Neuropediatrics, 1983b, 14, 213-219

Hughes JR, & Olson SF. An investigation of eight different types of temporal lobe discharges. Epilepsia, 1981, 22, 421-435

Hughes JR, & Park G. The EEG in dyslexia. In Kellaway P, Petersen I (Eds.). Clinical Electroencephalography in Children. Stockholm: Almqvist and Wiksell, 1968

Kellaway P. An orderly approach to visual analysis: Parameters of the normal EEG in adults and children. In Klass DW, Daly DD (Eds.). Current Practice of Clinical Electroencephalography. New York: Raven, 1979, pp 69-147

Kellaway P, & Crawley J. A Primer of Electroencephalography of Infants. Sections I and II. Methodology and criteria of normality. Bethesda, MD: NIH, 1964

Kellaway P, & Fox BJ. Electroencephalographic diaganosis of cerebral pathology in infants during sleep. I. Rationale, technique and the characteristics of normal sleep in infants. Journal of Pediatrics, 1952, 41, 262-287

Knobel M, Wolman MB, & Mason C. Hyperkinesis and organicity in children. Archives of General Psychiatry, 1959, 1, 310-321

Lenard HG, & Bell EF. Bioelectric brain development in hypothyroidism. Electroencephalography and Clinical Neurophysiology, 1973, 35, 545-549

Lombroso CT. Neurophysiological observations in diseased newborns. Biological Psychiatry, 1975, 10, 527-558

Lombroso CT. Quantified electrographic scales on 50 pre-term healthy newborns followed up to 40-43 weeks of conceptual age by serial polygraphic recordings. Electroencephalography and Clinical Neurophysiology, 1979, 46, 460-474

Lombroso CT. Neonatal electroencephalography, In Niedermeyer E, & Lopes da Silva F (Eds.). Electroencephalography. Baltimore: Urban and Schwarzenberg, 1982, pp 599-637

Lombroso CT, Schwartz IH, Clark DM, et al. Cteniods in healthy youths: Controlled study of 14- and 6-per-second positive spiking. Neurology, 1966, 16, 1152-1158

Maynard S, & Hughes JR. A distinctive electrographic entity: Bursts of rhythmical temporal theta. Clinical EEG, 1984, 15, 145-150

Metcalf DR. EEG sleep spindles ontogenesis. Neuropediatrics, 1970, 1, 428-423

Monod N, & Dreyfus-Brisac C. Prognostic value of the neonatal EEG in full term newborns. Handbook of Electroencephalography and Clinical Neurophysiology, 1982, 15(B), 89-100

Monod N, & Garma L. Auditory responsivity in the human premature. Biology of the Neonate, 1965, 8, 281-307

Obrist WD. Problems of aging. Handbook of Electroencephalography and Clinical Neurophysiology, 1976, 6A, 275-292

Pavy R, & Metcalfe J. The abnormal EEG in childhood communication and behavior abnormalities. Electroencephalography and Clinical Neurophysiology, 1965, 19, 414

Parmelee AH, & Stern E. Development of states in infants. In Clement CD, Purpura DP, Mayer F (Eds.). Sleep and the Maturing Nervous System. New York: Academic Press, 1972, pp 199-228

Peteršen I, & Eeg-Olofsson O. The development of the electroencephalogram in normal children from the age of 1 through 15 years. Nonparoxysmal activity. Neuropediatrics, 1971, 2, 247-304

Petre-Quadens O, & Jouvet M. Paradoxical sleep and dreaming in the mentally retarded. Journal of Neurological Sciences, 1966, 3, 608-612

Prechtl HFR. The behavioral states of the newborn infants (a review). Brain Research, 1974, 76, 185-212

Prechtl HFR, Theorell K, & Blair AW. Behavioral state cycles in abnormal infants. Developmental Medicine and Child Neurology, 1973, 15, 606-615

Reiher J, & Lebel M. Wicket Spikes: Clinical correlates of a previously undescribed EEG pattern. Canadian Journal of Neurological Sciences, 1977, 4, 39-47

Schulte FJ, Michaels R, Nolte R, et al. Brain and behavioral maturation in new-born infants of diabetic mothers. Part I. Nerve conduction of EEG patterns. Neuropediatrics, 1969, 1, 24-35

Schultz MA, Schulte FJ, Akiyama Y, & Parmalee AH Jr. Development of electroencephalographic sleep phenomena in hypothyroid infants. Electroencephalography and Clinical Neurophysiology, 1968, 25:351-358

Tharp BR. Neonatal and pediatric electroencephalography. In Aminoff MJ (Ed.). Electrodiagnosis in Clinical Neurology. New York: Churchill-Livingstone, 1980, pp 67-117

Tharp B. Neonatal electroencephalography. In Korbkin R, Guilleminault L (Eds.). Progress in Perinatal Neurology Vol. 1. Baltimore: Williams & Wilkins, 1981, pp 31-64

Varner J, Ellingson R, Danahy T, & Nelson B. Interhemispheric amplitude asymmetry in the EEGs of full-term newborns. Electroencephalography and Clinical Neurophysiology, 1975, 43, 846-852

Werner SS, Stockard JE, & Bickford RG. Atlas of Neonatal Electroencephalography. New York: Raven, 1977

Part II

Research

Abraham Towbin

7

Neuropathologic Correlates

Focal lesions in the brain cause corresponding functional neurological defects. This is well established in basic clinical-pathologic studies. In adults, acute new lesions in the brain — whether due to inflammation (infection), circulatory process (infarcts, hemorrhage), physical trauma, or other pathologic process — lead to varying loss or distortion of motor, sensory, or other neurological function. It is a basic axiom in pathology that when an organ is damaged, the severity of the damage determines the degree of consequent functional defect manifested. Massive lesions in the brain generally cause major loss of function. Lesser lesions, "small bites," cause lesser signs and symptoms. Small lesions, depending on their location, may be occult, latent, clinically silent; in other instances, small lesions manifest their presence by evoking minor neurological abnormalities, "soft signs."

When cerebral damage occurs, loss of neurological function may be transient, to a greater or lesser degree. With acute cerebral damage, with the center of the lesion devitalized and the surrounding margin of tissue compromised by edema and inflammation, loss of function is maximum. With survival, the devitalized center, being unable to regenerate, becomes contracted and scarred. In the periphery of the lesion the pathologic changes are largely reversible, so that, in time, much of the function returns. Commonly, the effects of such damage, small lesions that are minimized and sublimated, may become neurologically undemonstrable. This does not erase their presence, their significance. Return of function may be considered "within normal limits," but this does not take into account the subtle loss of versatility and acumen previously possessed, prior to the cerebral damage.

The interpretation of the effects of minor cerebral damage, "soft signs,"

SOFT NEUROLOGICAL SIGNS
ISBN 0-8089-1841-9

in an infant is encumbered by the fact that usually there is no individual baseline in assessing the neurological abnormalities. In adults there is a "before" and "after" status that can be applied in identifying the soft signs. In interpreting the significance of minor neurological abnormalities in infants, the usual test scheme of comparing the appearance (or disappearance) of soft signs with "normal" standard groups can be deceiving.

In adults, the pathology of cerebral damage — due to trauma, infection, vascular disease, neoplastic processes, and other pathologic processes — is generally well established, defined in standard reference literature. In contrast, information about the pathogenesis of neonatal nervous system damage is less well known to clinicians.

Recognizing the need for more valid information concerning perinatal brain injury and sequelant nervous system disability, the National Institutes of Health in 1959 formulated the Collaborative Perinatal Project, "Collaborative Study of Cerebral Palsy, Mental Retardation, and Other Neurologic and Sensory Disorders of Infancy and Childhood" (1965). The project was a study of 50,000 women and their offspring. Fifteen medical centers across the country participated, correlating perinatal data with follow-up pediatric neurological studies. Pathology studies, postmortem investigation of the neonatal deaths, provided information defining the nature of organic perinatal brain damage and its sequelae.

In practice, much of the pathology information that emerged from the Collaborative Perinatal Project and from later related research has not yet filtered down to the clinical practitioner. Research studies in recent decades, concerned with etiology and intermediate pathologic processes, manifestly have failed to reach the pediatric neurologist, psychiatrist, and psychologist. Often pediatric neurologists, although generally not knowledgeable about obstetrical mechanisms, express "expert opinion" about the cause of brain damage incurred during gestation and parturition. Most obstetricians have little follow-up information about neurological sequelae that develop in infants following complicated pregnancy and delivery. Likewise, pathologists have generally given short shrift to the study of fetal-neonatal brain damage and its sequelae.

Prior to the Collaborative Perinatal Project, pathology studies of brain damage in the fetus and newborn were long neglected, mainly because of laboratory technical difficulties. Brain tissue of the fetus and newborn is by nature soft and friable, gelatinous, sometimes diffluent. Pathologists in the past, limited to the use of small histologic sections, were confronted with insurmountable difficulties in attempting to demonstrate focal lesions in the newborn brain.

The technical breakthrough to overcome this problem, the development of an adequate methodology for studying the soft, gelatinous brain tissue, was accomplished by Yakovlev (1970) working in the Collaborative Perinatal Project. With the Yakovlev technique, the whole brain specimen is embedded in a plastic material (celloidin), then whole-brain histologic sections, cut serially, are produced, making it possible to identify with consistency focal lesions, large and small, and to establish their geographic relationship in the brain specimen (Figs. 7-1 through 7-3). For the first time, it became possible to study the incidence of the cerebral lesions, especially minimal lesions, and to project clinical correlations.

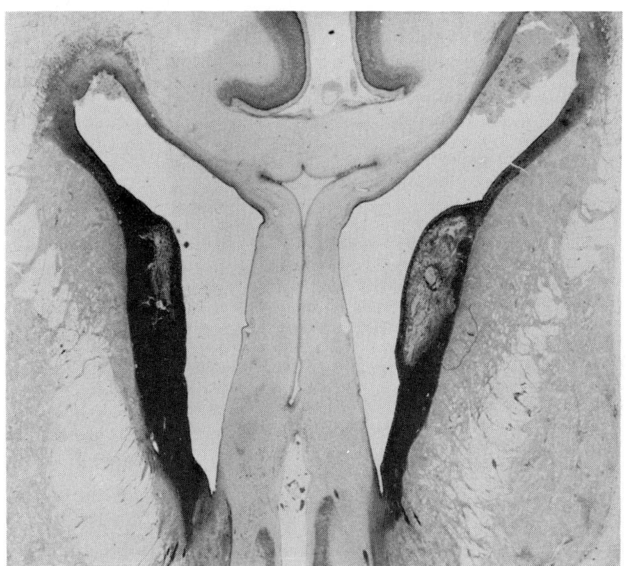

Figure 7-1. Premature brain, frontal section, the central portion of the cerebrum, through the septum and lateral ventricles. On the lateral aspects of the ventricles adjoining the basal ganglia (caudate) are bulging dark-staining structures, deposits of germinal matrix. On the right, the germinal matrix shows an area of rarifaction, a small acute infarct, with a dilated occluded vein. Clinical history of spontaneous delivery as 32 weeks' gestation due to premature detachment of the placenta; infant lived 2 days (W-73-61). (Reprinted from Towbin A. Cerebral intraventricular hemorrhage and subependymal matrix infarction in the fetus and premature newborn. American Journal of Pathology, 1968, 52, 121-129. With permission.)

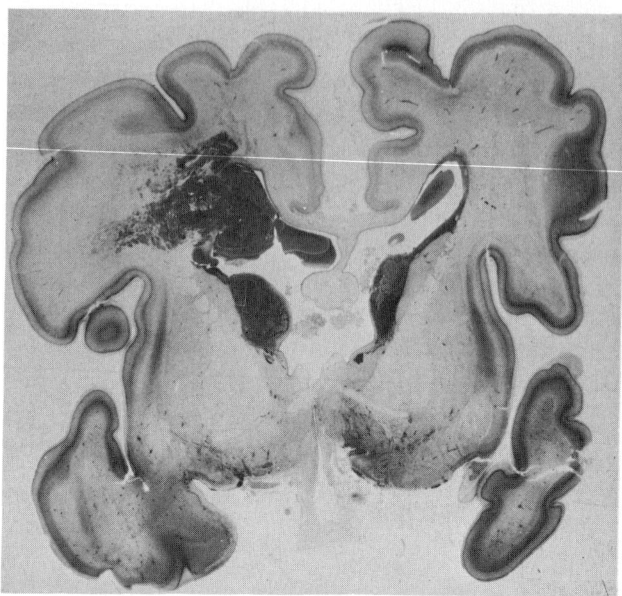

Figure 7-2. Massive acute deep cerebral infarction in a premature newborn. The area of infarction, deep in the upper portion of the left hemisphere, appears as dark confluent patches with infiltrating margins, obliterating the deep white matter and extending downward to involve the basal ganglia and germinal matrix tissue. On both sides, the germinal matrix deposit is effaced, replaced by a hemorrhagic mound of infarcted tissue bulging into the lower part of the cerebral ventricles. The case history indicated premature delivery at 35 weeks' gestation; the infant showed increasing generalized neurologic deterioration, with death at 23 hours (W-59). (Reprinted from Towbin A. Cerebral intraventricular hemorrhage and subependymal matrix infarction in the fetus and premature newborn. American Journal of Pathology, 1968, 52, 121-129. With permission.)

For the clinician, valid information about pathogenesis of cerebral damage in infants is a primary requisite in the interpretation of minor neurological abnormalities. It is necessary first to understand the underlying pathologic mechanisms that cause major lesions present in the newborn. Only with that can the nature and significance of minor cerebral lesions and their relation to soft signs be interpreted.

From neuropathologic studies in the Collaborative Perinatal Project and from other current investigations of fetal-neonatal disease, the following basic concepts have emerged.

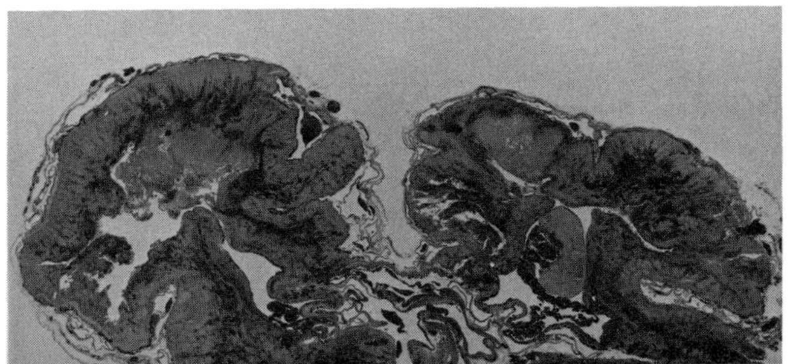

Figure. 7-3. Subacute cerebral damage in a term newborn. The deep periventricular strata in the cerebrum show far-advanced infarction, appearing as confluent pale areas surrounded by a jagged dark-staining border of congested tissue. Thrombosis of deep cerebral veins. Prenatal history of acute maternal illness, with vaginal bleeding, requiring hospitalization, 2 months before delivery (T-1). (Reprinted from Towbin A. Central nervous system damage in the human fetus and newborn infant. American Journal of Diseases of Children, 1970, 119, 529-542. With permission.)

Hypoxia

The most common cause of cerebral damage in the fetus and newborn is hypoxia. Many pathologic processes, complications of pregnancy and delivery, contribute to the development of hypoxia, inadequate oxygenation of the fetus and newborn (Csermely, 1972; Macgregor, 1960; Manterola, Towbin & Yakovlev, 1966; Potter, 1962; Towbin, 1966, 1968, 1969, 1970, 1971, 1978 a, b; Windle, 1968). Mechanical injury, especially spinal cord and brain stem damage, is also common in the newborn, but is of less significance than is hypoxia (Hellstrom & Sallmander, 1968; Towbin, 1964; Walter & Tedeschi, 1970). A host of other neonatal central nervous system disorders — genetic, metabolic, infectious, and toxic processes — make their appearance and, although much less frequent, these disorders often claim broader emphasis than do the effects of hypoxia, the process that underlies the bulk of neonatal neuropathologic case material (Windle, 1968).

Two Basic Forms of Hypoxic Brain Damage Occur in the Newborn

Deep cerebral damage occurs consistently in the premature fetus and newborn (Gröntoft, 1953; Macgregor, 1946; Towbin, 1968, 1970, 1971). *Corticalcerebraldamage*occursinthemature,atterm(Csermely,1972;Larroche,

1968; Okazaki, 1983; Towbin, 1968, 1970, 1971); in the monkey, exposure to hypoxia at term is associated with cortical damage (Myers, 1969).

Subacute Brain Damage Present at Birth; Prenatal Origin of Newborn Brain Damage

Newborn infants commonly harbor subacute, old, cerebral lesions, damage due to adverse gestational processes, damage incurred weeks or months prior to delivery (Fig. 7-3) (Goetzman, Lindenberg, & Ellis, 1984; Gröntoft, 1953; Macgregor, 1960; Manterola, Towbin, & Yakovlev, 1966; McGahan, Haesslein, Meyers, & Ford, 1984; Toverud, 1936; Towbin, 1968, 1970).

Biologically, the maternal-placental-fetal complex is delicately balanced, with a narrow margin of safety for the fetus. Maternal disease and local intrauterine disturbances that occur reverberate immediately in the fetus. Prologue to the stresses of birth are the hostile effects of intrauterine pathologic processes — organic cerebral attrition that the fetus commonly suffers in the wake of sublethal prenatal disturbances. As a consequence, in the newborn, brain damage often is present even though, clinically, the delivery is controlled and uncomplicated. Brain damage of subacute form, having its origin during a period prior to birth and developing silently, may evoke no neurological signs postnatally. Infants born with subacute or acute cerebral lesions may perform relatively well at birth, with neurological manifestations appearing months after birth. Thus, damage to the basal ganglia present at birth, later causing soft signs, or frank athetoid or other dyskinesia, cannot be recognized in the early infant period; small infants are naturally subject to wiggling, jerking, and purposeless movements.

Clinicians are generally not cognizant of the fact that newborn infants at times are born with subacute brain lesions, and automatically tend to ascribe infantile neurological disabilities to the events of labor and delivery, not taking into account adverse intrauterine processes, processes causing brain damage, that occur during pregnancy.

Transition Studies

These are studies that correlate acute cerebral damage present at birth with chronic lesions in the brain in cases of chronic neurological disability. The link between acute and chronic lesions lies in demonstrating intermediate lesions of subacute and chronic form pathologically in infants with manifest hypoxic or other complications during gestation and birth. For example, in hypoxic premature infants who live for a period of weeks or months, there are often areas of tan softening in the subependymal tissue of the cerebrum. The lesions, varying in size, are most frequent at the caudothalamic groove, near the deposits of germinal matrix. Correspondingly, deep subependymal periventricular chronic lesions are evident in infants who survive for a period, in cases of cerebral palsy (Fig. 7-4).

Central nervous system damage present in the newborn is the result of four main pathologic processes: hypoxia; mechanical injury; infectious disease; and genetic defects. By far, hypoxia is the most frequent process causing demonstrable cerebral abnormalities in the fetus and newborn.

HYPOXIC BRAIN DAMAGE

Although all the structures of the body are vulnerable to hypoxic injury during gestation and delivery, the most sensitive target proves to be the brain. Hypoxic brain damage is imprinted in the fetus and newborn when

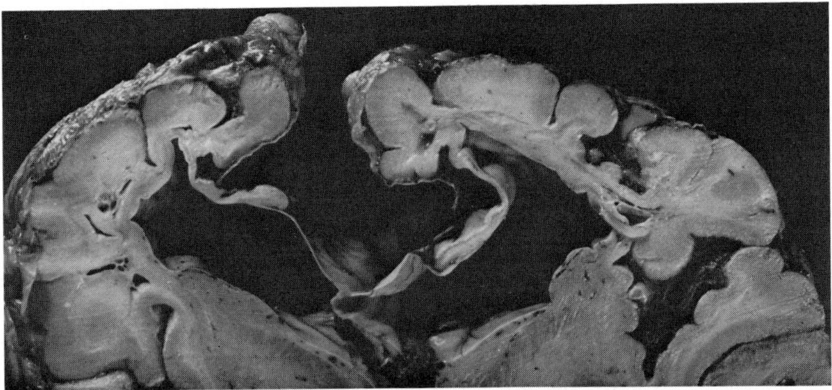

Figure 7-4. Cerebral lesions characteristic of cerebral palsy; old chronic residual lesions stemming from perinatal damage. Ventricles enlarged due to loss of substance in the periventricular white matter and basal ganglia, with scarring and cavitation. Seven-year-old with cerebral palsy and mental retardation. The pattern of damage is analogous to the subacute infarctional damage present in Figure 7-3 (CSS 5064). (Reprinted from Towbin A. The pathology of cerebral palsy. II. Archives of Pathology, 1955, 59, 529-552. With permission.)

complications occur during pregnancy and delivery. Complications due to maternal illness, placental disorders, umbilical cord entanglements with compression, exercise their damaging effects through the common denominator of fetal-neonatal oxygen deprivation, hypoxia. Postnatally, in the newborn, hypoxia is often due to antecedent brain damage, damage that compromises respiratory function. Apnea, episodic arrest of respiration, is particularly common in the premature. Pulmonary complication, the respiratory distress syndrome (hyaline membrane disease; pneumonia) may lead to hypoxic brain damage with varying lasting neurological disabilities.

Hypoxic complications during pregnancy and delivery vary in degree and duration. Fetal hypoxia often comes on gradually, with the mother at times reporting a loss of fetal activity, the syndrome of "fetus-in-coma." Severe, unremitting hypoxia leads to fetal or neonatal death. With less severe episodes of hypoxia, brain damage of less extent occurs and the fetus may survive, harboring subacute, old, "healed" lesions in the brain. Hypoxic complications during pregnancy and postnatally may be intermittent, with the brain accumulating a succession of cerebral lesions, leading to lasting neurological disabilities in those infants surviving.

Parenthetically, the relationship of prenatal hypoxia and kernicterus should be pointed out. There is increasing clinical and experimental evidence that hyperbilirubinemia is not a direct cause of cerebral damage. Kernicterus refers to yellow pigmentation of the basal ganglia and other neuronal assemblies, by bilirubin in cases of jaundice in the newborn, occurring predominantly in premature infants with Rh incompatibility or sepsis. The underlying cause of the cerebral damage in these cases is the occurrence of antecedent or concomitant perinatal hypoxia. The staining of the basal ganglia is secondary; the areas of cerebral tissue, previously devitalized by hypoxia, become passively stained by the yellow bilirubin pigment.

What is the pathogenesis of hypoxic cerebral damage, the step-by-step bodily changes that occur from the onset of oxygen deprivation to the time that acute damage is imprinted in the brain? Hypoxia leads to a consistent sequence of bodily changes in consecutive stages, with each stage precipitating the next (Towbin, 1968).

Hypoxia causes weakening of the heart muscle, myocardial fatigue, with resulting "forward" and "backward" heart failure. *Forward* failure, decreased profusion of blood through the arterial system, accounts for an initial shock-like collapse of bodily function. This may be rapidly fatal and pathologically there may be only minimal bodily changes. Infants who survive the acute shock effects of forward failure soon go into "backward" failure.

Backward failure results in blood being dammed back in the venous system of the body. Venous stasis with thrombosis (intravascular clotting during life) leads tc infarctional damage, focal and diffuse, devitalization of cerebral tissue with hemorrhage. Pathologically, the lesion may be massive, analogous to "stroke" damage in the adult. More often the lesions are circumscribed, small.

Pathologically, it is important to stress that the acute cerebral lesions in the newborn are of venous origin. The infarctional damage observed in the newborn cerebrum relates to the distribution of the venous drainage system and is not related geographically to the distribution pattern of cerebral arteries. Thromboses are found in veins, not in arteries, in the areas of infarction.

Basic Patterns of Fetal-Neonatal Hypoxic Cerebral Damage

With reference to gestational age, clinically and pathologically, it is important to realize that there are two basic patterns of hypoxic cerebral damage in the human fetus and newborn. In the *premature* fetus and newborn, prior to 35 weeks' gestation, hypoxic damage occurs primarily in the deep periventricular strata of the cerebrum, affecting the deep layers of white matter and adjoining basal ganglia (Fig. 7-2). In the *mature* fetus and newborn, the primary target for hypoxic damage is the cerebral cortex (Figs. 7-5 and 7-6).

Lesions in the premature cerebrum vary in extent, correlating with the severity of antecedent hypoxia. Minimal hypoxic cerebral damage in the premature fetus and newborn infant may appear as focal areas of infarction in the periventricular germinal matrix deposits (Fig. 7-1). Minimal infarctional lesions occur also in the surrounding deep white matter — small foci of necrosis known as periventricular leukomalacia.

Figure 7-2 illustrates the characteristic pattern of deep cerebral infarctional damage, a typical case, following severe hypoxia. The main damage appears at the core of the cerebrum, an area of hemorrhagic necrotic tissue with irregular penetrating margins, with the lesion adjoining portions of the basal ganglia and extending into the periventricular white matter. In some instances the infarctional damage extends through the hemispheric wall and into the cortex. Clinically, in the premature newborn with extensive deep cerebral hypoxic injury, with damage to the basal ganglia and neighboring structures, in the immediate postnatal period the picture is that of total

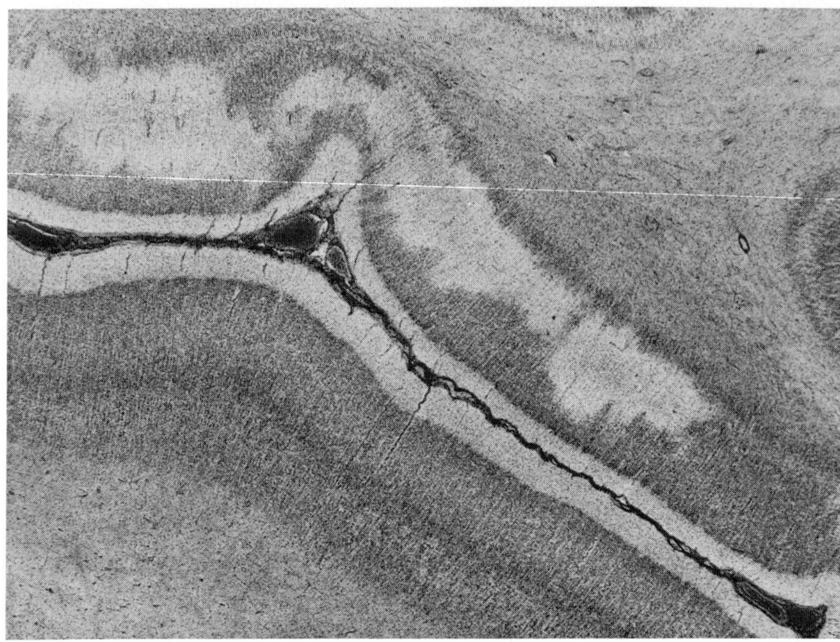

Figure 7-5. Minimal focal cortical damage in mature newborn cerebrum. Term pregnancy; fetal death prior to labor due to premature placental detachment. The lower right part of the illustration shows a cerebral convolution with well-preserved, laminated, six-layered cortex. The cerebral convolution in the upper part of the illustration shows confluent irregular pale patches, characteristic of acute hypoxic damage. It is noteworthy that neighboring the areas of cortical damage, there are small dilated meningeal veins containing thromboses (W-18). (Reprinted from Towbin A. Central nervous system damage in the human fetus and newborn infant. American Journal of Diseases of Children, 1970, 119, 529-542. With permission.)

neurological collapse, diffuse, floppy flaccidity, with depression of respiration and other vital function.

In the mature fetus and newborn, the hypoxic damage that occurs consistently in the cortex is pathologically analogous to the deep cerebral destruction that occurs in the premature infant — both are of venous infarctional nature. It is noteworthy that the pattern of hypoxic cerebral lesions in the mature newborn infant, mainly in the cortex, is much the same as that which occurs in adults exposed to hypoxia. Damage to the cortex and sub-

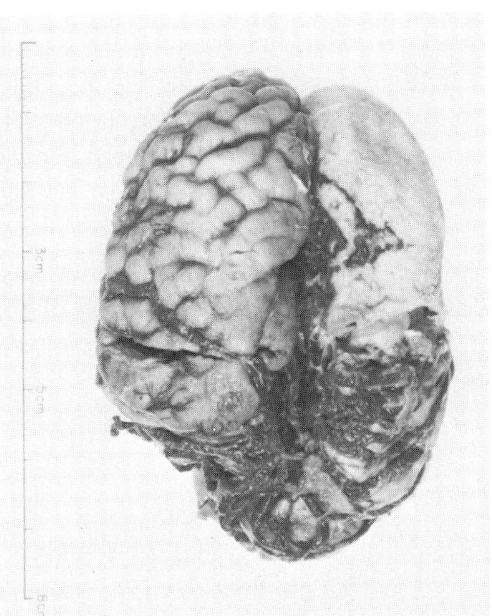

Figure. 7-6. Subacute hypoxic cortical infarction of right frontal lobe of the cerebrum in a mature newborn. At autopsy, the brain was small and in the area of infarction the convolutional pattern was wiped out and replaced by a smooth, leathery surface. The superficial cerebral veins were dilated and filled with thromboses. Maternal history of hepatitis during pregnancy (T-2). (Reprinted from Towbin A. Trauma in pregnancy — Injury to the fetus and newborn. In Tedeschi CG (Ed.). Forensic Medicine (vol. 1). Philadelphia: W.B. Saunders, pp 436-486, 1977. With permission.)

jacent tissue may be minimal (Fig. 7-5), or the infarctional destruction may extend widely, destroying major portions of the cerebrum (Fig. 7-6). Pertinently, however, the damage extending from the cortex does not reach the deep nuclear assemblies, does not encompass the basal ganglia.

Minimal cortical damage occurs in both diffuse and focal forms. In the diffuse pattern, varying numbers of neurons are injured or eliminated with blighting and depopulation of nerve cells more or less evenly spread through the cerebral cortex. In a more advanced form, cortical damage occurs as patchy infarctional laminar necrosis (Fig. 7-5).

In the fetus and newborn, the localization of cerebral damage, deep in the premature, cortical at term, is not a random occurence but is based on specific biologic factors (Towbin, 1970).

Germinal Matrix

In the premature, in the deep periventricular stratum, there are thick deposits of embryonic tissue, germinal matrix, bulging into the ventricles (Fig. 7-1). The deposits of germinal matrix are depots of building material, required for the future formation of the basal ganglia and other deep neuronal assemblies and for the development of the cerebral cortex. The matrix tissue, soft and friable, is manifestly vulnerable to hypoxia and readily undergoes infarctional disintegration. As the fetus matures, with histogenesis of the deep structures being completed, the germinal matrix is gradually used up; consequently, acute infarctional damage in the deep cerebral tissue at term does not occur.

Organogenesis

In the immature brain, between 22 and 35 weeks of gestation, growth momentum, and tissue differentiation is most active in the deep, periventricular structures, where elaboration of neurohistologic elements from the persisting deposits of germinal matrix is highly visible. In contrast, the cortical zone of the cerebrum at this time appears as a thin, compact, poorly vascularized ribbon, inert and rudimentary. During organogenesis, the parts undergoing active structural development are highly vulnerable to hypoxic infarctional injury. Later, as the fetus nears term and the germinal matrix becomes depleted, histogenesis at the core of the cerebrum declines, and the momentum of organogenesis shifts to the cerebral surface, where the cortex, maturing rapidly at term, becomes the main target of hypoxic-injury.

Vascular Development

Vascular development, particularly the elaboration of venous elements, directly influences the occurrence of infarction in the fetal-neonatal brain. In the premature, coincident with active organogenesis, vascularization of the deep cerebral structures proceeds early, providing a broad venous bed for the occurrence of thromboses, fostering deep cerebral infarction. At term, the cortex, previously essentially an avascular layer of tissue, rapidly undergoes differentiation and acquires a prominent venous drainage system; thrombosis of the newly formed surface veins results in cortical infarctional damage (Fig. 7-5).

Hypoxic exposure of the fetus and newborn results in four main types of nervous system disability — the tetralogy of cerebral palsy, mental retardation, epilepsy, and organic psychopathy. Generally, the pattern of nervous system disability can be correlated with the gestational age at the time of the hypoxic exposure. The two patterns of acute hypoxic cerebral damage, deep and cortical, correlate pathologically with equivalent chronic lesions, deep and cortical, and clinically with specific sequelant neurological manifestations. In the hypoxic premature, the specific occurrence of deep cerebral hypoxic damage, affecting basal ganglia, results in varying degrees of dyskinesia, with patterns of cerebral palsy, with manifestations of hypotonia or spasticity or athetosis.

Accordingly, cerebral palsy is known as the "disease of prematurity" — due to hypoxic damage to deep cerebral structures, basal ganglia, incurred in prematurely born infants due to deep cerebral damage in the premature fetus during gestation due to maternal illness, placental disorder, or other intrauterine pathologic processes. Manifestations of dyskinesia may be of major severity or minimal, expressed neurologically by the presence of relevant soft signs.

In the mature fetus and newborn, with hypoxia, with damage to the surface structures of the cerebrum, infants surviving develop sequelant cortical manifestations — mental retardation, epilepsy, and behavior disorders. It merits emphasis that hypoxic cerebral damage in the mature fetus and newborn affects the cortical strata, but does not extend to the basal ganglia, does not cause manifestations of cerebral palsy.

The occurrence of cerebral palsy is, in a sense, a time-marker. The presence of basal ganglia dysfunction, whether of major degree or limited to soft signs, reflects gestational damage prior to 35 weeks.

At times, cerebral palsy develops in infants born at term and clinically the manifest cerebral damage is erroneously attributed to faulty obstetrical management of the delivery. Often overlooked, or minimized, in such cases is the history of maternal illness, vaginal bleeding, or other early prenatal complications adversive to the fetus. In other instances, the intrauterine pathologic process causing fetal cerebral damage may be clinically silent.

In cases of cerebral palsy and other sequelae of perinatal injury, usually the record reveals a corresponding major gestational or birth complication, but not always. The enigmatic occurrence of cerebral palsy, mental retardation, and related cerebral dysfunctions in cases with a history of "uncomplicated gestation and delivery" requires comment. It should be emphasized that in some instances, pathologic intrauterine processes occur that are silent, producing no maternal symptoms.

What about cerebral palsy people who also have cortical manifestations of mental retardation and epilepsy? In pathologic studies of premature newborn brain damage, there are frequent cases in which the primary deep cerebral damage diffuses through the hemispheric wall, damaging the cortex. In such instances, with survival, it is expected that cerebral palsy, with superimposed disability of mental retardation and epilepsy will develop.

Clinically, in some cases, the pregnancy record indicates chronic maternal illness with ongoing adversive conditions for the fetus, extending from the premature period to term. These newborn infants, reflecting chronic intrauterine deprivation with malnutrition and chronic hypoxia, are often undersized, "dysmature." Such infants at times succumb during parturition. Autopsy studies of such cases reveal diffuse cerebral damage, deep and cortical, acute and chronic. Surviving infants commonly develop manifestations of cerebral palsy and cortical disabilities of epilepsy, mental retardation, and behavior disorders of varying severity. Clinical evidence of minimal brain dysfunction, abnormal EEG (without seizures), speech defects, and other soft signs are common in the low-birthweight newborn, both premature and dysmature (Hertzig, 1981; Renfield, 1975).

Severe hypoxia may lead to total necrosis of the cerebral structures, resulting in porencephaly or hydranencephaly, conditions in which all or a portion of the hemispheric wall is reduced to a thin sheet. Less severe hypoxic exposure causes correspondingly less extensive destruction, varying severity of scarring and cystic damage in the cerebrum, with the clinical consequence of mental retardation, cerebral palsy, and other major neurological disability. Mild hypoxia results in neuronal damage, focal or diffuse, with consequent neurological symptoms of a minimal or latent nature.

Clearly, the processes of hypoxic cerebral damage described here are not of an all-or-none character. In a broad perspective — from observations of hypoxic cerebral lesions in the newborn, lesions of varying severity, and the occurrence of corresponding chronic lesions in children with corresponding severity of cerebral palsy and other neurological disabilities — the conclusion is inescapable that minimal hypoxic lesions occurring in the fetal-neonatal period are responsible for the appearance later of lesser patterns of clinical disability, for varied subtle forms of attenuated, distorted CNS function, at times, soft signs.

Minimal hypoxic lesions in the deep cerebral structures are of very frequent occurrence in the human fetus and premature newborn, being evident at autopsy almost universally at 7 months' gestation. In pathologic studies, at the postmortem examinations of 140 premature newborn infants of 22-

35 weeks' gestation, deep cerebral infarctional damage, severe or minimal, was widely evident. In 48 percent of the cases, damage of severe to moderate degree was present. Significantly, in the other 52 percent of cases, acute hypoxic changes of minimal type were present, often diffusely spread through the germinal matrix and adjoining deep cerebral tissues, with venous stasis-thrombosis associated with focal necrosis and hemorrhage.

Hypoxic damage in the germinal matrix and deep white matter, even though the lesions appear minute, imposes an irrevocable loss of anlage elements and maturing tissue, creating a lasting handicap. These small foci of necrosis are the precursors of subacute and chronic lesions.

PHYSICAL INJURY

There remain many deeply rooted misconceptions regarding fetal-neonatal brain injury in clinical and lay literature. The concept that mental retardation, cerebral palsy, and other cerebral dysfunctions of the brain-injured child are due to "birth injury," to physical trauma incurred during the extraction of the fetus, still appears in the literature. The idea persists that the obstetrician's forceps, crushing the fetus head, is a major cause of newborn brain damage.

The occurrence of direct mechanical injury in the fetus and newborn, though of much less importance than hypoxic damage, is of some significance (Arey & Anderson, 1965; Pierson, 1923; Towbin, 1964; Ylppö, 1919). Direct injury to the skull, fractures due to application of obstetrical forceps, is in fact extremely rare. Intracranial hemorrhage, although more commonly due to hypoxic cerebral damage, may result from tearing of dural structures around the brain. This type of hemorrhage proves to be essentially an all-or-none phenomenon, at times being responsible for fetal-neonatal death, but it is of relatively limited importance compared to hypoxia as a cause of neurological sequelae.

The main form of physical trauma, as revealed in the Collaborative Perinatal Project investigations, is spinal cord and brain stem injury, incurred as the fetus is expressed through the birth canal and extracted at delivery (Towbin, 1964). Damage is due basically to stretch injury or to compression of the cord and brain stem incurred mainly through excessive traction and flexion of the fetal vertebral column in cephalic as well as breech delivery. Other factors of significance that contribute to injury include precipitous delivery, prematurity, primiparity, and intrauterine malposition of the fetus. Very small and very large fetuses are especially vulnerable to spinal injury.

Recent studies have increasingly called attention to the importance of endogenous spinal injury, damage incurred by the fetus prior to active labor or early in parturition. Malposition, as in face and brow presentation, or with transverse arrest, causing hyperflexion or hyperextension of the fetus, is a major case of endogenous spinal injury (Hellström & Sallmander, 1968). In breech delivery, endogenous spinal injury is frequent, with damage to the thoracic and lumbar spine due to hyperflexion during the descent of the fetus.

Spinal injury is common in the newborn, present in over 10 percent of cases examined at autopsy (Litzmann, 1880; Pierson, 1923; Towbin, 1964). With such injury, with damage to vital regulatory centers in the brain stem and cord, respiration may be depressed. Often this results in stillbirth or death soon after delivery. Or, the damaging effects may be indirect, the respiratory depression present leading secondarily to varying severity of cerebral hypoxic damage.

Spinal injuries at birth with evident vertebral fracture and dislocation and with mangling transection of the cord are infrequently encountered in the present day. However, a broad range of lesions, anatomically nontransectional, associated with varying damage to surrounding structures, does occur (Fig. 7-7) (Towbin, 1964).

At autopsy, the presence of spinal injury in the neonate is frequently indicated by epidural hemorrhage in the spinal canal; damage may extend outward involving the spinal skeletal and soft tissue structures. Tears in the dura and avulsion of spinal and cranial nerve roots may occur. The cord in spinal injury presents a gradient of lesions varying from frank laceration to focal hemorrhage and malacia and other parenchymal damage. Severe spinal injury may cause paraplegia from birth (Hellström & Sallmander, 1968). Damage to the spinal cord may be less crippling, of minor degree, and latent.

Ford (1960) pointed out that almost all case studies of spinal birth injury described in the literature refer to severe injuries; it follows necessarily, that clinically there must exist many with mild injuries who do not attract prominent attention, being without severe paralysis. Varied chronic sensory-motor disabilities, including hearing deficiency, disorders of deglutition, speech defects, and imbalance in eye muscle function, may result from perinatal injury to the brain stem with cranial nerve damage. As Ford has indicated, many cases of minor perinatal injury of the cord, with mild im-

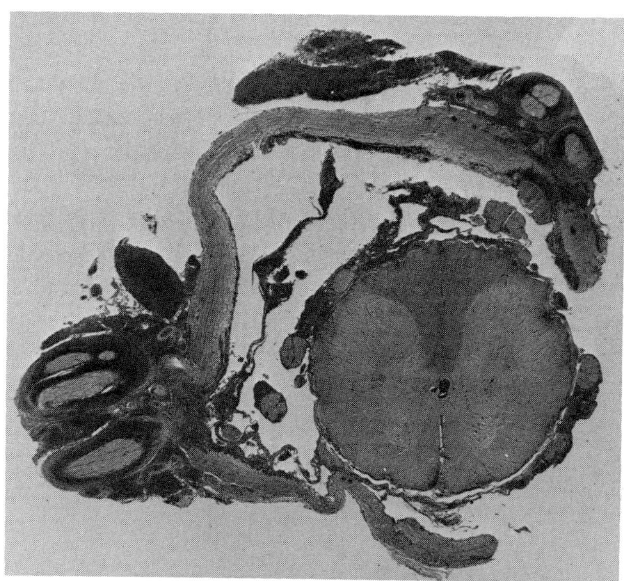

Figure 7-7. Spinal cord injury in the newborn. Histologic section transversely through the spinal cord shows disruption of the dura around the cord, with epidural hemorrhage and laceration and hemorrhage of the spinal nerve at its exit through the dura. Infant born at 37 weeks' gestation, Apgar score of four at 5 minutes; hypotonia and respiratory depression; death, 16 hours after delivery (W-107). (Reprinted from Towbin A. Spinal cord and brain stem injury at birth. Archives of Pathology, 1964, 77, 620-632. With permission.)

pairment of neurological dysfunction, go unrecognized. Children with this form of minimal neurological function are sometimes mistakenly considered to have mild cerebral palsy or are regarded as clumsy children.

INFECTIOUS DISEASES (Remington & Klein, 1983)

In the human fetus and newborn, of increasing importance clinically are two infectious processes, cytomegalic viral (CMV) encephalitis and Escherichia coli meningitis. While other infectious processes such as rubella and toxoplasmosis are of concern, in clinical practice it is the effects of CMV and E. coli infections that are currently the most serious problem.

Viral Infection

Cytomegaloviral disease, generally overlooked in the past, is now recognized increasingly in neonates; the infection is characterized by postnatal enlargement of the liver and spleen, hyperbilirubinemia, and characterized neurologically by lethargy and weakness.

The infection is caused by one of the five known herpes viruses in man. The cytomegalic virus-infected cell develops a large eosinophilic nuclear inclusion, and the nucleus and cytoplasm become increased in volume (cytomegaly). Pathologically, the virus infects the liver, kidney, brain, and other parenchymal organs.

The damage in the brain is primarily in periventricular structures (white matter and basal ganglia) and is ongoing during premature and term periods in fetal life. In some cases calcifications are evident in x-ray studies of the brain. Late sequelae consist of varying severities of microcephaly, often with dilated ventricles (hydrocephaly), with clinical mental retardation, spastic quadriplegia, deafness, and ocular involvement with strabismus, nystagmus, and other eye disorders.

Cytomegalic infection in women is of high incidence (50-70 percent have CMV antibodies serologically) but only in a small percent age of cases does the maternal infection become transmitted through the placenta and cause fetal-neonatal infection and organic damage during gestation. CMV is asymptomatic during gestation and the diagnosis is not made prior to delivery. The importance of CMV disease in the newborn was generally overlooked in the past and the diagnosis was missed clinically and pathologically. CMV is now considered the most frequent perinatal viral disease. It has been estimated to involve 8 per 1000 births and to be responsible for brain damage in 1 per 1000 births.

The prognosis in overt neonatal CMV infection is difficult to predict; over 70 percent of surviving infants present varying severities of spastic quadriplegia, mental retardation, and varied sensory defects.

Recent virologic and serologic studies of several thousand routine deliveries identified large numbers of infants born with unsuspected, clinically silent CMV infection. Many of these infants, asymptomatic at birth, developed some neurological abnormality, including mild mental retardation, deafness, and soft signs characteristic of minimal cerebral dysfunction.

The occurrence of other viral infections, such as rubella, that cause fetal-neonatal encephalitis is well known; such cases are episodic, rare. Infection with toxoplasma, a protozoan parasite, is widespread. Cases of overt neonatal infection lead to chronic sequelae of mental retardation, epilepsy, and other neurological defects, together with chorioretinitis. The effects of subclinical neonatal toxoplasmosis are not clear.

Bacterial Infection

Of the central nervous system bacterial infections most commonly encountered in the newborn, E. coli has become the most serious clinically. E. coli, gram-negative enteric bacilli, are currently responsible for the majority of cases of acute meningitis in neonates. Significant neurological sequelae of varying severity develop in 20-50 percent of infants who survive neonatal meningitis.

CONGENITAL MALFORMATIONS

Congenital malformations, as the term is generally used, implies the presence of abnormal structure stemming from genetic causes or due to induced environmental causes, teratogenic insults, during embryonic life, and does not apply to encephaloclastic processes, that is, breakdown of already-formed parts of the maturing fetal brain, as occurs with hypoxia or viral disease.

Congenital malformations of the central nervous system are of great variety but are relatively rare compared to the common encephaloclastic abnormalities due to hypoxia. Congenital malformations have been of wide interest clinically and pathologically. Detailed studies are extensively represented in the medical literature (Crome, 1972; Warkany, Lemire, & Cohen, 1981). It is not the province of this presentation to review these detailed studies.

Likewise the study of genetic, biochemical abnormalities, syndromes related to lipid metabolism, carbohydrate disorders, and disorders of amino acid metabolism that lead to mental retardation and other major and minor neurological findings are liberally presented in a host of current publications.

Clinically and pathologically, the more severe forms of central nervous system congenital disease, such as arhinencephaly, are generally readily identified. The importance of minimal cerebral malformations, such as cases with abnormalities in the pattern of cerebral convolutions, is a matter of conjecture. Very often cerebral malformations appear as constellations of changes effecting varied patterns of major functional defects, at times evoking only minimal manifestations, soft signs.

Clinically and pathologically, in the assessment of perinatal central nervous system abnormalities — whether due to hypoxia, physical injury, infection, or congenital defects — often the border line between what is physiological and what is pathological is not distinct. During the time of gestation the fetus is threatened by hypoxic, traumatic, infectious complications, all potentially brain-damaging or lethal. The period of gestation, climaxed by the events of birth, is the most hazardous experience to which most persons are ever exposed. For the fetus, premature or at term, during its marginal existence in utero and as it is pistoned down the birth canal and separated, hypoxic and mechanical injury to the central nervous system, in some measure, is inescapable.

Gestation and birth thus form an inexorable leveling mechanism; with the brain marred at birth, the potential of performance may be reduced from that of a genius to that of a plain child, or less. The damage may be slight, imperceptible clinically, or it may spell the difference between brothers, one a dexterous athlete and the other "an awkward child."

Substantially, it is said, all of us have a touch of mental retardation, cerebral palsy, or other blight, some more, some less, some with disability, some with soft signs—the endowment pathologically of gestation and birth.

REFERENCES

Arey JB, & Anderson GW. Pathology of the newborn. In Greenhill JP (Ed.). Obstetrics (13th ed.). Philadelphia: Saunders, 1965

Collaborative Perinatal Project. Collaborative study of cerebral palsy, mental retardation, and other neurologic and sensory disorders of infancy and childhood (Research Profile No. 11. Public Health Service Publication No. 1370). Bethesda, MD: National Institutes of Health, National Institute of Neurological Disease and Blindness, 1965

Crome L. Pathology of Mental Retardation. Baltimore: Williams & Wilkins, 1972

Csermely H. Perinatal anoxic changes of the central nervous system. Acta Paediatrica Academiae Scientiarum Hungaricae, 1972,13, 283-299

Ford FR. Diseases of the Nervous System in Infancy, Childhood, and Adolescence. Springfield, IL: Charles C. Thomas,1960

Goetzman BW, Lindenberg JA, & Ellis W. Documentation of perinatal brain injury. Pediatric Research, 1984, 18, 1366

Gröntoft O. Intracerebral and meningeal hemorrhages in perinatally deceased infants. Acta Obstetrica et Gynecologica Scandinavica, 1953, 3, 308-334

Hellström B, & Sallmander U. Prevention of cord injury in hyperextension of the fetal head. Journal of the American Medical Association, 1968, 202, 1041-1044

Hertzig ME. Neurological "soft" signs in low-birthweight children. Developmental Medicine and Child Neurology, 1981, 23, 778-791

Larroche JC. Nécrose cérébrale massive chez le nouveau-né. Biology of the Neonate, 1968, 13, 340-360

Litzmann CCT. Ein Beitrag zur Kenntnis des spinalen Lähmung bei Neugeboren. Archiv für Gynaekologie, 1880, 16, 87-106

Macgregor AR. The pathology of still-birth and neonatal death. British Medical Bulletin, 1946, 4, 174-178

Macgregor AR. Pathology of Infancy and Childhood: Part I. Disturbances of Prenatal Life. Edinburgh, Scotland: Livingston, 1960

Manterola A, Towbin A, & Yakovlev PI. Cerebral infarction in the human fetus near term. Journal of Neuropathology and Experimental Neurology, 1966, 25, 479-488

McGahan JP, Haesslein HC, Meyers M, & Ford KB. Sonographic recognition of in utero intraventricular hemorrhage. American Journal of Radiology, 1984, 142, 171-173

Myers RE. Atrophic cortical sclerosis associated with status marmoratus in a perinatally damaged monkey. Neurology, 1969, 19,1177-1188

Okazaki H. Fundamentals of Neuropathology. New York-Tokyo: Igaku-Shoin, 1983

Pierson RN. Spinal and cranial injuries of baby breech deliveries. Surgery of Gynecology and Obstetrics, 1923, 37, 802-815

Potter E. Pathology of the Fetus and the Infant. Chicago: Yearbook Publishers, 1962

Remington JS, & Klein JO. Infectious Disease of the Fetus and Newborn Infant (2nd ed.), Philadelphia: W.B. Saunders, 1983

Renfield ML. The small-for-dates infant. In Avery GB (Ed.). Neurology. Philadelphia: J.B. Lippincott Co., 1975

Toverud KU: Etiological factors in neonatal mortality, with special reference to cerebral hemorrhage. Acta Paediatrica Scandinavica, 1936, 18, 249-271

Towbin A. Spinal cord and brain stem injury at birth. Archives of Pathology, 1964, 77, 620-632

Towbin A. Massive cerebral hypoxic damage in the human fetus near term. In Luthy F, Bischoff A (Eds.). Proceedings of the Fifth International Congress of Neuropathology, Zurich, August 1965 (International Congress Series No. 100). Amsterdam: Excerpta Medica Foundation, 1966

Towbin A. Cerebral intraventricular hemorrhage and subependymal matrix infarction in the fetus and premature newborn. American Journal of Pathology, 1968, 52, 121-139

Towbin A. Central nervous system damage in the premature related to the occurrence of mental retardation. Fourth Multidisciplinary Conference on the Etiology of Mental Retardation (National Institutes of Health). Lincoln, Nebraska, 1970, pp 213-239

Towbin A. Mental retardation due to germinal matrix infarction. Science, 164, 156-161, 1969

Towbin A. Organic causes of minimal brain dysfunction. Journal of the American Medical Association, 1971, 217, 1207-1214

Towbin A. Obstetrical factors in fetal-neonatal visceral injury. Obstet Gynecol, 1978a, 52, 113-124

Towbin A. Cerebral dysfunctions related to perinatal organic damage: Clinical-neuropathologic correlations. Journal of Abnormal Psychology, 1978b, 87, 617-635

Walter CE, & Tedeschi CG. Spinal injury and neonatal death. American Journal of Obstetrics and Gynecology, 1970, 106, 272-278

Warkany J, Lemire RJ, & Cohen MM. Mental Retardation and Congenital Malformations of the Central Nervous System. Chicago: Yearbook Medical Publishers, 1981

Windle WF. The Albert Lasker Basic Research Award Lecture: Brain damage at birth. Journal of the American Medical Association, 1968, 206, 1968-1969, (excerpt)

Yakovlev PI. Whole brain histologic sections. In Tedeschi CG (Ed.). Neuropathology, Methods and Diagnosis. Boston: Little, Brown & Company, 1970

Ylppö A. Pathologisch-anatomische Studien bei Frügeboren. Zeitschrift für Kinderheilkunde, 1919, 20, 212-432

Paul L. Nichols

8

Minimal Brain Dysfunction and Soft Signs: The Collaborative Perinatal Project

The label "minimal brain dysfunction syndrome" (MBD) has been applied to "children of near average, average, or above average general intelligence with certain learning or behavioral disabilities ranging from mild to severe, which are associated with deviations of function of the central nervous system. These deviations may manifest themselves by various combinations of impairment in perception, conceptualization, language, memory, and control of attention, impulse, or motor function" (Clements, 1966, pp. 9-10). Children whose problems are due to severe neurological or sensory abnormalities or to cultural deprivation or emotional conditions are generally excluded. Prevalence estimates average around 5 percent of young school children, with boys affected at least 3 times as often as girls (Millichap, 1975; O'Malley & Eisenberg, 1973; Safer & Allen, 1976; Wender, 1971).

The concept of minimal brain dysfunction as a diagnostic entity is highly controversial (Schmitt, 1975). Minimal brain dysfunction has been considered synonymous with hyperactivity and learning difficulties, two of its most prominent features. For example, Schain (1977) concluded that "the terms 'learning disorders or disabilities,' 'hyperactive behavior disorders,' and 'minimal brain dysfunction' are interchangeable from a practical, clinical point of view.... They all refer to the same large group of children" (p. 25). Also, the term neurological soft signs is generally used only to designate minimal brain dysfunction (Touwen & Sporrel, 1979). More recently, this group of children has been labeled as having attention deficit disorder (American Psychiatric Association, 1980), and pharmaceutical companies advertising stimulant medication have switched from MBD to ADD.

Nichols and Chen (1981) reported the results of a large-scale study of MBD in the Collaborative Perinatal Project population. They concluded that the associations among neurological soft signs, hyperkinetic-impulsive behavior, and learning difficulties were so slight that the designation of a syndrome was unwarranted. Each symptom area, including neurological soft signs, was studied extensively in terms of association with other symptoms, antecedents, prediction, and familial associations. The results of their studies of neurological soft signs are summarized in this chapter.

THE COLLABORATIVE PERINATAL PROJECT

The data were taken from the Collaborative Perinatal Project (NCPP) of the National Institute of Neurological and Communicative Disorders and Stroke. Between 1959 and 1965 more than 44,000 women were registered in the NCPP, a prospective study of the relationship between perinatal problems and neurological and cognitive deficits in infancy and childhood. The total project population was over 53,000 because 6000 of the women registered during 1 or more subsequent pregnancies. Data were collected in 12 university medical centers on standardized forms at prenatal clinic visits, at admission for delivery, and during labor and delivery. Interdisciplinary project personnel examined the children neonatally and at specific intervals through the age of 8 years.

Nearly 95 percent of the women in the project were university hospital clinic patients, mostly from cities in the northeastern states. The ethnic distribution was 45 percent white, 47 percent black, 7 percent Puerto Rican, and the rest a variety of other groups. The NCPP population was characterized socioeconomically both at the time the women registered in the study and again when the children reached age 7. The median socioeconomic index score, based on combined data for education, occupation, and income, was lower for the NCPP population than for an age-matched sample of the U.S. population (Myrianthopoulos & French, 1968). The lower median score was related to the nonrepresentative ethnic distribution. Within ethnic groups the NCPP white and black populations were closer socioeconomically to age-matched U.S. white and black population samples.

The cohort for the present study was taken from 37,994 children who had neurological and psychological examinations and were given an IQ score at age 7. Excluded from this study were 1987 children whose ethnicity was not white or black, 1942 who were not in the first or second grade in school when tested, 3808 with IQs below 80, and an additional 368 with cerebral palsy or other major neurological abnormality. The "MBD cohort" consisted of the remaining 29,889 children.

NEUROLOGICAL SOFT SIGNS

Neurological soft signs were identified by neurologists who examined the project children at age 7. The 10 signs studied were poor coordination (abnormalities on tests of finger to nose, heel to knee, finger pursuit, rapid individual finger movements, or rapid alternating movements), abnormal gait (awkwardness when walking, running, walking on toes or heels, or hopping), impaired position sense (failure to touch index fingers with eyes closed or to specify direction of movement as toe was moved through small arc), nystagmus, strabismus, astereognosis (failure to distinguish by touch a bottle cap, nickel, and button), abnormal reflexes (hypoactive; increased or asymmetrical biceps, triceps, knee, or ankle jerk), mirror movements, other abnormal movements (fasciculations, myoclonus, tremor, athetosis, chorea, dystonia, ballismus, or tic), and abnormal tactile finger recognition (failure to identify 2 or more fingers that were lightly touched out of child's field of vision).

Some of the neurological items were coded dichotomously and others were coded 0-1-2, based on severity. For example, distinct lack of coordination such as dysdiadochokinesia (difficulty in executing rapid alternating movements) was coded 2, and generalized awkardness in fine motor tasks (such as tying shoe laces) was coded 1. Approximately two-thirds of the children judged to have poor coordination were given the 1 code. More than 90 percent of the children in the MBD cohort with abnormal gait were coded 1 for nonspecific awkwardness, and children whose difficulties were presumed to be due to a specific neurological defect were coded 2. (Recall that the MBD cohort excluded children with cerebral palsy and other major neurological abnormalities.) The majority of children with abnormal reflexes, astereognosis, and impaired position sense were coded 2 for "definite" (ranging from 70 percent for position sense to 90 percent for reflexes), and the rest were coded 1 for "suspicious." Table 8-1 shows the percentages of children within the 4 race-sex groups in the MBD cohort with each of the 10 soft signs. In this table, the 1 and 2 codes are combined.

Table 8-1
Percentages of Children in the Study Cohort with Neurological Soft Signs

Soft Sign	White Boys	White Girls	Black Boys	Black Girls	Total
Poor coordination	13.3%	6.9%	7.9%	4.1%	8.1%
Abnormal gait	6.3%	2.4%	3.1%	1.7%	3.5%
Impaired position sense	1.3%	1.3%	1.0%	0.6%	1.1%
Nystagmus	1.0%	0.9%	0.8%	0.5%	0.8%
Strabismus	7.6%	7.7%	8.4%	8.7%	8.1%
Astereognosis	1.0%	1.0%	0.7%	0.4%	0.8%
Abnormal reflexes	15.6%	14.6%	13.2%	13.0%	14.2%
Mirror movements	3.3%	2.6%	1.4%	1.0%	2.1%
Other abnormal movements	3.6%	1.9%	1.5%	0.7%	1.9%
Abnormal tactile finger recognition	11.6%	9.0%	18.0%	13.4%	12.9%

THE ASSOCIATION AMONG SYMPTOMS

To study the association among neurological soft signs and other symptoms of minimal brain dysfunction, correlation matrices were computed for the 10 soft signs and 16 other behavioral, cognitive, perceptual-motor and academic symptoms. The behavioral items, including hyperactivity, impulsivity, and short attention span, were adopted from 5-point ratings, completed by the examining psychologist following administration of the 7-year psychological test battery. Six cognitive and perceptual-motor variables included scores on the Bender-Gestalt, Draw-A-Person, and Auditory-Vocal Association (ITPA) tests, the WISC IQ, low verbal (relative to performance) IQ, and low performance (relative to verbal) IQ. Because the first three of these scores were highly correlated with IQ, performance on these tests was defined in terms of deviation scores relative to IQ. Performance on the Wide Range Achievement Test (WRAT) was the basis for three academic symptoms. Deviation scores for spelling, reading, and arithmetic were derived so each child could be compared to others in the same grade in school and with the same IQ. The 26 x 26 correlation matrices were calculated for each of the 4 race-sex groups, for samples from individual study centers, for samples of children with at least one symptom, and for samples of children with at least one "severe" symptom. A final matrix was calculated for the total MBD cohort. The correlational patterns in all groups were very consistent and similar to that in the total cohort, presented in Table 8-2. This matrix shows the expected

Table 8-2
Correlation Coefficients Among Individual Variables

	2	3	4	5	6	7	8	9	10	11	12	13	14	15	16	17	18	19	20	21	22	23	24	25	26
1. WISC IQ	-07	-11	-05	-20	-04	-14	-14	-01	-00	04	08	03	06	06	04	-02	-03	-01	-02	01	-04	-01	02	01	-15
2. Hyperactivity	—	-12	48	36	32	03	07	07	-05	-03	-00	03	-09	-06	-08	08	07	02	00	00	03	04	01	06	06
3. Hypoactivity		—	-04	05	02	34	34	-03	03	-00	02	-02	02	01	-03	01	01	01	01	00	02	04	01	01	-00
4. Impulsivity			—	30	33	-01	04	07	-05	-03	01	02	-06	-03	-05	06	05	02	-00	01	01	02	02	03	04
5. Short Attention Span				—	23	16	11	09	-07	-04	00	00	-10	-09	-13	06	05	02	02	01	03	03	01	04	07
6. Emotional Lability					—	-05	22	02	-03	-00	01	02	-02	-01	-05	04	04	01	02	01	02	03	02	03	02
7. Withdrawal						—	46	-01	01	-02	03	-02	-00	-01	-05	03	02	02	01	-01	03	01	01	02	03
8. Socioemotional Immaturity							—	-02	01	-01	04	-03	02	01	-03	04	02	02	01	00	01	02	01	04	02
9. Bender-Gestalt*								—	-21	-12	-03	03	-20	-16	-17	04	03	02	-00	01	03	01	01	01	10
10. Draw-A-Person*									—	02	01	00	12	07	05	-00	-00	-00	00	00	-01	01	02	-00	-03
11. Auditory-Vocal Association (ITPA)*										—	-14	12	19	23	20	00	-01	-00	01	01	-01	-01	02	02	-05
12. Low Verbal IQ											—	-09	-03	-05	-04	-01	-00	00	00	-01	00	-01	-01	-01	-01
13. Low Performance IQ												—	05	08	04	02	02	-00	00	-00	02	01	01	02	01
14. Spelling*													—	78	44	-02	-01	-01	-01	-01	-02	-03	-00	01	-09
15. Reading*														—	46	-01	-01	-01	-02	00	-01	-03	01	01	-07
16. Arithmetic*															—	-05	-03	-03	-02	-02	-03	-03	-02	-01	-09
17. Poor Coordination																—	28	11	03	05	07	14	14	17	03
18. Abnormal Gait																	—	07	03	05	06	11	09	13	03
19. Impaired Position Sense																		—	09	02	03	06	05	04	03
20. Astereognosis																			—	02	01	04	03	02	03
21. Nystagmus																				—	07	06	05	02	-00
22. Strabismus																					—	04	02	02	01
23. Abnormal Reflexes																						—	07	08	01
24. Mirror Movements																							—	09	-01
25. Other Abnormal Movements																								—	-00
26. Abnormal Tactile Finger Recognition																									—

*Deviation scores (corrected for IQ)

significant associations within each of the 4 symptom groups; for example, the correlation between poor coordination and abnormal gait was .28; between the Bender-Gestalt and Draw-A-Person deviation scores, -.21; hyperactivity and impulsivity, .48; and between spelling and reading deviation scores, .78. Of course, with such a large sample (29,889), these values are statistically significant at far less than the .001 level. In fact, a value of only .02 is significant at the .001 level.

These results suggest that within the large unselected NCPP population, the association among symptoms from different areas was very slight. This impression was confirmed by subjecting the matrix in Table 8-2 to a series of factor analyses (SPSS, PA2; Nie, Hull, Jenkins, et al, 1975). As expected, there was no MBD factor to which variables from the different areas were related. The same four factors were first to emerge in the total cohort analysis as in each individual race-sex group. Also, the results were essentially identical when orthogonal or oblique ($\delta = 0$) rotation was used: the correlation between factor loadings from the 2 methods in the total cohort analysis was .993.

Factor loadings of .10 or greater from the orthogonal rotation analysis in the total cohort are given for 4 factors in Table 8-3. The variables loading most highly on the 4 factors were (1) reading, spelling, and arithmetic deviation scores; (2) hyperactivity, impulsivity, short attention span, and emotional lability; (3) socioemotional immaturity, withdrawal, and hypoactivity; and (4) poor coordination and abnormal gait. The factors appear to reflect learning difficulties (LD), hyperkinetic-impulsive behavior (HI), immature behavior, and neurological soft signs (NS).

The factor analysis results were used to construct scales to measure MBD symptoms — not for a theoretical study of the underlying correlational structure in the MBD cohort. Linear functions based on the loadings of all symptoms were used to assign factor scores to each child. A factor score was the sum of terms consisting of a coefficient for each variable derived from the factor loadings, multiplied by an individual's standardized score for that variable.

The NS factor scores had a skewed distribution with a mean of 0.00 and standard deviation of 0.72. Two cutoffs were chosen to define abnormal groups, one including 8 percent of the cohort (score 1.00 or higher) and the other 3 percent (score 2.20 or higher). The study group consisted of 2331 children (two-thirds boys) with a variety of soft signs. The most frequent combinations of signs in these children were poor coordination (337), poor coordination and abnormal reflexes (312), poor coordination and abnormal gait (194), abnormal gait only (157), and poor coordination, abnormal gait,

Table 8.3
Factor Loadings of .10 or Greater in the Total Cohort Analysis

	Factor			
	I	II	III	IV
Hyperactivity	—	.71	—	—
Hypoactivity	—	—	.52	—
Impulsivity	—	.65	—	—
Short attention span	-.12	.49	.16	—
Emotional lability	—	.47	—	—
Withdrawal	—	—	.66	—
Socioemotional immaturity	—	.13	.67	—
Bender-Gestalt	-.24	.10	—	—
Draw-A-Person	.12	—	—	—
Auditory–Vocal Association	.28	—	—	—
WRAT Spelling	.85	—	—	—
WRAT Reading	.87	—	—	—
WRAT Arithmetic	.54	—	—	—
Poor coordination	—	—	—	.58
Abnormal gait	—	—	—	.43
Impaired position sense	—	—	—	.19
Nystagmus	—	—	—	.12
Strabismus	—	—	—	.13
Astereognosis	—	—	—	.10
Abnormal reflexes	—	—	—	.26
Mirror movements	—	—	—	.24
Other abnormal movements	—	—	—	.28
Abnormal tactile finger recognition	-.11	—	—	—
WISC IQ	—	-.13	-.22	—

and abnormal reflexes (95). At their 7-year neurological examination, nearly half (48.1 percent) were rated neurologically normal, 43.6 percent suspicious, and 8.3 percent abnormal. Children with severe neurological abnormality, such as cerebral palsy, were, of course, excluded from the MBD cohort.

RELIABILITY OF MEASUREMENT

Indirect indications of the reliability of the derived NS factors score came from quality control trials that were held for the 7-year neurological examination. A sample of 1045 children was reexamined by a neurologist from a different hospital 3 months after the original examination. The neurologist who first examined the child was present to discuss any differences. Although most of the children selected for reexamination had some positive findings initially, the visiting neurologists were unaware of the previous results. A preliminary report of these data indicated that the assessment of poor coordination, the most important item in the NS factor, differed significantly in 15 percent of the cases examined. For abnormal gait, the figure was 9 percent. Hospital differences in the diagnosis of these 2 symptoms, 1 or both of which was present in 85 percent of the NSs, were in fact considerable. The frequency of poor coordination among the study centers ranged from a high of 17 percent at Columbia-Presbyterian Medical Center in New York to a low of 2 percent in the children examined at the University of Tennessee College of Medicine in Memphis. Similarly, abnormal gait was diagnosed in nearly 6 percent of the children examined at Columbia-Presbyterian Medical Center and the University of Minnesota Hospital, but in fewer than 1 percent of those examined at the University of Tennessee College of Medicine.

The frequencies of abnormal NS factor scores within the study centers reflected, of course, these variations. For example, only 1.7 percent of the children from Memphis were in the NS group, compared to 16.5 percent of those from New York (Columbia). The reexamination results indicated that the differences in frequency were largely the result of variations in examiner threshold by study center. To solve any potential problems in data analysis and interpretation that these variations could cause, the associations between the NS factor score and antecedent variables were always calculated separately within each sample and the results combined, and study centers were included as control variables in multivariate analyses.

ASSOCIATIONS WITH ANTECEDENT VARIABLES

A major advantage of studies using the NCPP population is the overwhelming amount of prospectively ascertained information collected in socioeconomic and medical history interviews, prenatal examinations, labor and delivery observations, and follow-up examinations of the children. For this study, a total of 249 variables passed an initial screening for associations with neurological soft signs.

For a more detailed second screening, series of 2 x 2 contingency tables were combined by a procedure described by Nichols and Chen (1981).

Briefly, the factor score was dichotomized; NS (score ≥ 1.00) versus no NS. Dichotomous antecedents, for example diabetes in pregnancy, were tested directly. Continuously distributed antecedents were divided into two categories, for example very young versus all other mothers.

Within each institutional subsample, each association was tested separately for each race-sex group. The individual results were then combined, both for race-sex totals and for the entire sample. To calculate combined χ^2s, the difference in frequency of an MBD symptom between the two antecedent conditions was determined. This difference was weighted by the number of cases per subsample having the antecedent condition under study. This weighting procedure resulted in χ^2 values nearly identical to those produced with the more familiar Cochran (1954) technique, and permitted direct estimates of empiric "relative risks" (the ratio of the frequency of NS in a specified group to the frequency in the rest of the MBD cohort). The procedure was then repeated for the "severe" 3 percent cutoff (factor score ≥ 2.20).

About half of the antecedents (128 of 249) screened using this procedure were significantly associated with the presence of neurological soft signs ($p < .05$). These variables were grouped into demographic and maternal (23), pregnancy and delivery (14), neonatal and infancy (41), preschool (19), and medical history and concomitant (18). Within each of these 5 epochs, multivariate discriminant analyses were performed so that variables with the largest independent associations could be identified. The multivariate analyses compared the NS study group (N = 2331) to a control group (N = 12,511) with normal scores on all 3 MBD factor scores — neurological soft signs, learning difficulties, and hyperkinetic-impulsive behavior. In the following sections, the variables that were significant in the multivariate analyses will be mentioned, and one or two of the most significant variables in each epoch will be discussed in some detail.

Demographic and Maternal Characteristics

Socioeconomic information was obtained from NCPP participants at 2 time periods — during prenatal interviews, and again when the children reached 7 years of age. Most of the maternal variables, including reproductive history, age, height, and weight, were obtained during prenatal interviews. The multivariate analysis indicated that, compared to the normal control group, the NS children were characterized by the following: longer histories of maternal cigarette smoking, taller mothers, less maternal educa-

Table 8-4
Frequencies and Relative Risks for Neurological Soft Signs Among Children Whose Mothers Had a Long History of Cigarette Smoking

		Neurological Soft Signs			Relative Risk
Group	(N)	Observed	Expected	Relative Risk	for "Severe" NS
White boys	(1515)	241	187.1	1.29*	1.48*
White girls	(1468)	121	103.6	1.17	1.35
Black boys	(869)	59	68.3	0.86	1.18
Black girls	(936)	38	38.4	0.99	0.79
Total	(4788)	459	397.4	1.15†	1.33*

*$p < .001$
†$p < .01$

tion, more changes in residence, lower socioeconomic index scores, fewer working mothers (prenatal interview), more retarded younger siblings, more parental consanguinity, more children adopted at 7 years, more prior fetal deaths, and more mental illness in siblings.

Observed and expected frequencies of neurological soft signs are shown in Table 8-4 for children whose mothers reported a cigarette smoking history of 10 years or longer. Expected frequencies were determined from all other children and considered the race, sex, and hospital of birth of the exposed children. Relative risks for NS and "severe" NS (the 3 percent cutoff) are shown; if values were determine from the χ^2 tests. These low, but statistically significant risks are typical of the associations between prenatal or perinatal antecedents that were found in this study.

Another maternal characteristic related to neurological soft signs was height. The relative risk for NS among children whose mothers were tall (at least 5'8") was 1.31 ($p < .001$). The increased risk was consistent within the four race-sex groups but statistically significant only for black boys.

Pregnancy and Delivery Complications

Antecedent variables representing pregnancy and delivery complications were derived from prenatal examinations and interviews and recorded labor and delivery room events. Most of the variables screened from these periods had no relationship to neurological soft signs. The seven variables retained in the multivariate analysis indicated that, compared to the normal control group, the NS children had lower fetal heart rates during the second

Table 8-5
Frequencies and Relative Risks for Neurological Soft Signs Among Children Who Had a Short Umbilical Cord

		Neurological Soft Signs			Relative Risk
Group	(N)	Observed	Expected	Relative Risk	for "Severe" NS
White boys	(256)	46	29.4	1.57*	1.75†
White girls	(313)	29	19.8	1.46†	1.01
Black boys	(246)	18	17.7	1.02	0.80
Black girls	(408)	22	15.6	1.41	0.82
Total	(1223)	115	82.5	1.39¶	1.21

*$p < .01$
†$p < .05$
¶$p < .001$

stage of labor, shorter umbilical cords, and a higher incidence of chorionitis. Pregnancy characteristics of the mothers of affected children included more cigarette smoking, more hospitalizations, more low hematocrit readings, and more diabetes.

Smoking during pregnancy is obviously related to the variable discussed in the previous section, length of smoking history. The frequency of neurological soft signs ranged from 7.2 percent among 15,448 children whose mothers did not smoke at all during pregnancy to 12.5 percent among 447 children whose mothers smoked 2 or more packages of cigarettes per day ($p < .001$). Associations of this magnitude are not useful for prediction because of the overlap between the groups. They are, however, useful in identifying possible risk factors for further study.

Another significant variable from this period was a short umbilical cord (less than 40 cm or 2 standard deviations below the NCPP population mean). Observed and expected frequencies of NS among these children are shown in Table 8-5. The risk across race-sex groups was 1.39 ($p < .001$), with the greatest risk among white boys.

The Neonatal and Infancy Periods

This group of variables included neonatal observations, abnormalities noted on the neonatal or 1-year summary protocols, mental and motor performance and behavior at 8 months, and measurements of height, weight, and head circumference through the first year. Neurological soft signs were more strongly related to these variables than were learning difficulties or hyperkinetic-impulsive behavior.

Just as all tall mothers had more children with neurological soft signs than did shorter mothers, the longest infants, measured at birth, 4 months, or 8 months, were also at increased risk. For example, a group of 486 children whose length at 4 months was at least 2 standard deviations above their race-sex group mean had a relative risk of 1.30 ($p < .05$).

Other neonatal and infancy variables that characterized the NS children in the multivariate analysis were low Bayley motor score at 8 months, delayed motor development at 1 year, strabismus at 1 year, erythroblastosis, low weight at 4 months, low head circumference at 1 year, neonatal seizures, multiple apneic episodes, minor genitourinary malformations, neonatal brain abnormality, one-minute Apgar score below 4, and neonatal nerve abnormality.

The best discriminator between the NS and control groups among these variables was the Bayley motor score at 8 months. The NCPP children were given the research version of the Bayley Scales of Infant Development (Bayley, 1969). The motor scale consisted of 43 items; the mean raw score (total number of items passed) was 33. Observed and expected frequencies of NS among children whose scores were under 25 (the lowest 3 percent of scores in the study cohort) are shown in Table 8-6. Abnormal NS scores were nearly twice as frequent as expected ($p < .001$), and the increases were significant for each race-sex group. Abnormal NS scores ranged from 17 percent among these children down to only 6 percent among

Table 8-6
Frequencies and Relative Risks for Neurological Soft Signs Among Children Who Had Low Bayley Motor Scores at 8 Months

		Neurological Soft Signs			
Group	(N)	Observed	Expected	Relative Risk	Relative Risk for "Severe" NS
White boys	(248)	68	32.4	2.10*	2.17*
White girls	(191)	28	14.3	1.96*	2.23†
Black boys	(202)	24	15.8	1.52†	1.14
Black girls	(170)	16	7.5	2.12 ¶	2.40†
Total	(811)	136	70.0	1.94*	1.95

*$p < .001$
†$p < .05$
¶$p < .01$

children whose Bayley scores were 40 or higher (about 6 percent of the cohort).

Neonatal brain abnormality was diagnosed by a senior pediatrician after reviewing the nursery record for signs of seizures, clonic spasms, hypertonia, hypotonia, hyperactivity, lethargy, paralysis-paresis, or asymmetrical or abnormal reflexes. Only 87 of the cohort children had a "definite" brain abnormality, and in this small group, NS was more frequent than expected (14 observed, 6.5 expected, $p < .01$). A much larger group of children ($N =$ 2742, or 9 percent of the study cohort) received a "suspect" brain abnormality diagnosis. These children had a slightly increased risk of NS (1.25, $p < .01$).

Among children with low birthweight relative to their race-sex mean (approximately 2600 g for white boys, 2500 g for white girls, 2400 g for black boys, and 2300 g for black girls), the frequency of NS was significantly increased (1.33, $p < .001$). In the multivariate analysis, however, birthweight was no longer significantly related to NS after correlated variables (especially weight at 4 months) were simultaneously considered.

Preschool Characteristics

The children in the NCPP were given cognitive and motor tests at age 4, after which the examining psychologists completed behavior ratings. In this section, associations between these 4-year measures and neurological soft signs at age 7 will be summarized.

Compared to the control group, the NS children performed more poorly on the following tests: hopping, Porteus maze IV, Stanford-Binet IQ, copy cross, copy square, copy circle, line walk, stringing beads, ball catch, and Graham block sort test. Their behavior was characterized by hyperactivity, emotional lability, short attention span, emotional flatness (the emotionality rating was split into 2 variables, and more of each extreme was found among the NSs), and more ratings of suspicious or abnormal behavior. In addition, the NSs were more often left handed and were heavier than the control group. These 19 variables all made significant ($p < .05$) independent contributions in the multivariate analysis.

The 2 best discriminators, failure on the hopping and Porteus maze tasks, are similar to the two 7-year variables that loaded most highly on the NS factor — poor coordination and abnormal gait. The NS children tended to have similar fine and gross motor problems at age 4. The hopping task required the child to execute a well-balanced hop on one foot. Two trials per foot were allowed. Estimated relative risks for NS among children who failed on the right foot were nearly identical to those for children who failed on the left foot. Results for the former will be presented. Failure was twice as common among boys as among girls, and more than twice as common among whites (25 percent) as among blacks (11 percent). Observed and expected frequencies for NS are shown among children who could not hop at age 4 (see Table 8-7). The risks for "severe" NS (the extreme 3 percent of factor scores) were increased to a greater degree than were those for the more broadly defined cutoff (the extreme 8 percent). The hopping task was failed by 41 percent of the NS children and only 14 percent of the comparison group.

The Porteus maze IV test required the child to draw a line between 2 boundaries outlining a figure. More than one-fourth of the whites and one-half of the blacks in the cohort failed the test (a deviation of more than 1.5 inches outside the boundary). The increased frequencies of NS among these children is shown in Table 8-8. The estimated risks for the total sample, as well as for the 4 race-sex groups, were all highly significant.

Several behavior ratings at age 4 were related to neurological soft signs at age 7. Children rated on a 5-point scale of level of activity as (4) *unusual amount of activity and restlessness, very seldom able to sit quietly* , or (5) *extreme overactivity or restlessness* had significantly more NS than expected (Table 8-9). The overall risk for NS was 1.72, and for "severe" NS, 1.92 (both $p < .001$). Since hyperkinetic-impulsive behavior at age 7, one of 3 MBD symptoms studied, was slightly more frequent than expected among children with soft signs, associations such as these with 4-year behavior are not surprising. In an additional multivariate analysis, the NS group was

Table 8-7
Frequencies and Relative Risks for Neurological Soft Signs Among Children Who Could Not Hop at Age 4

		Neurological Soft Signs			
Group	(N)	Observed	Expected	Relative Risk	Relative Risk for "Severe" NS
White boys	(1810)	349	194.7	1.79 *	2.37 *
White girls	(906)	104	54.5	1.91 *	2.42 *
Black boys	(841)	108	58.4	1.85 *	2.06 *
Black girls	(390)	30	14.2	2.11 *	2.20†
Total	(3947)	591	321.9	1.84 *	2.31 *

* $p < .001$
† $p < .05$

Table 8-8
Frequencies and Relative Risks for Neurological Soft Signs Among Children Who Failed the Porteus Maze IV at Age 4

		Neurological Soft Signs			Relative Risk
Group	(N)	Observed	Expected	Relative Risk	for "Severe" NS
White boys	(1856)	361	194.0	1.86 *	2.50 *
White girls	(1521)	157	95.3	1.65 *	1.84 *
Black boys	(3133)	274	175.0	1.57 *	1.75 *
Black girls	(3238)	157	92.1	1.70 *	2.06 *
Total	(9748)	949	556.4	1.71 *	2.07 *

*$p < .001$

confined to children with normal scores on the other 2 MBD factors: HI and LD. Some 4-year behavior ratings, including hyperactivity and emotional lability, were still significant discriminators between the control group and children with only neurological soft signs. In other words, there was an excess of abnormal 4-year behavior ratings among NS children whose behavior at age 7 was rated normal.

Concomitant and Medical History Variables

When the NCPP children reached 7 years of age, their neurological examination, from which the soft signs in the current study were derived, included a complete physical examination. Children's health histories from

Table 8-9
Frequencies and Relative Risks for Neurological Soft Signs Among Children Rated Hyperactive at Age 4

		Neurological Soft Signs			Relative Risk
Group	(N)	Observed	Expected	Relative Risk	for "Severe" NS
White boys	(1136)	229	128.9	1.78 *	2.07 *
White girls	(727)	74	47.4	1.56 *	1.68 †
Black boys	(888)	104	64.0	1.64 *	1.87 *
Black girls	(773)	55	29.1	1.89 *	1.73 †
Total	(3524)	463	269.4	1.72 *	1.92 *

*$p < .001$
†$p < .05$

ages 1 to 7 were reviewed and recorded on a summary protocol. Physical measurements were also taken. The association between the medical history and concomitant variables and neurological soft signs will be summarized in this section.

One important discriminator between the NS and control groups was difficulty with right-left identification. Because this variable itself has been considered by some to be a neurological soft sign, an association with the derived NS score is not surprising. The relative risk for an abnormal NS score among the children who failed to perform all of these commands correctly — show me your *right* hand; show me your *left* eye; put your *right* hand on your *left* eye; put your *left* hand on your *right* ear—are shown in Table 8-10. All comparisons were significant at the .001 level, and the relative risks, especially for "severe" NS, were consistent for the four race-sex groups.

The multivariate analyses showed that NS children were heavier at age 7 than the control group. They also had more diagnoses of cranial nerve abnormality, refractive error, amblyopia, other eye conditions, skin conditions and infections, asthma, and German measles. The NS children had more left and variable hand dominance and more variable overall dominance than did the control group. Many of the diagnosed conditions were infrequent but associated with high relative risks for NS. For example, 53 of 128 children in the cohort with a specific cranial nerve abnormality (mostly the seventh nerve, affecting facial muscles, or the twelfth, affecting muscles in the tongue) had neurological soft signs, compared to only 12 expected ($p < .001$).

A more frequent condition, affecting 7 percent of the white children and 11 percent of the black children in the cohort was refractive error, including

Table 8-10
Frequencies and Relative Risks for Neurological Soft Signs Among Children Who Had Difficulty with Right–Left Identification at Age 7

		Neurological Soft Signs			Relative Risk for "Severe" NS
Group	(N)	Observed	Expected	Relative Risk	
White boys	(1498)	292	162.5	1.80 *	2.00 *
White girls	(1177)	119	73.8	1.61 *	2.18 *
Black boys	(1663)	191	98.7	1.94 *	1.99 *
Black girls	(1515)	94	47.8	1.96 *	2.01 †
Total	(5853)	696	382.8	1.82 *	2.03 *

* $p < .001$
† $p < .01$

Table 8-11
Frequencies and Relative Risks for Neurological Soft Signs Among Children with Refractive Errors

		Neurological Soft Signs			Relative Risk
Group	(N)	Observed	Expected	Relative Risk	for "Severe" NS
White boys	(512)	109	66.0	1.65 *	2.00 *
White girls	(529)	62	36.8	1.69 *	1.61
Black boys	(720)	82	54.3	1.51 *	1.48
Black girls	(795)	54	30.6	1.76 *	1.65
Total	(2556)	307	187.7	1.64 *	1.72 *

*$p < .001$

loss of acuity (below 20/30), hyperopia, or astigmatism. These children's increased risk for neurological soft signs is shown in Table 8-11. Refractive errors were also associated with increased frequencies of learning difficulties and hyperkinetic-impulsive behavior.

FAMILIAL ASSOCIATIONS

Although there have been a few anecdotal reports of a genetic predisposition to poor coordination in children (Gordon, 1977), detailed family studies of neurological soft signs are rare. Because many mothers registered in the NCPP for more than one pregnancy, and many reported relatives also in the project, large samples of siblings and cousins could be studied for familial associations. Also, there were 55 twins among the 2331 NS chidren (more than expected, because twins had a slightly increased relative risk for NS [1.33, $p < .05$]).

For twins, siblings, and cousins, all NS children were identified, and the observed and expected frequencies of affected project relatives calculated. Thus in families with two affected children, each was counted as both an index and secondary case. This procedure is unbiased in studies such as the NCPP, in which families with more than one affected child are not more likely to be identified than are families with none or one affected (i.e., ascertainment of the NCPP study children was complete). As usual, expected frequencies were based not only on the child's race and sex, but also on the collaborating NCPP hospital in which he or she was examined. Results of these analyses are summarized in Table 8-12. The twin data, confined to the 40 affected whose zygosity was determined and whose co-twin was

Table 8-12
Frequencies and Relative Risks for Neurological Soft Signs Among Twins, Siblings, and Cousins of Affected Children

		Neurological Soft Signs		
Relationship to Proband	**Number of Relatives**	**Affected**	**Expected**	**Relative Risk**
Monozygotic twin	12	8	1.4	5.88*
Dizygotic twin, total	28	8	3.5	2.27†
Same sex	17	6	2.3	2.64†
Opposite sex	11	2	1.2	1.61
Full sibling	830	124	93.9	1.32¶
First cousin	842	110	95.5	1.15

*$p < .001$
†$p < .05$
¶$p < .01$

also in the study cohort, suggested a familial association. The frequency of NS among monozygotic twins affected was 5.9 times the expected value; for the dizygotic twins, 2.6 times. Among 830 project siblings of children with NS, 124 also had NS, compared to 94 expected ($p < .01$). Although the increased risk was not great, there were about 30 percent more affected children than expected.

With only a 30 percent risk to siblings of those affected, little increase in the risk to cousins would be expected under any hypothesis to explain the family resemblance. Nevertheless, the cousin data were suggestive of a familial association: among 842 first cousins of affected children, 110 had NS, compared to 96 expected ($p = .08$, one-tail).

Altogether, these analyses indicate a significant familial component to neurological soft signs, and the estimated risks to relatives of affected children are compatible with a genetic influence. According to the polygenic model of inheritance, siblings of more "genetically loaded" children should be at higher risk than siblings of other affected children. Table 8-13 shows that the risk to siblings of children with "severe" NS (the extreme 3 percent of the distribution of scores) was indeed higher than for siblings of children with scores between the 92nd and 97th percentiles (1.52 versus 1.22).

The results of an additional analysis suggest a familial association between minor and major neurological abnormalities. The frequency of abnormal NS scores was examined among 69 cohort children who had non-cohort NCPP siblings given a diagnosis of cerebral palsy at age 7. Just as siblings of children with "severe" NS were at higher risk than siblings of

Table 8-13
Frequencies of Neurological Soft Signs Among Siblings of Affected Children

Condition in Proband	Number of Siblings	Neurological Soft Signs		
		Affected	Expected	Relative Risk
"Mild" NS	551	71	62.3	1.22
"Severe" NS	279	48	31.6	1.52 *
Cerebral palsy	69	16	7.0	2.29 *

* $p < .01$

children with fewer soft signs (Table 8-13), siblings of children with CP were at an even higher risk. There were more than twice as many cases of NS as expected among the siblings of the children with cerebral palsy (16 affected, 7 expected, $p < .01$). Familial incidence has been reported in some cases of cerebral palsy with unknown etiology (Bundey & Griffiths, 1977).

The polygenic model has been used to account for sex differences in the frequencies of some conditions. The less frequently affected sex is assumed to be more genetically loaded, and siblings of these affected children, or girls in the case of NS, should be at increased risk. The risks to siblings of affected girls and boys, however, were very similar: 1.34 for siblings of boys and 1.28 for siblings of girls. Therefore, polygenic inheritance with different thresholds by sex does not appear to explain why boys have more neurological soft signs than girls.

The importance of the familial associations compared to the demographic, maternal, pregnancy, delivery, neonatal, and infancy factors identified earlier was assessed with a multivariate analysis on the subsample of NS children having a sibling in the cohort. The most important socioeconomic and early predictors were entered into a discriminant function analysis with a new variable added: presence of a sibling with neurological soft signs. A subsample of 642 NS children was compared to 3299 children with no MBD symptoms. The top 4 discriminators between the 2 groups and their standardized coefficients (a statistic measuring the relative importance of the discriminators) were delayed motor development at 1 year (.22), Bayley motor score at 8 months (-.21), head circumfrance at 1 year (-.20), and siblings with neurological soft signs (.19). This analysis shows that even after controling for a child's early status, an affected sibling is still a significant discriminator between children with and without neurological soft signs at age 7.

SUMMARY

Neurological soft signs were identified in a sample of 29,889 children whose mothers registered for prenatal care in the Collaborative Perinatal Project. Children who had IQ scores below 80 or severe neurological abnormalities were not included. Each child was given a score on a factor-analytically derived dimension, the most important components of which were fine and gross motor incoordination and abnormal gait. The NS group was defined as children with scores in the top 8 percent of the distribution. For some analyses, the top 3 percent of scores were considered "severe" NS.

Slight associations were found between NS and 2 other similarly derived dimensions: learning difficulties and hyperkinetic-impulsive behavior. Among 249 antecedent variables screened for associations with neurological soft signs, the most important discriminators between the NS children and a symptom-free control group were later performances and conditions, for example, failure on hopping and Porteus maze tasks at age 4.

The NS children differed in size from the comparison group. During the first year of life, the NSs were tall, and they also had tall mothers. Although they were lighter during the first year, the NSs were heavier at ages 4 and 7 than were children in the comparison group. Other early antecedents of NS included poor performance on the Bayley Motor Scale at 8 months and maternal smoking during pregnancy. A significant familial association for neurological soft signs was found, and the frequencies of NS among relatives were compatible with a weak genetic influence.

Although this study identified some early antecedents of soft signs, most of these antecedents were not good predictors. Their identification will be useful in the formation of specific etiological hypotheses. The finding of many significant associations is consistent with the notion that neurological soft signs have multiple etiologies.

ACKNOWLEDGMENT

Portions of this chapter are taken from Nichols PL, & Chen TC. Minimal Brain Dysfunction: A Prospective Study, and are reproduced with the permission of the publisher, Lawrence Erlbaum Associates, Hillsdale, NJ.

REFERENCES

American Psychiatric Association. Diagnostic and Statistical Manual of Mental Disorders (3rd ed.). Washington, DC: Author, 1980

Bayley N. Manual for the Bayley Scales of Infant Development. New York: Psychological Corporation, 1969

Bundey S, & Griffiths MI. Recurrence risks in families of children with symmetrical spasticity. Developmental Medicine and Child Neurology, 1977, 19, 179-191

Clements SD. Minimal brain dysfunction in children (NINDB Monograph No. 3, U.S. Public Health Service Publication No. 1415). Washington, DC: U.S. Government Printing Office, 1966

Cochran WG. Some methods for strengthening the common χ^2 tests. Biometrics, 1954, 10, 417-451

Gordon NS. The clumsy child. In Drillien CM, & Drummond MB (Eds.). Neurodevelopmental Problems in Early Childhood: Assessment and Management. Oxford: Blackwell Scientific Publications, 1977

Millichap JG. The Hyperactive Child with Minimal Brain Dysfunction. Chicago: Year Book Medical Publishers, 1975

Myrianthopoulos NC, & French KS. An application of the U.S. Bureau of the Census socioeconomic index to a large, diversified patient population. Social Science and Medicine, 1968, 2, 283-299

Nichols PL, & Chen TC. Minimal Brain Dysfunction: A Prospective Study. Hillsdale, NJ: Erlbaum, 1981

Nie NH, Hull CH, Jenkins JG, et al. SPSS: Statistical Package for the Social Sciences (2nd ed.). New York: McGraw-Hill, 1975

O'Malley JE, & Eisenberg L. The hyperkinetic syndrome. In Walzer S, & Wolff PH (Eds.). Minimal Cerebral Dysfunction in Children. New York: Grune & Stratton, 1973

Safer DJ, & Allen RP. Hyperactive Children: Diagnosis and Management. Baltimore: University Park Press, 1976

Schain RJ. Etiology and early manifestations of MBD. In Millichap JG (Ed.). Learning Disabilities and Related Disorders: Facts and Current Issues. Chicago: Year Book Medical Publishers, 1977

Schmitt BD. The minimal brain dysfunction myth. American Journal of Diseases of Children, 1975, 129, 1313-1318

Touwen BCL, & Sporrel T. Soft signs and MBD. Developmental Medicine and Child Neurology, 1979, 21, 528-530

Wender PH. Minimal Brain Dysfunction in Children. New York: Wiley-Interscience, 1971

Ellen D. Rie

9

Soft Signs in Learning Disabilities

The presumption that children with learning disabilities suffer from deblitating weaknesses in the central nervous system led to the search for neurological manifestations of the disorder. In the hope of confirming the hypothetical neurological impairment and for the purpose of establishing a diagnostic procedure offering hard evidence of the syndrome, researchers studied the relationship between learning disabilities and neurological soft signs for well over 2 decades. Because of serious definitional and methodologic problems, often encountered in clinical studies with children, but particularly evident here, the results have been both confusing and controversial and no conclusive relationship has been established. For learning disabled children, the controversial findings diminished the predictive potential and clinical significance of these signs. Yet, periodic reports, some attesting to the association between soft signs and learning disabilities (LD) while others not, continue to surface.

The waning, but recurrent reference to and interest in neurological soft signs, partly due to the assumption that LD children fail to learn because of central nervous system impairments, suggests that the issue is not a closed one. It is well known that damage to the brain can affect a broad range of adaptive behaviors (Boll, 1977) and that motor-sensory manifestations of the damage have been postulated (Ingram, 1973). The consideration of and search for the understanding of the relationship between neurological status and learning in children clearly hold promise for shedding light not only on the learning process itself but also on the intimate interaction between the brain and human behavior.

The purpose of this chapter is to give a brief historical account of the concept of learning disabilities and to readdress the major issues and concerns involved in understanding the role of neurological soft signs in the

SOFT NEUROLOGICAL SIGNS
ISBN 0-8089-1841-9

diagnosis of this syndrome. It is hoped that this review will generate renewed interest in the study of the relationship between these signs and impaired learning in children.

A BRIEF HISTORY OF THE CONCEPT OF LEARNING DISABILITIES

The Categorization of Deviant Children

When the French government asked Alfred Binet, at the turn of the century, to develop procedures to identify mentally retarded children, two major developments took place. First, the concept of individual differences among children gained attention, and second, the need for a more refined diagnostic system for the evaluation of child psychopathology was recognized. Binet and his colleague, Theodore Simon, believed that intelligence could be measured by assessing the ability to make sound judgments. Previous measures of intelligence explored sensory-motor skills and reaction time. Instead, Binet and Simon constructed an instrument that would measure problem solving abilities. The Stanford-Binet ultimately came to be used not only to identify retarded children but also to determine intellectual differences among all children. This measure of individual differences accentuated and called attention to the absence of specific diagnostic entities for children. A great effort was made in the first decade of the century to correct this situation.

Work on the refinement of the categorization of childhood psychopathology continued well into the 1920s and 1930s, and by the 1950s specific entities became well established. Defective children came to be categorized as schizophrenic, autistic, culturally deprived, mentally retarded, and brain damaged (Birch, 1965).

Brain Damage and Behavior

In the 1920s, as attention to individual differences, differential diagnosis, and refined labeling in children increased significantly, a worldwide epidemic of encephalitis took its toll on children. Survivors of the epidemic were reported to have symptoms of restlessness, clumsiness, and disinhibited motor activity (Bond, 1932; Hohman, 1922). These observations led to the speculation that brain damage might be the causal factor in learning and behavior disorders in children. Several years later, Kahn and Cohen (1934) hypothesized a causal relationship between brain damage and learning disability after noting that children with demonstrable brain damage exhibited problems in learning. These observations were followed by those of Strauss and Werner (1942), who found that brain injured retarded children had unique abnormalities in cognitive functioning when compared with non brain damaged retardates. In particular, they observed specific symptoms of perseveration, focus on small detail, inconsistent responses to the same stimulus, and forced responsiveness (Strauss & Werner, 1943). As a result of these findings, the practice of labeling children with these symptoms as brain damaged, with no further evidence of brain damage, became established. The term *minimal* was suggested by Knobloch and Pasamanick (1959) to indicate that the impairment was limited and/or mild.

The expression "damage," offensive to both the clinician and the parent, was highly criticized. In response to the criticism, Clements and Peters (1962) recommended the term *dysfunction* in lieu of "damage." Of the ten common characteristics of children with "minimal brain dysfunction," three were: specific learning defects in the presence of normal intelligence, equivocal neurological signs, and coordination deficits. Despite the specification of characteristics, judgments regarding the presence or absence of these symptoms were difficult to make and diagnosis depended on the subjective predilections of the clinician rather than on uniform methods and standards for measurement. The demand for rigorous, neurological evidence of brain impairment grew. Wolff and Hurwitz (1973), for example, stated that the validity of the minimal brain damage syndrome (MBD) must be derived from the evaluation of the functional significance of neurological soft signs.

Studies directed at finding neurological evidence of brain damage, for confirmation of the diagnosis, prospered in the 1960s and 1970s, but no consistent finding ensued. Kalverboer (1975) criticized the MBD studies because of biased groups, dubious criteria for brain damage, lack of standardization for neurological assessment, built-in correlations among tests, and poorly defined soft signs. Eventual disenchantment with the medical diagnosis, in concert with the growing involvement on the part of parents and schools, led to a more practical, less subjective movement. Barton Schmitt (1975) reflected the widespread opinion that "MBD is an invalid wastebasket diagnosis ... It is time to discard this term."

The Shift from MBD to Learning Disability

In response to the disenchantment with the MBD label and with the subjective diagnostic procedures employed in the clinic, educators and parents increased their involvement in the identification process and in plans for intervention. Educators turned their attention to psychoeducational models (Myklebust, 1967) and to attempts to define learning disability in terms of ratios or quotients. Parents organized to focus attention on the problem and proposed the term learning disability in lieu of MBD. Meanwhile, the clinical psychologist attended to the clinical interpretation of test responses, studied test profiles for clues, and depended on symptomatology known to characterize adult organics, for diagnosis. As did the physician, the psychologist had a difficult time supporting the methods empirically. Interest in a neuropsychological approach (Reitan, 1967; 1968), one that had the potential for bridging the gap among medicine, psychology and education, emerged in the late 1960s. The neuropsychological model, largely influenced by the Russian psychologists, Luria and Vygotsky, and by Pribram in the United States, gained both impetus and prominence in the 1970s (Amante, 1976; Boll, 1977; Gaddes, 1968; Klonoff, 1971; Mattis, French, & Rapin, 1975; Myklebust, Bannochie, & Killen, 1971; Selz & Reitan, 1979). Though very much alive today as evidenced by the interest in and promotion of the Reitan and Luria neuropsychological batteries, the neuropsychological approach does not enjoy widespread use or appeal. Current federal and state mandates preclude the use of neuropsychological batteries. These batteries are cumbersome and costly procedures requiring special training, and that they correlate highly with IQ, because they are not truely diagnostic.

As the shift from a medical to an educational diagnosis took place in the 1960s, the term MBD was slowly but surely replaced by the more acceptable designation, learning disability. The new label, nonetheless, carried with it the implication of an underlying neurological impairment. Parents of disabled children organized and established *The Association for Children with Learning Disabilities* in 1962 and the label was firmly established when Kirk and Bateman (1963) adopted its use.

Definition by Law

The search for a systematic and operational method for the diagnosis of learning disabilities found its way from the physician's office to Congress.

In 1967, in an attempt to provide an all inclusive definition of learning disabilities, the National Advisory Committee on Handicapped Children defined the syndrome in the following manner:

> Children with Specific Learning Disabilities exhibit a disorder in one or more of the basic psychological processes involved in understanding or in using spoken or written language. These may be manifested in disorder of listening, thinking, talking, reading, writing, spelling or arithmetic. They include conditions which have been referred to as perceptual handicaps, brain injury, minimal brain dysfunction, dyslexia, developmental aphasia, etc. They do not include learning problems which are due primarily to visual, hearing, or motor handicaps, to mental retardation, emotional disturbance, or to environmental disadvantage.

In 1968, the Journal for Children with Learning Disabilities was published and in 1975 Public Law 94-142, legalizing the syndrome of LD and mandating service for disabled children, was signed. The definition proposed by the National Advisory Committee on Handicapped Children cited above was modified slightly but adopted when the federal guidelines for the evaluation of LD were published in 1977. A notable exclusion in this definition was any reference to neurological impairment. Because learning problems due to visual and hearing handicaps, emotional disturbance, or to environmental disadvantage were excluded, besides familial-genetic predispositions or simply normal individual variability, the only other etiology would seem to be that of a neurological impairment.

The "Specific" Learning Disability

It is not known to this author how the descriptive term *specific* became attached to learning disability. The federal and many state definitions include this appendage. It would appear that the addition of the term was designed to suggest that the child's learning problems were circumscribed, delimited, and possibly extrinsic to high level cognitive functioning. It was important to the parent to perceive the disability as a problem resolved by special teaching methods and not one pervasively and inherently symptomatic of some subnormal condition. The finding in early studies of LD children of average or better IQs stregthened the notion of "normalcy." The Association for Children with Learning Disabilities, for example, advertises to the public that great men like Einstein and Edison were learning disabled. The unchallenged argument that LD children had normal or higher general intelligence gave educators the theoretical basis for an educational diagnosis. By comparing IQ and achievement, a simple solution to a very complex problem was found. The feeling was, and still is, that the larger the difference between achievement and general intelligence the greater the disability. Because of this premise, the notion of diagnosis by discrepancy between achievement and IQ was formulated.

While socially acceptable, the assumption that general intelligence is unaffected by the neurological defect causing the learning problem defies not only logic but both theory and fact. Luria (1973), in concert with Ukhtomsky's concept of a "working constellation" conceived of the brain "as a complex functional system which includes joint work of different levels and areas, each of which plays its own role." He further stated that "the most complex forms of human actions require the participation of all brain systems...." Performance on tests of intelligence certainly require high level functioning and consequently would be vulnerable to the same conditions as those affecting learning.

If one were to suspect some global reduction in general intelligence as the result of impairment in the brain why is this reduction not reflected in research studies of LD children? First, samples of LD children were not from homogeneous populations. All too often children with behavioral and psychological problems or those with hyperactivity were identified as LD. This questionable practice had the effect of obscuring the findings on tests of intelligence inasmuch as there is reason to suspect that hyperactive children do not necessarily suffer from neurological deficits. Dalameter and Lahey (1983) in a study of the physiological correlates of conduct problems found that hyperactivity and conduct were "intertwined." The inclusion of neurologically normal children could have had the effect of inflating the mean IQs for the sample at large. Secondly, children in the lower IQ ranges, e.g., below 85, often were systematically excluded from samples of LD children, artificially forcing the mean score upwards. Another reason for the apparent contradiction between theory and finding is that the IQ may not be a sufficiently refined and subtle instrument to reflect differences. The achievement tests appear to be better able to detect the child's real level of performance. For example, children with congenital hydrocephalus who were managed successfully medically and who performed on an average level on tests of intelligence were found to show deficits in verbal reasoning, fine motor skills, memory, speed of information processing, and in visuospatial problem solving (Prigatano, Zeiner, Pollay, & Kaplan, 1983).

The intelligence test did not reflect these problems quantitatively, but qualitatively these children learn differently from their normal counterparts. The authors concluded that one must go beyond IQ to understand the cognitive deficits of these children. A similar argument could be made for LD children.

Quite apart from logical and theoretical arguments regarding the intellectual status of LD children reports of mean IQ reveal a startling pattern. By the 1970s, when selection procedures were more carefully conceived, even with the exclusion of children with IQs below 85, the majority of researchers reported mean IQs of LD samples in the low 90s (Rie, 1980). Mean scores in the low 90s may indeed reflect a global effect on intelligence of the primary disability. Should this prove to be the case, the current basis for identification of LD children, the discrepancy between IQ and achievement, would certainly be invalid.

Diagnosis by Law

While the federal regulation defines LD, it does not address itself to the issue of the method of differential diagnosis except to state generally that a severe discrepancy between achievement and intellectual ability must be demonstrated (Procedures for Evaluating Specific Learning Disabilities, Federal Register, 1977, p. 65083). Criteria for degree and determination of discrepancy were not provided by this publication. As a consequence, individual states undertook to delineate standards and guidelines for diagnosis for themselves. In Ohio, for example, the Guidelines for the Identification of Children with Specific Learning Disabilities (1983) states that the child should have "a severe discrepancy between achievement and ability which adversely affects his or her educational performance to such a degree that special educational and related services are required." The guideline further states that a discrepancy score of two or greater than two between intellectual ability and achievement in one or more of the skill areas is required for identification. The discrepancy score is calculated in the following manner: From the score obtained from the measure of intelligence minus the mean of the test and divided by the standard deviation of the test, the score obtained by following the same procedure for the test of achievement, is subtracted. If a child's IQ were 110 (110 minus 100 divided by 15), and his achievement in reading were, in terms of standard scores, 80 (80 minus 100 divided by 15) his discrepancy score would be two and he would qualify for special schooling as a LD student. It is important to recognize that the discrepancy score of two is not a magic number; it is an arbitrary one that reflects the extent to which individual states are willing to support disabled children. That this procedure or ones similar to it are technically flawed is well documented (Telzrow, 1984). Not only are test scores themselves somewhat unreliable, the statistical maneuvers render them even more so. One unfortunate outcome is the overidentification of high IQ and the underidentification of low IQ children (Telzrow, 1984).

THOUGHTS ON THE CURRENT SITUATION

One of the unfortunate outcomes of the change from a purely medical diagnosis of MBD to the statistical, educational diagnostic scheme is that the expertise of both physician and clinical psychologist is largely ignored. These professionals play an alarmingly minor role in the diagnosis and treatment of learning disabilities at the present time. To reduce the LD entity to difference scores is a reductio ad absurdum and the dynamic investigation of a complex anomaly has been legalistically stifled.

The treatment of learning disabled children as a homogeneous group, whose IQ is higher than its achievement, does disservice to the child especially in regard to treatment. For example, a 9-year-old child, brought to the author's attention recently was found to have mastered the basic skills at grade level. His teacher, however, complained that this young man had a miserable time with the application of his learning to problem solving. A comprehensive examination revealed a substantive impairment in concept formation, in verbal mediational skills, and in motor coordination. By most means of evaluation this child was learning disabled. But, because the discrepancy formula did not take into account his pattern of disability, this very high risk child was not eligible for tutorial help. His achievement was too high for his average IQ. The teacher wisely retained him in the hope of giving him more time to mature. Learning disabled children constitute a heterogeneous group and efforts at subcategorization are essential if we are to develop intervention techniques helpful to them.

Cruickshank (1983) applauds some recent developments in the field of learning disabilities. He cited the careful and well thought out approach to research by the International Academy for Research in Learning Disability and the Scientific Studies Committee of the Association for Children with Learning Disabilities. Despite these positive directions, Cruickshank (1983) wrote that "the field of learning disabilities in the United States is in a mess."

HISTORY OF SOFT SIGNS

Introduction

The scientific investigation of neurological soft signs (NSS) in learning disabled children started about 20 years ago. It was initiated in response to the criticism that MBD children should not be labeled as such in the absence of demonstrable brain damage and in an effort to obtain independent, measurable, objective, and standardized signs pathognomonic of the disorder. It was felt that the isolation of predictive soft signs would confirm brain damage in much the same way as hard signs did.

Research, however, was hampered by two major obstacles. First, no acceptable norms for soft signs existed. Attempts at standardization often failed because the plasticity of the growing child did not lend itself to reliable and valid measurements. The performance of children on these tasks was too variable for any degree of confidence. Moreover, the assessment of the presence or absence of these signs proved to be difficult; interexaminer reliability tended to be below acceptable levels. More importantly, the decision as to what constituted a soft sign varied from study to study, often idiosyncratic to the author. Even when soft signs could be measured relatively reliably, one was at a loss about how to interpret the results.

In addition to the problem of what to test, how to measure it reliably, and how to interpret the performance, the characteristics of LD samples in terms of age, sex, selection criteria, and degree and type of deficit made comparisons and replication almost impossible (Erickson, 1977). Difficulties in selecting homogeneous samples because of mixed populations resulted in findings that were inconsistent.

Defining Soft Signs

At the turn of the century neurologists applied the expression "eqiuvocal" to describe neurological signs suggestive only of neuropathology. They observed that these equivocal signs had a transient quality but persisted over the years (Kennard, 1960). The term equivocal came to be used to describe LD children. Other terms such as nonoptimal (Touwen & Prechtl, 1970) and paraclassical (Satz & Fletcher, 1980) refer to similar phenomena. Kennard (1960) and Bender (1956) both felt that soft signs were associated with complex rather than simple motor responses and can be characterized as nonfocal as opposed to focal, as they have little localizing value (Golden, 1982).

The NSS generally considered in studies of LD children are those involving fine or gross motor movements, asymmetries, dyskinesia, visual-motor coordination, sensory integration, laterality, right-left discrimination, and general clumsiness. On occasion, speed of performance, articulation, and ocular movements are included. Motor items often tested are diadochokinesia, hand-finger immobility, and balance. Sensory items regularly checked are graphesthesia, astereognosis, and finger localization. Less frequently, visual or hearing impairments, strabismus, and nystagmus are listed as neurological indicators of learning disabilities.

Touwen and Prechtl (1970) regarded clusters of signs rather than single signs as more valuable for clinical interpretation. They suggested that signs associated with neurological entities should be treated as a cluster. The entities they thought important in the neurological evaluation of children were hemisyndrome, dyskinesia, associated movements, difficulties in coordination, sensory disturbances, and clumsiness.

Twitchell, Lecours, Rudel, and Teuber (1966) concluded that motor defects were common in children with minimal brain damage. They attributed the significance of these signs to their persistence into ages when they usually disappear in normal children. More recently, Lucas (1980), in reference to motor development, cautioned that there is much variability among individual children in patterns of neurological integration and skillfulness and that differences in muscular control and coordination can be due to a variety of mechanisms. Yet, he acknowledges that damage to the central nervous system can affect motor functioning. He cautioned that individual variability "should not be overidentified as pathologic."

Review of Past Research

One of the first major studies of the relationship between neurological soft signs and learning and behavior disorders was conducted by Kennard in 1960. She concluded that equivocal signs of central nervous system dysfunctions must be true signs of organic disease because they appear consistently in a given individual and are of a similar pattern among groups of patients. Finding that equivocal signs correlated positively with the clinical diagnosis of pathology, she stressed their importance in diagnosis.

A lengthy assessment of soft neurological signs appeared in Clements and Peters' (1963) study of minimal brain dysfunction. They suggested that the total number of soft signs is more predictive of MBD than are individual signs. Boshes and Myklebust (1964) studied children with reading problems and found no relationship between NSS and reading. However, they concluded that the differences between the experimental and control groups were qualitative not quantitative and that the signs have value in the detection of qualitative differences. Boshes and Myklebust (1964) contended that the child with minimal neurological problems is different in psychological organization from the normal population.

While Lucas, Rodin, and Simson (1965) did not find a relationship between abnormalities on the neurological exam and disturbed behavior, they felt that a neurological dysfunction might underlie the hyperactive syndrome. Hertzig, Bortner, and Birch (1969) took a stronger position after studying children educationally designated as brain damaged. They found that these children "do in fact have clear evidence of central nervous system abnormality, though of great neurological heterogeneity." Soft signs involving disturbance of balance, coordination, and speech were more frequently occurring while those least frequently occurring were abnormalities of position sense.

In a comprehensive study, Rutter, Graham, and Yule (1970) found higher frequencies of left handedness, developmental abnormalities, cranial signs, abnormal coordination, power, tone, and reflexes, and marked neurological abnormalities in children independently diagnosed as neurologically impaired than in controls. Soft signs were grouped into three categories: (1) signs of developmental delay; (2) signs due to neurological and nonneurological factors; and (3) slight abnormalities. The authors cautioned that the value of the signs depends to a great extent on the judgments of the examiners, and that the total composite neurological score is not a useful screening instrument.

Werry, Minde, Guzman, Weiss, Dogan, and Hoy (1970) compared 20 hyperactive, disturbed children with nonhyperactive neurotics and controls. Finding that hyperactive children had significantly more neurological abnormalities than the other two groups, they speculated that hyperactivity is likely to be an organic syndrome, most likely a biologic variant. The principal differences found were in signs reflecting sensori-motor incoordination. Wolff and Hurwitz (1973) studied choreiform movements in normal children. Although they spoke of the predictive value of this sign they were careful to convey the dangers of using soft signs for the diagnosis of MBD.

One of the few studies to use learning disabled children specifically compared two groups of boys, disabled and normal controls. Using a point scale to indicate degree of presence or absence of 80 signs, Peters, Romine, and Dykman (1975) reported that 44 signs significantly discriminated between the groups. The authors argued for validity of the neurological examination in the selection of learning disabled children.

Rie, Rie, Stewart, and Rettemnier (1978) examined 80 LD children for soft signs, general intelligence, age, and sex. The data were subjected to a factor analysis and the following conclusions were drawn. Total number of soft signs was not predictive of learning disability; hyperactivity and LD were not related; the signs tended to be age related; and neurological signs requiring complex responses were the most predictive of learning disability. While motor coordination that involved reflexive action was not associated with organicity, motor coordination involving ccomplex, integrative actions were. A general ability factor was associated with the absence of signs while a verbal-motor and a visual-motor factor contained very different patterns of signs. Of note was the finding that LD children with language impairment (low verbal scores) had most difficulty with signs involving verbal directions, while the converse was true of the organics whose deficit was in the visual-perceptual realm. Rie et al emphasized the importance of the age factor.

One of the latest studies of neurological status in learning disabled children (Johnston, Starke, Mellits, & Tallal, 1981) compared language impaired and normal children. It was found that the impaired group was less efficient in tasks involving rate of movement, perception of dichaptic stimuli, and left-right discrimination. A discriminant analysis classified correctly 87 percent of the population into their respective groups. These data are comparable to those of Rie et al, who also found that right-left discrimination was a problem for language impaired subjects.

For as many investigators as there were who found some association between soft signs and learning disability there were an equal number contesting the finding. Kenny and Clemmens (1971) evaluated 100 children with learning and/or behavioral problems. No significant relationship between the neurological examination and the disability was found. They concluded that neurological evaluations were unproductive. Kinsbourne (1973) was among the first to argue publicly against correlational findings and suggested that the neurological examination is not relevant to the association area of the cortex where reading takes place. In a similar vein, Barlow (1974) questioned the extension of a statistical relationship to the prediction of individual performance.

Adams, Kocsis, and Estes (1974) tested children with learning disabilities and found that they could not be reliably distinguished from normal controls despite having found that graphesthesia and diadochokinesia were more prevalent in the disabled group. After an exhaustive study of 575 children, Stine, Saratsiostis, and Mosser (1975) concluded that neurological signs are not predictive of a particular form of behavior. Neurological signs were found in both normal and disabled children.

Erickson (1977) examined 155 second grade children and found that reading-disabled groups and control groups, matched for sex and IQ, did not differ on neurological test items. She reported correlations between neurological items and mental age and IQ, however.

Significance of Research

It is difficult to abstract salient points from these studies. Criteria defining experimental and control groups differed from study to study and soft signs utilized not only differed in type and in method of measurement but also in number. A few investigators focused solely on choreiform movements (Wolff et al, 1973) while others tested a wide range of motor-sensory items (Johnston et al, 1981; Rie et al, 1978). A few recurring themes, however obscure, merit mentioning.

No particular sign or group of signs shows a consistent relationship with learning disabilities. Differences in sample characteristics and/or in heterogeneity within a sample are partly responsible for the inconsistent findings from study to study. Another major obstacle in interpreting these data involves the signs themselves. Walking a straight line is a very different skill from skipping, in degree of complexity. Sensory functions differ from motor functions; some neurological items require both visual and auditory skills for solution while other items involve one skill more than the other. Some require complex and integrated neural actions while others are more reflexive in type. A better sorting of neurological items into discrete categories and organization according to level of difficulty and standardization for age is required for further research.

The careful selection of discrete and homogeneous samples, in combination with standardized and classified soft signs, is a prerequisite for reliable and valid measurements. It is when these procedures are pursued diligently that robust relationships can be expected. The phenomenon every clinician has observed for many years, that children who have grave difficulty learning a variety of cognitive tasks, who otherwise appear healthy, are much more likely to show minor motor-sensory dysfunctions than normal ones, should be measurable. When the learning problem is specified and when the motor-sensory tasks are delineated according to level of difficulty, to age appropriateness, and to type and category, research findings will become more meaningful.

Some Tentative Generalities

A few recurring themes, however tentative and obscure, merit mentioning. One is the way in which soft signs are related to age. In both the disabled and in the general population they tend to disappear with increasing age (Dykman et al, 1971; Peters et al, 1975; Rie et al, 1978). In the disabled group, however, there is some evidence to suggest a delay in their time of disappearance (Dykman et al, 1971; Peters et al, 1975). There is, however, so much individual variability among children at any given age that it is difficult to assess whether the deviancy is normal for that child or whether it represents some tacit abnormality (Lucas, 1980). Differences between LD and normal controls are more likely to occur at the younger ages than at the older ages (Peters et al, 1975), suggesting that the signs are more discriminating during the latency period than later. Should soft signs persist well beyond the age when they normally disappear, they might be suggestive of a neurological impairment, according to some investigators (Twitchell et al, 1966).

At this time there is insufficient evidence to conclude that total number of signs is predictive of a learning disability. Brain damaged retarded children are known to have a greater number of signs than normal but the findings in the LD studies are conflicting. Sample heterogeneity, variability of the individual child, spurious measurement, and the use of nonmeaningful reflexive signs probably confounded these investigations. As with the limitations of a single sign, such as choreiform movements, which has been studied extensively but to no definite conclusion, total number, however appealing, simply does not distinguish reliably between pathologic and normal groups. When samples are both more homogeneous and select, total number may eventually prove be indicative of neurological impairment. In the clinical setting, many but not all learning disabled children look more clumsy, have more problems with right-left discrimination, skipping, etc. than expected. A recent evaluation of a very disabled 16-year-old LD boy seen in this author's clinic showed very few of the classic signs of MBD on either neuropsychological or cognitive tests. The only indications of central nervous system dysfunction were his inability to skip, mixed dominance, and right-left disorientation. Whereas few or no signs does not negate a learning disability, it is possible that many signs can be very suggestive of one.

As Bender (1956), Kennard (1960), and Clements (1966) noted many years ago and as Rie et al (1978) demonstrated more recently, the most revealing signs are those requiring integrated motor acts. Kennard (1960) recognized that equivocal signs represented complex responses, and suggested that unlike the "voluntary activity" associated with the sensorimotor cortex, they represent patterns of learned responses. She stated that "finger tapping, hopping, graphesthesia and left-right discrimination all require complex and coordinate adjustments...."

Another generalization from the research findings is that soft signs appear to be positively related to general intelligence (Kennard, 1960; Erickson, 1977; Rie et al, 1978). Even after children with IQs below 90 were excluded from the study, Erickson (1977) found a positive correlation between total neurological score and IQ in second grade children. Peters et al (1975) detected that number of signs and IQ were related even in children with IQs between 75 and 90. A significant correlation between IQ and performance on the Physical and Neurological Examination for Soft Signs, an official battery of the National Institute of Mental Health, was found by Holden, Tarnowksi, and Prinz (1983).

The growing awareness of the heterogeneity of LD children in recent years has led to the recognition of the importance of subtyping. Children with language deficits, thought to be at greater risk for underachievement than those with visuoperceptual deficits (Rie and Rie, 1979), have been found to have difficulties with right-left discrimination (Rie et al, 1978; Sutherland, Kolb, Schoel, Whishaw, & Davies, 1982). Interestingly, Stine, Saratsiotis, and Mosser (1975) found that the most common neurological finding in LD children was error of body movement following a verbal command. These errors were also associated with underachievement. Findings on laterality, however, tend to be much more ambiguous. Several studies pointed to a higher incidence of problems of lateral dominance in LD than in normal controls (Benton, 1959; Harris, 1957) while others found no such relationship (Belmont & Birch, 1965; Bettman, 1967; Connolly, 1983). Connolly (1983) stressed that LD children did not have problems with mixed or lateral dominance any more than generally found. She did find, however, a greater incidence of left eye dominance in the LD group.

If one were to ask if motor clumsiness is indicative of LD the response would be no. There is too much individual variability among children and the assessment of clumsiness is too subjective a judgment for clinical usefulness. Although sometimes seen in LD children, as Illingworth (1968; 1980) stated on several occasions, clumsiness may be due to a variety of factors, especially normal variation or family feature.

Interestingly 2 or more nonfocal signs were found in less than 5 percent of children between the ages of 8 and 12 (Birch, Richardson, Horobin, et al, 1970) Yet, Hertzig (1982) found that the number of children exhibiting 2 or more signs did not differ in a 4 year pre-post testing. She discussed the stability of signs over a 4-year period and found that patterns of consistency and inconsistency varied from sign to sign and that children in the lower IQ groups showed more inconsistency over time than did brighter children. Both positive and negative findings of astereognosis and double simultaneous stimulation were found to be highly stable. Hertzig argued that these patterns illustrated disorganization in the central nervous system and were not merely a function of developmental lags.

THE STANDARDIZATION OF NEUROLOGICAL SOFT SIGNS

Much of the criticism of studies of soft signs in LD children centers around the lack of standardization and the absence of normative data on the signs themselves. One of the first batteries was published in 1962 when Clements and Peters listed 80 signs ranging from simple reflexive acts such as pupillary reaction to light to integrated motor acts such as skipping. In 1975, Peters et al (1975) described more completely each item in this battery and offered a standard format for administration. This was one of the first attempts at standardizing a very large battery of soft signs.

In 1973 Close organized a neurological battery for use in drug research. That battery was published by the Early Clinic Drug Evaluation Unit of the National Institute of Mental Health in 1976 as the Physical and Neurological Examination for Soft Signs (PANESS). In 1983, Levine, Meltzer, Busch, Palfrey, and Sullivan published The Pediatric Early Elementary Examination (PEEX).

In the Peters et al study, 44 of the 80 items discriminated between LD and normal control 9-year-old boys. At older ages (10 or more) only 11 items significantly discriminated between the 2 groups. Items of fine motor coordination, symmetrical associated movement, dysgraphia, and inability to converge the eyes were the discriminating items with the older boys.

Items discriminating at the .01 level of significance in the younger group were: head rotation, copy finger movements, hop on one foot, skip, foot tapping, associated movements, finger-nose test, finger pursuit, diadochokinesia, clipping paper together, plantar sensitivity, right-left confusion, inability to wink, frown, and tongue strength and waggle. Interexaminer reliability was 84 percent. It is to be noted that these data are based on the performance of boys, and their clinical usefulness is limited to that sex.

The PANESS contains 43 items divided according to type. The first 8 concern integrated motor acts such as touch finger to nose. Items 9 through 16 test graphesthesia (palm tracing) while items 17 to 20 measure stereognosis (object recognition). Balance, cortical sensibility (e.g., face or hand brushed with cotton, eyes closed), persistence measurements (stick out tongue, etc.), and repetitive movements (e.g., tapping), constitute the remainder of the test. As did Peters et al (1975), Werry and Aman (1976) report high reliability of the items. However, they cautioned that the high reliability was due in part to the large number of absent signs. No differences were noted among normal, hyperactive, and neurologically impaired children. The authors warned that despite its official status the PANESS should be regarded as an experimental instrument with unproven value as a diagnostic or predictive instrument. The conclusion reached was that there were too many noncontributory items in this battery. However, the number of children tested was very small.

In an even stronger statement, Camp, Bailer, Press, and Winsberg (1977) found a developmental trend after examining 111 normal and 32 behaviorally deviant boys. These researchers found a striking pattern in the 9-year-olds. The normal 9-year-old boys had significantly more soft signs than did the hyperactive ones. Unlike the previous researchers, Camp et al (1977) questioned the reliability of measurement of the items and criticized the directions for administration. They discouraged the clinical use of this instrument.

Holden et al (1983) had kinder words for the PANESS. Although they found variability across conditions, they felt that total score was a relatively stable indicator of overall performance. Test-retest reliability results were a bit ambiguous and the authors reported fewer reliable results when different examiners were used than when the same examiner was used. They also reported that there might be some practice effect. These authors argue for further investigations of the battery and suggest, rightly so, that brain damaged rather than hyperactive children should be used as the criterion group because the case for homogeneity of hyperactive children "has not been supported."

To meet the need for reliable and valid procedures to evaluate children between the ages of 7 and 9, The Pediatric Early Elementary Examination: Studies of a Neurodevelopmental Examination for 7 to 9 Year-Old Children, was developed by a team at The Children's Hospital in Boston (Levine et al, 1982). The major purpose of this examination was to provide the pediatrician with a systematic approach to the evaluation of learning disabilities. The authors note that the primary care pediatrician relies on subjective impressions or on fragmented assessment procedures. The objectives of the PEEX were to establish norms for 7- to 9-year-old children, to encourage health care providers to take a role in the diagnosis of "low serverity disabilities," to uncover areas of concern in a child's development, and to increase the role of the pediatrician in the diagnosis of LD in children. Seven neurodevelopmental areas were surveyed: minor neurological indicators (associated movements, extinction of simultaneous stimuli, finger agnosia, left-right discrimination, visual tracking, and dysdiadochokinesis), temporal-sequential and visual-spatial orientation, auditory-language function, fine and gross motor function, memory, and other functions. The least reliable area was that of minor neurological indicators but agreement of rating was reported to be 87 percent. One hundred eighty seven normal children and 59 LD children were evaluated. The researchers found as did others that natural variation in the distribution of weaknesses was evident on this battery. Another finding, consistent across batteries, was the high correlation among "areas of concern" and IQ and achievement. Not suprisingly, together with the auditory-language area, minor neurological indicators appeared to exert the greatest influencing on IQ. Since the learning disabled group exhibited a greater number of "areas of concern" than did the normals, the writers speculated that isolated areas of developmental dysfunction are not particularly debilitating but the multiple areas of dysfunction are associated with learning problems. Although the PEEX measures broader functions than most soft sign batteries, many of the tasks in areas other than "minor neurologic indicators" overlap with and are perceived by others as soft signs.

On the PEEX all of the minor neurological indicators except stimulus extinction were significantly higher in the LD than in the normal groups. Although the authors found this comprehensive battery a useful beginning in the assessment of children for developmental and learning problems, they caution that a potential disadvantage lies in misinterpretation of data and they express concern over the amount of time necessary for administration.

CONCLUSIONS

The great number of children found in regular classes in the United States who fail to learn within expected time intervals is testament to the need for the continued refinement of categories of disability. That they fail for many reasons, environmental, genetic, physiologic, traumatic and combinations thereof, is well known. The emergence of the LD syndrome in the middle of this century inspired professional as well as political actions. These actions resulted in the educational identification and treatment of the disorder. Programs for LD children exist in virtually every public school in the country today. Yet, in the absence of systematic program evaluation, it is difficult to assess the efficacy of special classes or individual tutoring for LD children and to determine the degree to which they may or may not be beneficial. Individual educational planning, designed especially for the LD child, is a noteworthy endeavor, but as Cruickshank (1983) warned, decisions about children can be arbitrary and dogmatic even in the face of legal restraints.

Unfortunately, Public Law 94-142 has put the public schools in a precarious position. Should the classroom teacher wish to refer a child with behavioral or learning problems for a more comprehensive evaluation than can be performed in the schools, at least in Ohio, the school would be obligated according to this law to pay for the outside services. As a consequence, schools are reluctant to go beyond the services available to them within the school system.

In some ways, medicine and clinical psychology have shirked their responsibility to the LD child. With the exception of the neuropsychological movement, the contributions of medicine and clinical psychology have been at an impasse in recent years. What is urgently needed is research on both the subdivision of the broad category of learning disabilities into discrete types and developmental norms for motor-sensory skills in children. After these two procedures are completed, it will be possible to determine the motor-sensory correlates of learning disabilities. These two tasks are especially suited to medicine and psychology but they can also be approached through a multidisciplinary effort.

Knowledge of soft signs and their relationships to learning in childhood has the potential for reducing diagnostic error. The child who fails in school, who is otherwise psychologically healthy, and who manifests one or more of the more complex soft signs is highly likely to suffer from a learning disability. Understanding the signs could be a helpful source of information, combined with educational and neuropsychological data for the determination of the "type" of disability. With this knowledge, programs truly facilitative can be established for each child.

REFERENCES

Adams RM, Kocsis RE, & Estes RE. Soft neurological signs in learning disabled children and controls. American Journal of Diseases in Children, 1974, 128, 614-618

Amante D. A neuropsychodiagnostic model. International Journal of Neuroscience, 1976, 6, 189-195

Barlow CF. Soft signs in children with learning disorders. American Journal of Diseases in Children, 1974, 128, 605-606

Belmont L, & Birch HG. Lateral dominance, lateral awareness, and reading disability. Child Development, 1965, 36, 57-71

Bender L. Psychopathology of Children with Organic Brain Disorders. Springfield, IL: Charles C. Thomas, 1956

Benton AL. Right-left Discrimination and Finger Localization. New York: Paul B. Hoeber, 1959

Bettman JW, Stern EL, Whitsel LS, & Gofman HF. Cerebral dominance in developmental dyslexia. Archives of Ophthalmology, 1967, 76, 722-729

Birch HG. The problem of "brain damage" in chidren. In Birch HG (Ed.). Brain Damage in Children: The Biological and Social Aspects. Baltimore:Williams and Wilkins, 1964

Birch HG, Richardson SA, Horobin G, et al. Mental Subnormality in the Community: A Clinical and Epidemiologic Study. Baltimore: Williams and Wilkins, 1970

Boll TJ. A rationale for neuropsychological evaluation. Professional Psychology, 1977, February, 64-71

Bond E. Postencephalitic, ordinary and extraordinary children. Journal of Pediatrics, 1932, 1, 311-314

Boshes B, & Myklebust HR. A neruological and behavioral study of children with learning disabilities. Neurology, 1964, 14, 7-12

Camp JA, Bialer I, Press M, & Winsberg BG. The physical and neurological examination for soft signs (PANESS): Pediatric norms and comparisons between normal and deviant boys. Psychopharmacology Bulletin, 1977, 13, 39-41

Clements SD, & Peters JE. Minimal brain dysfunction in the school-age child. Archives of General Psychiatry, 1962, 6, 185-197

Clements SD. Minimal brain dysfunction in children. NINDB Monograph No. 3, Department of Health, Education, and Welfare, Washington, DC, 1966

Close J. Scored neurological examination. Psychopharmacology Bulletin, Special Issue, Pharmacotherapy of Children, 1973, 142-148

Connolly B. Lateral dominance in children with learning disabilities. Physical Therapy, 1983, 63(2), 183-187

Cruickshank WM. Straight is the bamboo tree. Journal of Learning Disabilities, 1983, 16(4), 191-196

Delameter AM, & Lahey BB. Physiological correlates of conduct problems and anxiety in hyperactive and learning-disabled children. The Journal of Abnormal Child Psychology, 1983, 11(1), 85-100

Dykmen RA, Ackerman PT, Clements SD, & Peters JE. Specific learning disabilities: An attentional deficit syndrome. In Myklebust HR (Ed.). Progress in Learning Disabilities, Vol. II. New York: Grune & Stratton, 1978, pp. 56-93

Erickson M. Reading disability in relation to performance on neurological tests for minimal brain dysfunction. Developmental Medicine and Child Neurology, 1977, 19, 768-775

Gaddes WH: A neuropsychological approach to learning disorders. Journal of Learning Disabilities, 1968, 1(9), 46-57

Golden G. Neurological correlates of learning disabilities. Annals of Neurology, 1982, 12(5), 409-481

Harris AJ. Lateral dominance, directional confusion and reading disability. Journal of Psychology, 1957, 44, 283-294

Hertzig M. Stability and change in nonfocal neurologic signs. Journal of the American Academy of Child Psychiatry, 1982, 21(3), 231-236

Hertzig M, Bortner M, & Birch H. Neurologic findings in children educationally designated as "brain-damaged." American Journal of Orthopsychiatry, 1969, 39(3), 437-466

Hohman LB. Postencephalitic behavior disorders in children. Johns Hopkins Hospital Bulletin, 1922, 33, 372-375

Holden EW, Tarnowski KJ, & Prinz RJ. Reliability of neurological soft signs in children: Reevaluation of the PANESS. Journal of Abnormal Child Psychology, 1982, 10(2), 163-172

Illingworth RS. Delayed motor development. Pediatric Clinics of North America, 1968, 15(3), 569-580

Illingworth RS. Developmental variations in relation to MBD. In Rie HE, & Rie ED (Eds.). Handbook of Minimal Brain Dysfunctions. New

York: John Wiley and Sons, 1980, pp. 522-567

Ingram TT. Soft signs. Developmental Medicine and Child Neurology, 1973, 15, 527-530

Johnston RB, Stark RE, Mellits ED, & Tallal P. Neurological status of language-impaired and normal children. Annals of Neurology, 1981, 10(2), 159-163

Kahn E, & Cohen LM. Organic driveness: A brain stem syndrome and an experience. The New England Journal of Medicine, 1934, 210, 748-756

Kalverboer AF. A Neurobehavioral Study in Pre-school Children. Clinics in Developmental Medicine No. 54. London: Spastics International Medical Publications, 1975, pp. 85-99

Kennard M. Value of equivocal signs in neurologic diagnosis. Neurology, 1960, 10, 753-764

Kenny TJ, & Clemmens RL. Medical and psychological correlates in children with learning disabilities. The Journal of Pediatrics, 1971, 78, 273-277

Kinsbourne M. School problems. Pediatrics, 1973, 52, 697-710

Kirk SA, & Bateman B. Diagnosis and remediation of learning disabilities. Exceptional Child, 1962, 29, 73-78

Klonoff H. Factor analysis of a neuropsychological battery for children aged 9 to 15. Perceptual and Motor Skills, 1971, 32, 603-616

Knights RM, & Tymchuk AJ. An evaluation of the Halstead-Reitan Category Test for Children. Cortex, 1968, 4, 403-414

Knobloch H, & Pasamanick B. Syndrome of minimal cerebral damage in infancy. Journal of the American Medical Association, 1959, 170, 184-1387

Levin MD, Meltzer LT, Busch B, et al. The pediatric early elementary examination: Studies of neurodevelopmental examination for 7 to 9 year old children. Pediatrics, 1983, 71(6), 894-903

Lucas A, Rodine E, & Simson C. Neurological assessment of children with early school problems. Developmental Medicine and Child Neurology, 1965, 7, 145-156

Lucas A. Muscular control and coordination. In Rie HE, & Rie ED (Eds.). Handbook of Minimal Brain Dysfunctions. New York: John Wiley and Sons, 1980, pp. 233-253

Luria AR. The Working Brain: An Introduction to Neuropsychology. Harmondsworth, Middlesex: Penguin, 1973

Mattis S, French JH, & Rapin I. Dyslexia in children and young adults: Three independent neuropsychological syndromes. Developmental

Medicine and Child Neurology, 1975, 17, 150-163

Myklebust H. Learning disabilities in psychoneurologically disturbed children: Behavioral correlates of brain dysfunctions. In Hoch P, & Zubin J (Eds.). Psychopathology of Mental Development. New York: Grune & Stratton, 1967

Myklebust H, Bannochie M, & Killen J. Learning disabilities and cognitive processes. Progress in Learning Disabilities, Vol. 11. New York: Grune & Stratton, 1971, pp. 213-251

Ohio Guidelines for the Identification of Children with Specific Learning Disabilities, Columbus, Ohio, 1983

Peters JE, Romine RA, & Dykman RA. A special neurological examination of children with learning disabilities. Developmental Medicine and Child Neurology, 1975, 17, 63-78

Prigatano GP, Zeiner HZ, Pollay M, & Kaplan RJ. Neuropsychological functioning in children with shunted uncomplicated hydrocephalus. Child's Brain, 1983, 10,112-120

Procedures for Evaluating Specific Learning Disabilities, Federal Register, 1977, p. 65083

Reitan RM. Psychological assessment of deficits asssociated with brain lesions in subjects with normal and subnormal intelligence. In Khanna JL (Ed.). Brain Damage and Mental Retardation: A Psychological Evaluation. Springfield, IL: Charles C. Thomas, 1967, pp. 47-87

Reitan RM. Manual for administration of neuropsychological test batteries for adults and children. Published by author, Indianapolis, 1969

Rie ED. Effects of MBD on learning, intellective functions, and achievement. In Rie HE, & Rie ED (Eds.). Handbook of Minimal Brain Dysfunctions. New York: John Wiley and Sons, 1980, pp. 272-298

Rie ED, & Rie HE. Reading deficits and intellectual patterns among children with neurocognitive dysfunctions. Intelligence, 1979, 3, 383-389

Rie ED, Rie HE, Stewart S, & Rettemnier S. An analysis of neurological soft signs in children with learning problems. Brain and Language, 1978, 6, 32-46

Rutter M, Graham P, & Yule W. A Neuropsychiatric Study in Childhood. Clinics in Developmental Medicine Nos. 35/36. London: Heinemann Medical Books, 1970

Satz P, & Fletcher JM. Minimal brain dysfunction: An appraisal of research concepts and methods. In Rie HD, & Rie ED (Eds.). Handbook of Minimal Brain Dysfunctions. New York: John Wiley and Sons, 1980, pp. 667-715

Schmitt BD. The minimal brain dysfunction myth. American Journal of Diseases in Children, 1975, 129, 1313-1318

Selz M, & Retan R. Rules for neuropsychological diagnosis: Classification of brain function in older children. Journal of Consulting and Clinical Psychology, 1979, 47(2), 258-264

Stine O, Saratsiotis J, & Mosser R. Relationships between neurological findings and classroom behavior. American Journal of Diseases in Children, 1975, 129, 1036-1040

Strauss AA, & Werner H: Disorders of conceptual thinking in the brain-injured child. Journal of Nervous and Mental Disease, 1942, 96, 153-172

Strauss AA, & Werner H. Comparative psychopathology of the brain-injured child and the traumatic brain injured adult. American Journal of Psychiatry, 1943, 99, 835-838

Sutherland R, Kolb B, Schoel W, et al. Neuropsychological assessment of children and adults with Tourette syndrome: A comparison with learning disabilities and schizophrenia. In Friedhoff A, & Chase TN (Eds.). Gilles de la Tourette Syndrome. New York: Raven Press, 1983 pp. 311-322

Telzrow CF. Best practices in reducing error in learning disability qualification. Best Practices Manual of the National Association of School Psychologists, 1984

Touwen B, & Prechtl H. The Neurological Examination of the Child with Minor Nervous Dysfunction. Clinics in Developmental Medicine No. 38. London: Spastics International Medical Publications, 1970, pp. 83-91

Twitchell T, LeCours A, Rudel R, & Teuber H. Minimal cerebral dysfunction in children: Motor deficits. Transactions of the American Neurological Association, 1966, 91, 353-355

Werry JS, Minde K, Guzman A, et al. Studies on the hyperactive child VII: Neurological status compared with neurotic and normal children. American Journal of Orthopsychiatry, 1970, 42, 441-451

Werry JS, & Aman MA. The reliability and diagnostic validity of the physical and neurological examination for soft signs (PANESS). Journal of Autism and Childhood Schizophrenia, 1976, 6(3), 252-262

Wolff P, Hurwitz I. Functional implications of the minimal brain damage syndrome. Seminars in Psychiatry, 1973, 5(1), 105-115

Jan Catherine Reeves
John Scott Werry

10

Soft Signs in Hyperactivity

The history of hyperactivity has been reviewed by Ross and Ross (1982) and Werry and Campbell (1986) among others. Any review of soft neurological signs in hyperactivity is fraught with historical difficulties in the evolution of thinking about this disorder, moving from "organic driveness," through minimal brain damage, the hyperkinetic syndrome, and Attention Deficit Disorder. These evolving, and often interchangeably used, labels, are often further confused by terms such as learning disabilities and psychiatric disabilities in general.

Though never exactly precisely defined, any hope of specificity was laid to rest by the introduction of the concept of minimal brain dysfunction (MBD) introduced by Clements and Peters (1962). This embraced an organic and syndromal view of hyperactivity, with heavy emphasis being placed on associated neuropsychological and cognitive symptomatology. However, the description of symptomatology was vague and all encompassing. The NIH commissioned monograph by Clements (1966), by nominating hyperactivity as the core symptom of MBD, opened a Pandora's box and, as a result, much of the clinical literature on hyperactivity since that time has been based on vague, poorly defined notions, with hyperactivity being variously called a syndrome, a symptom, and even a non-entity or social plot (see Werry & Campbell, 1986).

Much of the early research on hyperactivity was based on the idea that etiology was somehow attributable to brain damage, and the presence of EEG abnormalities in some hyperkinetic children and an observed increase in the frequency of neurological soft signs added fuel to this fire. Despite this, any association between brain damage and hyperactivity is, at best, infrequent and elusive (Rutter, 1982; Werry, 1979). More recently, under the

SOFT NEUROLOGICAL SIGNS
ISBN 0-8089-1841-9

influence of Virginia Douglas (Douglas & Peters, 1979), research has focused on the symptoms of short attention span, distractibility, and impulsiveness, associated with hyperactivity, and recognition of this core symptomatology is reflected in the change of name in 1980 in the new DSM-III Classification to Attention Deficit Disorder (ADD). The fact that ADD can now be diagnosed without the presence of hyperactivity reflects the radical change in direction, away from neurological concepts, that has taken place in the space of 2 decades.

METHODOLOGIC ISSUES IN EVALUATING STUDIES

Diagnosis and Diagnostic Methods

The major pitfall to any review of soft signs in hyperactivity lies in diagnosis. Barkley (1982) reviewed 210 studies of hyperactivity and found that few stated any assessment diagnostic criteria or other details defining adequate methodology. As a result, there are considerable discrepancies in approach to diagnosis across studies and countries (see Trites, 1979). Until the advent of DSM-III in 1980, Americans had favored the vague all encompassing notion of hyperactivity espoused by Clements, which led to this diagnosis being common in the U.S. However, the McGill group of Weiss and colleagues (Weiss & Hechtman, 1979; Werry, Weiss, & Douglas, 1964) and subsequently English psychiatry (e.g., Rutter & Shaffer, 1980; Schachar, Rutter, & Smith, 1981), insisted on the diagnosis being confined to those children who showed "pervasive" hyperactivity, with clear evidence of hyperkinesis in most, if not all, environments. Partly because of this, the English made the diagnosis infrequently and considered the disorder uncommon (Rutter, 1982). This was further compounded by the insistence of the English that most cases of hyperactivity were in fact Conduct Disorder or, in short, antisocial/conduct type symptoms, which overrode a diagnosis of "hyperactivity." An epidemiologic analysis using Conners Teacher Questionnaire by Glow (1980) showed this latter fact to account for most of the discrepancies between U.S. and U.K. figures.

Thus, as a minimum, studies should clearly define diagnostic criteria as follows:

1. Specific descriptors of hyperactivity: Ideally these should be operationally defined and more recent studies should use DSM-III. Symptoms should at least be clearly described, with their method of assessment

stated. Problems with attention and impulse control should be the main or primary symptoms (see Douglas & Peters, 1979).

2. Parent and teacher reports of restlessness, overactivity, short attention span, and impulsiveness, formalized in standardized parent and teacher questionnaires: There are now several such measures with established reliability and validity, for which published norms are available, and that have scales that will discriminate hyperactive from normal children, e.g., Conners Parent and Teacher Questionnaires (Goyette, Conners, & Ulrich, 1978; Trites, 1979), Revised Behavior Problem Checklist (Quay, 1983). To be judged hyperactive a child should score at least two standard deviations above the mean for his or her age.
3. Durational criteria: Symptoms should be present for at least 6 months, with age of onset in early childhood.
4. Pervasiveness criteria: There should be clear evidence of the disorder in more than one environment.
5. Cultural criteria: For the behavior to be considered significant when occurring in different cultural subgroups, emphasis must be placed on a preschool history of hyperkinesis and a significant difference between the child and his or her siblings or peers (see Klein & Gittelman-Klein, 1975).

Other Descriptive Data

1. The age range of subjects: This should be specified in all studies.
2. Intelligence: This should be specified and ordinarily only children of normal intelligence should be included.

Associated or Exclusionary Criteria

Exclusion criteria, if any, should be mentioned: Ideally there should be an absence of gross neurological abnormality or unequivocal evidence of brain damage and psychotic children should be excluded.

Current and Previous Medication

Mention should be made in all studies of the current medication status of the subjects. Whether or not they have been free from medication for a period prior to the study is important information as most psychotropic drugs are known to affect findings at neurological examination.

Normal Control Groups

An important area of consideration is the use of physically and behaviorally normal control groups. Groups should be matched for age, sex, and socioeconomic status.

Contrast Groups

It is important also to use other diagnostic groups if one is to establish whether positive neurological findings are unique to hyperactive children or are a feature of psychiatrically disturbed children in general, as compared to normal controls. The etiological and diagnostic importance of positive neurological findings in hyperactive children will depend upon whether, as a group, they have significantly more neurological abnormalities than other deviant groups.

Neurological Examination

Of prime importance is the use of a systematized neurological examination, of demonstrated reliability, where the individual items to be examined are clearly specified and where there is a standard format for administration and scoring. Such an examination should have clinical validity; i.e., be able to discriminate effectively between pathologic and normal samples, and satisfactory interrater reliability needs to have been established. Few such systems of examination exist, let alone subject to reliability and validity studies. Ideally, an examination should be conducted with the examiner blind to the subject's diagnostic status. One, the Physical And Neurological Examination for Soft Signs (PANESS) (Close, 1973), has been shown to have problems with scoring, nonoccurring signs, and inadequate item content, but appears to be reasonably reliable (Camp, Bialer, Sverd, & Winsberg, 1978; Werry & Aman, 1976), especially as revised by Holden, Tarnowski, and Prinz (1982).

Rutter looked extensively at the issue of reliability within a specially developed neurological examination (Rutter, Graham, & Yule, 1970). He was able to show that items relating to sensorimotor coordination, constructional ability, and speech and language can all be assessed with good reliability.

However, the absence of adequately proven methods of neurological examination is a serious problem in most studies to be discussed.

STUDIES OF SOFT SIGNS IN HYPERACTIVITY

Acceptable Studies

For the purpose of this chapter, and because MBD is covered elsewhere in the book, we have confined the review to such papers that mainly emphasize the symptoms of hyperactivity as primary, recognizing, as Barkley (1982) points out, that few of these papers enable any reviewer to be sure that the conclusions to be made can be said with certainty to apply to hyperactivity as now defined in ADD or to hyperactivity uncontaminated by Conduct Disorder. While no study fits all of the above mentioned criteria, several come close and can be adjudged acceptable. There are 12 studies in this group.

Sandberg, Rutter, and Taylor (1978), in their study of psychiatric clinic attenders, compared 7 children with a diagnosis of hyperkinetic syndrome to 22 children with Conduct Disorder. The hyperkinetic syndrome was diagnosed in accordance with the multiaxial scheme based on the Ninth International Classification of Disease (Rutter, Shaffer, & Shepherd, 1975). They used a systematized examination of 16 tests of sensorimotor coordination, with demonstrated reliability and the ability to discriminate between normal children and those with learning and behavior problems. The hyperkinetic children differed significantly from the Conduct Disorder group in having a greater number of abnormalities on the neurological examination ($p < .05$). This study, although well designed and controlled, suffers from the weakness of very small sample size.

Interestingly, in the same study the authors compared seven children with "generalized hyperactivity" as defined by high scores for hyperactivity on Connors Parent and Teacher Questionnaires and direct observation measures, with a group matched for age, IQ, and psychiatric diagnosis. The generalized hyperactivity group was heterogenous as to the diagnosis. Their results showed that the children who were generally hyperactive had more abnormal findings on neurological examination and this difference reached the 5 percent level of significance, offering, as the authors suggest, some support for the possible validity of a less common syndrome of generalized overactivity, but again the sample size was very small.

Werry, Minde, Guzman, Weiss, Dogan, and Hoy (1972) compared 20 hyperactive children of normal intelligence with a group of 20 neurotic children and 20 normal children matched for age, sex, IQ, and socioeconomic status. The clinical diagnosis of hyperactivity was arrived at by using two psychiatrists and a standard diagnostic interview supported by teacher ratings and, in some, classroom observation. A wide range neurological examination consisting of 140 signs, including the "equivocal" ones, was used. Attempts were made to establish the inter-examiner reliability of elicitation, and rating, of the individual signs and, at an 80 percent level of examiner agreement, only 3 of the 140 signs fell below this level. The signs were rated on a four point scale of severity. Attempts to keep the two examiners blind were not successful because of obvious differences in the groups and chance remarks by the children. Their results showed that half the signs were absent altogether and that only 17 of the 70 signs that occurred did so in more than 10 percent of the 60 children. Ten of the 17 signs proved more common in the hyperactive group ($p = 0.05$), than in the neurotic or normal groups. Eight out of ten of the reliable signs that discriminated between the two groups, were assessing sensorimotor coordination. The cut-off point, that best discriminated between the hyperactive group and the others, was three or more minor signs. There was no difference between groups in major neurological signs, EEG abnormalities, or medical history.

Wikler, Dixon, and Parker (1970) confirmed Werry et al's findings of increased soft signs in hyperactives as compared to normal control children. Twenty-four behaviorally disordered children of normal intelligence and free of medication were classified as hyperactive (n = 11) or nonhyperactive (n = 9), on the basis of a checklist and psychiatrists' reports. Using an examination for soft signs for which training sessions had been held, the patient group was tested and compared to a group of matched controls. Formal interrater reliability was not reported, although checks were made by the senior author when signs were elicited. The examiners were apparently not blind to group membership. Significantly more soft signs were found in the patient group compared to the controls, but there was no significant difference in the total number of soft signs between the hyperactive and nonhyperactive patient groups as well as their respective control subgroups. However, there was a significantly greater number of soft signs in each of the patient subgroups than in their respective control subjects. Although this is one of the methodologically stronger papers in this review, it is noteworthy that several items on the hyperactivity checklist used by these authors would not nowadays be considered pathognomonic of hyperactivity (e.g., has poor manners; is extremely bossy).

In an investigation of hyperkinesis as rated on behavioral scales only, Sandberg, Wieselberg, and Shaffer (1980) studied 226 boys from inner London primary schools. They divided the children into 2 groups, according to whether or not they scored in the top 10 percent on the scales of hyperactivity and conduct disturbance on either the Conners or Rutter Teacher Questionnaires. Using the same reliable neurological exam as that described above (Sandberg et al, 1978) they found no relationship between the scores in the top 10 percent of the scales and number of neurological abnormalities. When those scoring high on hyperkinesis alone were compared with the children scoring high on Conduct Disorder scales, the presence of neurological abnormalities did not distinguish between the two groups. It is important to note that this was not a diagnosed sample of Attention Deficit Disorder and clinical ratings were not used. The authors themselves comment that the scales taken singly do not discriminate well between children showing hyperkinetic behavior and conduct disturbance.

In a study by Mikkelson, Brown, Minichiello, Millican, and Rappoport (1982), PANESS scores of 30 hyperactive boys were compared to those of 40 enuretic, 11 encopretic and enuretic, and 22 normal controls. Diagnoses of the hyperactives were based on scores greater than two standard deviations from the norm on factors I and IV of the Conners Teacher Rating Scale, plus clinical confirmation of hyperactivity. Acceptable reliability of PANESS scores was obtained by two physicians in a counterbalanced retesting of 10 hyperactive children. The examiners were not blind to diagnosis. A strong negative correlation was found between age and PANESS scores, there being a significant tendency for younger children to have higher scores. Results showed that age adjusted mean PANESS score of the hyperactive group was significantly higher than both the control and enuretic groups. However, age adjusted scores for the latter two groups showed no significant differences. Within the enuretic group, those children who were also encopretic had significantly more soft signs than the rest of the enuretic group.

The authors conclude that the PANESS may be a valid measure of the level of neurodevelopmental maturity rather than a specific diagnostic instrument. The implication for hyperactivity being that disorder may reflect a delay in central nervous system development and is perhaps etiologically related to such neurodevelopmental immaturity.

A similar relationship between age and PANESS scores was found by

Camp et al (1978). This study differs, however, from that of Mikkelsen et al above in the apparent inability of the PANESS to differentiate hyperactives from normals. Camp et al administered the PANESS to 32 hyperactive boys, diagnosed by clinical evaluation and parent and teacher rating scales. However, the names and nature of the scales is not specified and no norms are provided. The hyperactives were compared with 111 normal children. They found no significant difference between the 2 groups except that the 9-year-old hyperactives did better than their age-matched normal counterparts.

Apart from drug condition not being reported, and raters in this study also being nonblind, there is no obvious explanation for the discrepancy of these findings, but Camp's study used large sample sizes. The authors concluded that the PANESS did not have adequate clinical validity, though it is also possible that there were, in fact, really no differences in the two groups.

An earlier study by Werry and Aman (1976) that investigated the reliability and diagnostic validity of the PANESS concluded that the system of examination was very reliable largely because most of the signs did not occur! They compared ten hyperactive children with five with major neurological impairment and six normal children. All children were free of medication at the time of testing and the examiners were blind to diagnosis. The number of signs occurring differed only slightly over groups but the median number of signs was greatest in the neurologically impaired group, while the hyperactive children had a higher median score than the normals. However, the amount of overlap between groups was considerable and while this is supportive evidence for increased soft signs in hyperactives as compared to normal children, the sample size was very small indeed.

Levine, Busch, and Aufseeser (1982) studied Attention Deficit Disorder in children referred to a clinic because of school problems. Using parent and teacher questionnaires, which were developed by the author, and which had been previously standardized on community samples, a child qualified for inclusion in the ADD group if he satisfied two of three criteria. The first was a score on the parent questionnaire that was approximately two standard deviations below the community mean. The second criterion was a score less than a specified cut-off point on the teacher questionnaire, but the degree of statistical deviance was not stated. A multidisciplinary team consensus of significant attention deficit provided the third criterion.

Six hundred and forty-six children were studied and of these 220 qualified for the ADD group, the remaining 426 had learning problems without ADD.

Although all children underwent neurodevelopmental examinations, including assessment of soft signs, it is not clear who carried out these examinations or whether a systematized approach was used, and no interrater reliability was reported.

Twenty-eight percent of the attention deficit group had two or more synkinesias compared to only 12 percent of the remainder of the clinic sample ($p < .01$). There was a trend ($p < .05$) toward greater delay in growth and fine motor function in the ADD group. Of those in the ADD group two-thirds were reported to have specific learning disabilities.

What seems remarkable in this paper is the large number of children in the ADD group. Information obtained in the same study regarding preschool and current behavior problems showed that the attention deficit group had a much greater number of behavioral problems than the comparison group and that these problems were more severe. It is likely that this sample also included a large number of children with Conduct Disorders and that the findings regarding neurologic status should not be construed as applying to a pure ADD sample.

Quinn and Rappoport (1974) reported the neurological status and minor physical anomaly scores of 81 hyperactive boys. They were diagnosed using the composite concepts of several investigators of that period and had to be distractible or restless at home, and at school, for at least 2 years. Although the list of soft signs evaluated is detailed, it is not clear by whom the examination was carried out, and there is no report of any reliability studies. Their results showed the mean number of soft signs was 3.41 (range 0-11) and soft signs were positively associated with the degree of hyperactivity as measured by the Conners Teacher Questionnaire. There was no correlation found between minor physical anomalies and number of soft signs.

In an extensive neuropsychiatric study of hyperkinetic disorders in 7-year-olds, Gilberg, Calstrom, and Rasmussen (1983) studied 18 children who were rated hyperkinetic in 3 surroundings, i.e., in a child psychiatric examination, during a neurological examination, and according to the mother. This group was called "generally hyperkinetic." Twenty-nine children showed evidence of attention deficits in two of the three situations and were called the "cross situational" group. These two groups were compared to each other and to a group of 50 normal children. The neurological examination is not described but included an assessment of soft signs. Comparisons between groups revealed that the "generally hyperkinetic" children had significantly more neurological abnormalities than the "cross situationally" hyperkinetic group, and that this group in turn had significantly more soft signs than the normal group. Both of these were significant at the .001 level. However, it is important to note that this was not a diagnosed sample of Attention Deficit Disorder and included children with a variety of psychiatric diagnoses, including MBD and mental retardation. One would therefore expect that a higher incidence of soft signs would be reported than would be found in a "pure" ADD sample.

Denckla and Rudel (1978) studied 48 boys of normal intelligence diagnosed as hyperactive based on scores of at least 16 on the hyperactivity scale of both the Conners Parent and Teacher Questionnaires. They were compared to an unmatched control group of 50 normal boys. The neurological examination included a timed coordination battery, but reliability studies were not performed and the examiner was not blind to diagnosis. Nine discriminating variables produced a highly significant degree of dissimilarity between the hyperactive subjects and controls, with overflow movements and heel-toe walking making the greatest contribution to the discriminant function scores. Synkinetic and mirror movements differentiated hyperactive boys from controls at all ages. Furthermore, when attempts to classify children according to membership of the hyperactive or normal group were made, on the basis of discriminant function scores, 88.8 percent were correctly classified. The authors coined the phrase "developmental delay" to describe the lack of age-related maturation in the coordination of hyperactive children.

Hertzig, Bortner, and Birch (1969) investigated the incidence of soft signs in a group of 90 brain damaged children attending a special education facility and compared this group to 15 normal controls. The examiner was blind to diagnosis and attempted to identify the hyperkinetic behavior disorder within the examination setting, noting impulsiveness, restlessness, and inattention. Hard and soft signs were considered separately in the results. Twenty-nine percent of the brain damaged group had hard signs compared to none of the controls, whereas 90 percent of the brain damaged group exhibited soft signs compared to 33 percent of the controls; the most common signs being disturbances of balance, coordination, and speech. No control had more than one soft sign. Nineteen of the brain damaged children were considered hyperkinetic and this group had a significantly greater frequency of soft signs than the nonhyperkinetic children in the brain damaged group. However, this increased frequency of soft signs was not associated with any particular set of signs. The fact that this sample was medically diagnosed as brain damaged makes it difficult to apply these findings to the general population of hyperkinetic children who are not in special educational placement.

Methodologically Unacceptable Studies

There are four other studies that indicate an increase of soft signs in hyperkinetic children but that have serious methodologic problems: Nahas and Krynicki (1978), Anderson (1963), Kenny, Clemmens, Hudson, Lentz, Cicci, and Nair (1971), and Satterfield, Cantwell, Saul, and Yusin (1974).

In their investigation of EEG abnormalities in children with psychiatric disorders, Nahas and Krynicki (1978) compared a group of 41 MBD children with impaired impulse, attention, or motor function, with 28 learning disordered MBD children, 24 with adjustment reaction and 20 with behavioral problems. All were given an examination for soft signs, with the adjustment reaction group having the lowest number of neurological abnormalities (3/24), the MBD learning group having the highest number of soft signs (17/28), while the MBD group with impulse and attentional difficulties fell midway between (16/41).

Although these results are in the expected direction thay can be questioned on a number of counts. The diagnostic groups were very loosely defined, although they clearly contained some children with ADD. No systematized neurological examination was used, interrater reliability was not reported, and examiners were not blind to diagnosis.

Anderson (1963) investigated 30 hyperkinetic children with apparently no gross neurological deficits, although 13 had a history of at least 1 convulsion and 7 were actually being treated for epilepsy! The neurological examination was abnormal, in some respect, in all but one child, with positive pyramidal tract signs and choreiform or mirror movements being the most common. However, the lack of any defined diagnostic criteria, systematized neurological examination, or control group, combined with the unusually high frequency of coexistent epilepsy and hence of major brain disorder, means little weight can be attached to these findings.

Kenny et al (1971) studied 100 children referred to a clinic because of hyperactivity. After medical evaluation they were divided into 3 groups. In the first group, 41 children had primary diagnosis of MBD, 35 in the second group were intellectually subnormal, and the third group consisted of 18 emotionally disordered children. The age range was 2-16 years. All children underwent a neurological examination with emphasis on soft signs. But it does not appear to have been systematized and reliability studies were not done. Results of the neurological examination were reported for the total group of children and not for particular diagnostic groups. Although 48 children had evidence of soft signs, there was no significant relationship, using chi square test, among the neurological examination,

EEG findings and the final diagnosis.

In an uncontrolled study by Satterfield et al (1974), 125 hyperactive boys diagnosed by behavioral criteria, using parent and teacher questionnaires, were given a structured neurological examination by one of the authors, who was blind to the results of psychological testing. No cut-off criteria were reported for the questionnaire diagnosis of hyperactivity and reliability studies were not carried out. Their results that 54 percent of the sample exhibited one or more neurological abnormalities are therefore open to question.

STUDIES OF DRUG EFFECTS UPON SOFT SIGNS IN HYPERACTIVITY

Four studies have addressed the issue of soft signs and their relationship to drug treatment in hyperactives. Shekim, Dekirmenjian, and Chapel (1979) investigated urinary MHPG (3-methoxy-4-hydroxy-phenethyleneglycol, a norepinephrine metabolite) excretion and response to d-amphetamine in 15 drug-free hyperactive children, of normal intelligence, diagnosed in accordance with DSM-II as hyperkinetic reaction of childhood. Each child was given a 32 item PANESS but no details are reported regarding who administered the examination, nor whether reliability studies were performed. The raters were presumably not blind and no control group was used for the PANESS. The nine children who responded to d-amphetamine tended to be younger and had significantly higher mean PANESS scores ($p < .002$) than the six nonresponders. The age difference was not significant but the authors commented that the higher PANESS scores may have been a result of the apparent developmental trend in the PANESS. Bearing in mind the obvious weakness in this study it is difficult to attach great significance to these findings.

Sattterfield, Cantwell, Saul, Lesser, and Podosin (1973) investigated the use of EEG recordings and neurological abnormalities as predictors of response to methylphenidate in hyperactive boys. Fifty-seven hyperactive boys were diagnosed by two child psychiatrists using a structured interview as described by Rutter and Graham (1968). Parent and teacher rating scales were also obtained, but these were not specified apart from test-retest correlation and no cut-off point was used to confirm the diagnosis. Before treatment, a neurological examination for soft signs, based on that of Paine and Oppé (1966) was conducted. Some aspects of the examination were structured but formal tests of limb coordination were not performed, instead casual observation of shoe-lace tying was rated. It is not clear who carried out the examinations and reliability studies were not performed. Forty-nine percent of the subjects had no neurological abnormalities, while 51 percent had 1 or more minor neurological signs. When the subjects were ranked on the extent of abnormality of the EEG and the number of soft signs, there was a high correlation between the degree of neurological and EEG abnormalities and drug response, thus suggesting a better response to stimulants in those children with a greater number of soft signs and an abnormal EEG.

Lerer and Lerer (1976) investigated the effects of methylphenidate on the soft signs of 40 hyperactive children, referred because of behavioral difficulties, and selected because of the presence of 3 or more neurological abnormalities. Although the type of abnormality was not specified, those with gross neurological dysfunction were not included. In a double blind placebo controlled design the children were divided into a drug and placebo treatment group. Children were examined for soft signs pretreatment and then 30 and 60 days after treatment with methylphenidate or placebo. Those in the placebo group were then switched to methylphenidate and reexamined for soft signs. A child was considered improved if two or more neurological abnormalities showed complete resolution on repeat testing. After 60 days, 16 of the 20 drug treated children had improved, compared with none on placebo, and when the placebo group was given methylphenidate, 13 out of 20 showed improvement after 60 days. These results are highly significant but should be viewed with extreme caution in view of the numerous methodologic flaws in this study. For example, no standardized neurological examination was used, the initial examination was not performed blind, although repeat testing was, and no interrater reliability was established. Also relevant is the fact that no control group was used, either deviant or normal.

Noting the findings of Lerer and Lerer, and in an attempt to examine the reproducibility of soft signs over time, McMahan and Greenberg (1977) conducted serial neurological examinations on 44 hyperactive boys undergoing a double blind placebo controlled drug study. Using a systematic neurological examination, which included assessment of soft signs, the boys were examined 5 times during an 8 week treatment course by a pediatrician who was blind to knowledge of the subjects' drug state. They found that the number of soft signs occurring at each examination was variable, within subjects and across treatment groups. In some cases signs changed from positive to negative, and in others the change was in the opposite direction, with the direction of change being apparently random and quite unaffected by drug treatment.

In contrast to Lerer and Lerer's study, the authors felt there was no evidence to suggest any drug effect. More importantly, almost all other studies reviewed here have assessed soft signs on the basis of only one examination and this study makes the point that not only are soft signs unreliable over time, but their clinical significance is difficult to interpret, there being no indication that they have any value in assessing response to treatment.

Despite the innovative design of this study and the interesting findings, it is open to criticism on methodologic grounds in that no reliability studies are reported for the neurological examination and diagnostic criteria for hyperactivity are not specified except that the children were described as overly active in school.

CONCLUSIONS AND CLINICAL IMPLICATIONS

It is difficult to draw conclusions with any degree of certainty because of the heterogeneity of diagnostic selection criteria used in the various studies and criticized in detail already. Apart from this being a major problem, lack of uniformity in the use of neurological examinations, not to mention the paucity of studies using a standardized examination with established reliability and validity, further impeded the accuracy with which conclusions regarding soft signs can be drawn. This is compounded by the lack of agreement between researchers as to what constitutes a soft sign, and hence there is considerable variability among studies with regard to the neurological abnormalities investigated.

Subject to these caveats, the majority of studies have found an increased number of soft signs in hyperactive children as compared with normal children (see Table 10-1). However, it is unclear whether this difference holds, and is more or less so, when hyperactives are compared with other diagnostic groups, matched for sex and chronologic and mental age, i.e., developmental age.

With regard to which soft signs occur with greater frequency in hyperactives, there appears to be some measure of agreement between studies. As can be seen from Table 10-1, in those studies where soft signs of higher frequency have been specified, the great majority fall into the category of delays in sensorimotor coordination and speech. Werry and Aman (1976) found that the cut-off point that best discriminated between the hyperactive group and others was three or more soft signs. No doubt some of the poorly

Review of Research on Neurological "Soft Signs" in Hyperactive Children

Authors	Number of Hyperactive Children	Diagnosis	Contrast Group	Neurological Examination (I Reliability II Raters Blind)	Results Soft Signs (SS)	Soft Signs with Increased Frequency Among Hyperactives
Sandberg et al, 1978	7	Multiaxial classification (Rutter et al, 1975), Conners TQ.	Conduct disorder N = 22	I. Interrater II. ?*	SS ↑ in HA†, $p < .05$	?
Werry et al, 1972	20	Assessment by two psychiatrists, teacher ratings, classroom observation.	Neurotics N = 20 Normals = 20	I. Interrater II. No	SS ↑ in HA, $p < .05$	Hand and finger coordination, supination–pronation, standing on one foot, hopping on one foot, immature speech, ability to stand still.
Wikler et al, 1970	11	>12⁄18 items on HA checklist and psychiatric interview	Normals N = 24 Non-HA patients N = 9	I. Signs checked by senior author. II. ?	HA *v* normals, $p<.01$ Non-HA *v* normals, $p < .01$ HA *v* Non-HA, p = NS	Equivocal Babinski, dysdiadochokinesis, disturbances of gait, coordination and muscle tone ↑ in patient group. Overflow movements ↑ in normals.
Mikkelsen et al, 1982	30	2 SD from norm on Factors I or IV of Conners TQ and inpatient evaluation.	Eneuretics N = 40 Normals N = 22	I. Interrater II. ?	Total PANESS score HA *v* normals, $p<.01$ HA *v* eneuretics, $p < .05$ Eneuretics *v* normals, p = NS	?
Werry & Aman, 1976	10	Psychiatric evaluation Conners TQ.	Neurologically impaired N = 5 Normals N = 6	I. Interrater II. Yes	SS neurological group > HA HA > normals. Large amount of overlap between groups.	?
Camp et al, 1978	32	Psychiatric evaluation and parent and teacher rating scales.	Normals N = 111	I. ? II. ?	No difference between groups.	?
Quinn & Rapoport, 1974	81	Distractibility and restlessness at home and school for 2 yrs; parent, teacher, and physician assessments of hyperactivity.	No	I. ? II. ?	SS correlated with Factor IV (hyperactivity) of Conners TQ, $p < .02$.	?

Table 10-1 *continued*
Review of Research on Neurological "Soft Signs" in Hyperactive Children

Authors	Number of Hyperactive Children	Diagnosis	Contrast Group	Neurological Examination (I Reliability II Raters Blind)	Results Soft Signs (SS)	Soft Signs with Increased Frequency Among Hyperactives
Denckla & Rudel, 1978	48	>16/27 on HA Factor of Conners PQ and TQ.	Normals N = 50	I. ? II. ?	SS ↑ in HA, $p < .001$.	Synkinetic and mirror movements, heel–toe walking.
Anderson, 1963	30	Not specified.	No	I. ? II. ?	Neurological exam abnormal in some respect in 29/30.	Choreiform or mirror movements N = 29. Poor muscle coordination N = 27. Positive pyramidal tract signs N = 18. Slow speech development N = 15.
Levine et al, 1982	Attention deficit group N = 220	Multidisciplinary team assessment, parent and teacher questionnaires.	Learning problem group N = 426	I. ? II. ?	SS ↑ in attention deficit group, $p < .01$	Multiple synkinesias (2 or more), delay in gross motor function, delay in fine motor function.
Gilberg et al, 1983	18	Not a clinically diagnosed ADD sample. Generalized hyperkinesis in in 3 settings.	Normals N = 50	I. ? II. ?	SS ↑ in attention deficit group, $p < .01$	?
Holden et al, 1982	?	Various diagnoses in sample. N = 28. Conners PQ.	No	I. Test–retest Interrater II. ?	PANESS total score correlated with HA factor of Conners PQ, $p < .001$.	?
Hertzig et al, 1969	Brain damaged children N=90, including 19 hyperkinetic behavior disorder.	Assessment of hyperkinesis, distractibility, within examination setting.	Normals N = 15	I. ? II. Yes	SS ↑ in HA *v* rest of brain damaged group, $p < .01$. HA *v* normals, $p < .01$.	Abnormalities of balance, coordination and speech.
Nahas & Krynicki, 1978	MBD N = 69	MBD with learning disorders N = 28. MBD with disordered attention, impulse or motor function N = 41.	Adjustment reaction N = 20. Behavior disorder N = 20	I. ? II. ?	SS in MBD learning group > MBD attention group > behavior disorder group >adjustment reaction group. $p < .01$.	?
Kenny et al, 1971	100 referred for hyperactivity.	MBD N = 41. Mental retardation N = 35. Emotional problems N = 18.	No	I. ? II. ?	No difference between diagnostic groups in number of SS.	?

*? indicates no data given.

controlled and coordinated movement is due to impulsivity, but there would seem to be a residual core pathology of impaired motor performance. It is not clear what this association actually means in relation to normals and other diagnostic groups. It is not specific to ADD.

Rutter et al (1970) found that 14 percent of normal 10-11-year-olds showed mirror movements. Similarly, Wolff and Hurwitz (1966) found that 11 percent of normal children had choreiform movements.

As delayed coordination and speech is a normal finding in young children it can only be considered significant when viewed in relation to the child's developmental and mental age. The presence of soft signs in hyperactives does not necessarily indicate brain damage as these have not been consistently linked with EEG abnormalities or abnormal medical histories indicative of brain damage. Psychiatric disorders, especially Conduct Disorder, mental retardation, and specific maturational disorders can produce a similar clinical picture. One can only conclude that apart from suggesting a delay in central nervous system maturation, the significance of soft signs in hyperactivity is otherwise unknown.

It would seem that soft signs have no predictive value for drug treatment in hyperactives and McMahan and Greenberg (1977) have highlighted the problem of lack of reliability of soft signs over time. Future research needs to focus on longitudinal studies and address the issue of the stability of soft signs, while identifying factors associated with their persistence or disappearance. In the meantime their role in the long term is unknown.

In view of the uncertain etiologic, diagnostic, prognostic, and pharmacotherapeutic value of soft signs in hyperactivity, it seems only right to conclude that apart possibly from pin pointing specific problems (e.g., dyspraxia), not peculiar in any way to hyperactivity, soft signs have yet to demonstrate any clear clinical utility in hyperactivity (ADD).

ACKNOWLEDGMENT

Preparation of this paper was supported in part by a grant from the Medical Research Council of New Zealand to Professor Werry.

REFERENCES

American Psychiatric Association. Diagnostic and Statistical Manual of Mental Disorders, 3rd edition. Washington DC: Author, 1980

Anderson WW: The hyperkinetic child: A neurological appraisal. Neurology, 1963, 13, 968-973

Barkley RA. Guidelines for defining hyperactivity in children: Attention deficit disorder and hyperactivity. In Lahey BJ, & Kazdin AE (Eds.). Advances in Clinical Child Psychology. (Vol. 5). New York: Plenum Press, 1982, pp. 137-180

Camp JA, Bialer I, Sverd J, & Winsberg BG. Clinical usefulness of the NIMH physical and neurological examination for soft signs. American Journal of Psychiatry, 1978, 135(3), 362-364

Clements SD. Minimal Brain Dysfunction in Children (National Institute of Neurological Diseases and Blindness Monograph No. 3). Washington, DC: Department of Health, Education and Welfare, 1966

Clements S, & Peters J. Minimal brain dysfunction in the school-age child. Archives of General Psychiatry, 1962, 6, 185-197

Close J. Scored neurological examination. Psychopharmacology Bulletin: Special Issue, Pharmacotherapy of Children, 1973, 142-148

Denckla MB, & Rudel RG. Anomalies of motor development in hyperactive boys. Annals of Neurology, 1978, 3(3), 231-233

Douglas VI, & Peters KG. Toward a clearer definintion of the attention deficit of hyperactive children. In Hale G, & Lewis M (Eds.). Attention and Cognitive Development. New York: Plenum Press, 1979

Gilberg C, Carlstrom G, & Rasmussen P. Hyperkinetic disorders in seven-year-old children with perceptual, motor and attentional deficits. Journal of Child Psychology and Psychiatry, 1983, 24(2), 233-246

Glow RA. A validation of Conners TQ and a cross-cultural comparison of prevalence of hyperactivity in children. In Burrows GD, & Werry JS (Eds.). Advances in Human Psychopharmacology (Vol. 1). Greenwich, CT: JAI Press, 1980, pp. 303-322

Goyette CH, Conners CK, & Ulrich RF. Normative data on Revised Conners Parent and Teacher Rating Scales. Journal of Abnormal Child Psychology, 1978, 6, 221-236

Hertzig ME, Bortner M, & Birch HG. Neurologic findings in children educationally designated as "brain-damaged." American Journal of Orthopsychiatry, 1969, 39(3), 437-446

Holden EW, Tarnowski KJ, & Prinz RJ. Reliability of neurological soft signs in children: Reevaluation of the PANESS. Journal of Abnormal Child Psychology, 1982, 10(2), 163-172

Kenny TJ, Clemmens RL, Hudson BW, et al. Characteristics of children referred because of hyperactivity. Journal of Pediatrics, 1971, 79(4), 618-622

Klein DF, & Gittelman-Klein R. Problems in the diagnosis of minimal brain dysfunction and the hyperkinetic syndrome. International Journal of Mental Health, 1975, 4, 45-60

Lerer RJ, & Lerer MP: The effects of methylphenidate on the soft neurological signs of hyperactive children. Pediatrics, 1976, 57(4), 521-525

Levine MD, Busch B, & Aufseeser C. The dimension of inattention among children with school problems. Pediatrics, 1982, 70(3), 387-395

McMahon SA, & Greenberg LM. Serial neurologic examination of hyperactive children. Pediatrics, 1977, 59(4), 584-587

Mikkelsen EJ, Brown GL, Minichiello MD, et al. Neurologic status in hyperactive, enuretic, encopretic, and normal boys. Journal of the American Academy of Child Psychiatry, 1982, 21(1), 75-81

Nahas AD, & Krynicki N. Discriminant analysis of EEG in children with situational, learning and impulse disorders. Neuropsychobiology, 1978, 4, 74-85

Paine RS, & Oppé TE. Neurological Examination of Children. Clinics in Developmental Medicine No. 20/21. London: Spastics International Medical Publications & Wm. Heinemann, 1966

Quay HC. A dimensional approach to children's behavior disorder: The Revised Behavior Problem Checklist. School Psychology Review, 1983, 12, 244-249

Quinn PO, & Rappoport JL. Minor physical anomalies and neurologic status in hyperactive boys. Pediatrics, 1974, 53(5), 742-747

Ross DM, & Ross SA. Hyperactivity: Research, Theory and Action (2nd ed). New York: Wiley, 1982

Rutter M. Syndromes attributed to "Minimal Brain Dysfunction" in childhood. American Journal of Psychiatry, 1982, 139(1), 21-33

Rutter M, & Graham P. The reliability and validity of the psychiatric assessment of the child. I Interview with the child. British Journal of Psychiatry, 1968, 114, 581-592

Rutter M, Graham P, & Yule W. A Neuropsychiatric Study in Childhood. Clinics in Developmental Medicine No. 35/36. London: Heinemann, 1970

Rutter M, & Shaffer D. DSM-III: A step forward or back in terms of the classification of child psychiatric disorders? Journal of the American Academy of Child Psychiatry, 1980, 19(3), 371-394

Rutter M, Shaffer D, & Shepherd M. A Multi-axial classification of child psychiatric disorders. Geneva: World Health Organization, 1975

Sandberg ST, Rutter M, & Taylor E. Hyperkinetic disorder in psychiatric clinic attenders. Developmental Medicine and Child Neurology, 1978, 20, 279-299

Sandberg ST, Wieselberg M, & Shaffer D. Hyperkinetic and conduct problem children in a primary school population: Some epidemiological considerations. Journal of Child Psychology and Psychiatry, 1980, 21, 293-311

Satterfield JH, Cantwell DP, Saul RE, et al. Response to stimulant drug treatment in hyperactive children: Prediction from EEG and neurological findings. Journal of Autism and Childhood Schizophrenia, 1973, 3(1), 36-48

Satterfield JH, Cantwell DP, Saul RE, & Yusin A. Intelligence, academic achievement, and EEG abnormalities in hyperactive children. American Journal of Psychiatry, 1974, 131(4), 391-395

Schachar R, Rutter M, & Smith A. The characteristics of situationally and pervasively hyperactive children: Implications for syndrome definition. Journal of Child Psychology and Psychiatry, 1981, 22, 375-392

Shekim WO, Dekirmenjian H, & Chapel JL. Urinary MHPG excretion in minimal brain dysfunction and its modification by d-amphetamine. American Journal of Psychiatry, 1979, 136(5), 667-671

Trites RL (Ed.). Hyperactivity in Children: Etiology, Measurement, and Treatment Implications. Baltimore: University Park Press, 1979

Weiss G, & Hechtman L. The hyperactive child syndrome. Science, 1979, 205, 1348-1345

Werry JS. Organic factors. In Quay HC, & Werry JS (Eds.). Psychopathological Disorders of Childhood (2nd ed.). New York: John Wiley & Sons, 1979

Werry JS, & Aman MG. The reliability and diagnostic validity of the physical and neurological examination for soft signs (PANESS). Journal of Autism and Childhood Schizophrenia, 1976, 6(3), 253-262

Werry JS, & Campbell SB. Attention Deficit Disorder. In Quay HC, & Werry JS (Eds.). Psychopathological Disorders of Childhood (3rd ed.). New York: Wiley, 1986

Werry JS, Minde K, Guzman A, et al. Studies on the hyperactive child-VII: Neurological status compared with neurotic and normal children. American Journal of Orthopsychiatry, 1972, 42(3), 441-451

Werry JS, Weiss G, & Douglas V. Studies on the hyperactive child I — some preliminary findings. Canadian Psychiatric Association Journal, 1964, 9, 120-130

Wikler A, Dixon JF, & Parker JB. Brain function in problem children and controls: Psychometric, neurological, and electroencephalographic

comparisons. American Journal of Psychiatry, 1970, 127(5), 94-105
Wolff PH, & Hurwitz J. The choreiform syndrome. Developmental Medicine and Child Neurology, 1966, 8, 160-165

Heinz F.R. Prechtl

11

Choreiform Movements

Choreiform or choreatiform movements in children were described in 1959 by Prechtl and Stemmer in a paper first published in German, which appeared later in English (1962). The phenomenon of short, irregular muscle twitches was discovered during routine EEG recordings in children 7-14 years of age who were referred to a neurologist mainly because of learning and behavior problems. Although these movements in a way resembled abnormal movements seen in patients with chorea minor, our cases did not suffer from this disease. A systematic investigation of a group of 50 children, aged 9-12 years, was then carried out, the subjects being solely selected on the basis of the presence of choreiform movements. Other neurologic conditions or mental defects were excluded. However, in the selection of the children the fact was overlooked that the group was biased towards cases with learning and behavior problems. This was later discovered in larger investigations in local school populations when a close relationship between the occurrence of choreiform dyskinesia and school performance was lacking. It was therefore decided to study a new large group of schoolchildren. This time the selection was made on the basis of a representative sample from the population of a middle sized Dutch town (Arnhem). The results were reported in the thesis of the late Dr. Tiny Stemmer but have never been published in English.

DEFINITION

Choreiform movements have been described: "these movements are slight and jerky and occur quite irregularly and arrhythmically in different muscles. They are characterized by their sudden occurrence and short dur-

SOFT NEUROLOGICAL SIGNS
ISBN 0-8089-1841-9

ation, distinguishing them clearly from slow tonic athetoid movements" (Prechtl & Stemmer, 1962). This description has been corroborated by electromyographic investigations. With surface as well as with needle electrodes, brief discharges of about 500 milliseconds duration occur irregularly either in a relaxed (and electrically silent) muscle or are superimposed on the background activity during contraction. They then exceed the background in amplitude.

Choreiform twitches may occur in trunk, proximal and distal limb muscles, the eye muscles and tongue, and can be seen as muscle artifacts in the EEG recording, originating from the musculus temporalis and the neck muscles.

TESTING PROCEDURE

As the choreiform twitches can most clearly be seen if the muscles are contracted, it is advisable to standardize the testing procedure. A convenient way is to ask the patient to stand as still as possible with the feet together, the arms horizontally elevated and stretched out in front, the fingers of both hands maximally extended and spread. The eyes should be closed and the tongue stuck out. This posture should be held for 20-30 seconds. To test for the presence of choreiform movements in the eye muscles, the eyes are then opened and the patient asked to fixate the finger top of the examiner, which is held up half a meter in front of the patient's eyes.

SCORING

Between the absence of any choreiform jerks and severe choreiform dyskinesia there is a smooth continuum in the quantitative expression of choreiform movements. In order to obtain a quantification of the phenomenon the following scoring system has been developed.

O (no): No choreiform movements or spurious movements, i.e., 1 or 2 within 30 seconds.
1 (mild): Up to 5 isolated twitches of small amplitude per 30 seconds.
2 (moderate): Up to 10 twitches, sometimes in bursts, amplitude of displacement of hands 3 centimeters or more per 30 seconds.
3 (severe): continuous twitches of large amplitude per 30 seconds.

A distinction can be made between involvement of proximal (trunk, face, shoulder) muscles and distal (hand, finger) muscles. Sometimes only one of the two groups is involved, although usually they can be seen in both.

The reliability of the assessment has been tested for interscorer agreement by Stemmer who found a correlation coefficient of r = 0.92 (N = 132) and by Rutter et al (1966) who reported an agreement of 57 percent (N = 79). The latter was a mixture of interscorer agreement and test-retest reliability (up to 1 month interval). Stemmer found a replication of her findings in the same children seen after an interval of 1-2 weeks of r = 0.69 (N = 798). It may be concluded that the assessment of choreiform movements is sufficiently reliable (Rutter et al, 1966).

INCIDENCE OF CHOREIFORM MOVEMENTS

All investigators of choreiform movements agree on the difference in the incidence of choreiform movements found between boys and girls and on the close relationship between incidence and age.

The difference in the incidence of choreiform movements between boys and girls is 4:1 or 3:1 (Rutter et al, 1966; Stemmer, 1964; Wolff & Hurwitz, 1966). Stemmer found only 6 out of 1995 girls who showed severe choreiform movements. Among 3889 boys, 107 had severe choreiform movements.

Choreiform movements are never seen in children younger than 2-3 years (Dijkstra, 1960). In a kindergarten population severe choreiform movements were found in 4.5 percent of boys at 4 years, in 5.1 percent at 5 years, and 9.4 percent at 6 years (Stemmer, 1964). In an elementary school population, between 6 and 14 years of age, the incidence varied from 3.6 percent at 6 years to 5.1 percent at 8 years and declined afterwards to 1 percent at 12 years. None were found in 13- and 14-year-olds. However, at secondary schoolage (12-18 years), the incidence of severe choreiform movements in 12-year-old boys was 5.3 percent, at 13 years it was 2.2 percent, at 14 years 1 percent, and at 15 years 0.6 percent. None of the 16-18-year-old secondary schoolboys had such dyskinesia. This is probably due to the selection in the school because a representative sample of 727 boys undergoing their first medical examination for the military service (10 percent of total) showed an incidence of choreiform movements of 0.7 percent.

The findings indicate an age related change in the incidence of choreiform movements in children attending normal schools. There is a rise until 8 years and a rapid decrease with the onset of puberty at about 12 years.

A different result was obtained in children from special schools for mental and physical handicaps. Among 144 boys, 19 (13.2 percent) suffered severe and 17 (11.8 percent) moderate choreiform movements. These findings are substantiated by the study of Wolff and Hurwitz (1966) who also found a significantly higher incidence of choreiform movements among children in special schools and among juvenile delinquents in the USA and Japan. Rutter et al (1966) report that among 98 patients in a special school at Aberdeen, 30 percent had marked choreiform movements.

PATHOPHYSIOLOGY OF CHOREIFORM MOVEMENTS

From electromyographic recordings of choreiform twitches it must be concluded that groups of motoneurons fire spontaneously in an irregular fashion, even in a relaxed muscle. This requires a degree of instability of motoneuron membrane potentials that is not found under normal conditions. It is not known what the origin of this instability is.

Choreiform movements can transiently occur during fever. They may also even be present in adults after intensive muscle contraction, e.g., in the arm and fingers after carrying a heavy suitcase. In this situation one may assume a process similar to that seen in posttetanic potentiation. However, it seems unlikely that similar mechanisms are present in children with choreiform dyskinesia.

ETIOLOGY

The various attempts to clarify the etiology of choreiform dyskinesia have so far only produced conflicting evidence. The original idea (Prechtl & Stemmer, 1962) of a major role for birth asphyxia could not be confirmed in later investigations. From prospective studies it seems more likely that many unfavorable pre and perinatal conditions may contribute to the etiology but further studies are necessary to investigate this problem in more detail. A major difficulty is formed by the long latency in the development of choreiform dyskinesia, which is mostly not clearly expressed before school age.

Retrospective studies based on parental reports of the obstetric history provided negative results but the low reliability of such data has been well documented.

An interesting observation was made by Stemmer who examined the 53 6-14-year-old siblings of 30 children with marked choreiform movements. The incidence of choreiform movements was significantly higher in siblings ($p < 0.05$) than in age-matched controls drawn from the same population. It is therefore not unlikely that genetic factors may also contribute to the etiology of choreiform dyskinesia.

RELATIONSHIPS WITH OTHER VARIABLES

If choreiform movements are considered as a sign of minor neurologic dysfunction, they should frequently occur in conjunction with other minor neurologic signs. From clinical experience this is certainly the case but, with the exception of the Rutter et al's (1970) Isle of Wight-study, reports of systematic studies on representative samples are lacking. A rigorous standardization of the neurologic examination techniques (see Touwen, 1979) is mandatory in such investigations.

The close relationship with learning and behavioral problems originally suggested was based on errors in the selection of cases.

There are, however, a number of close relationships with specific behavioral variables. The writing of children with marked choreiform twitches in the fingers is clumsy in all individuals studied. When they are drawing a straight line, the involuntary jerks produce "spikes," which interrupt the continuity of the line, which is in fact a convenient test of the interference often found in writing.

A similar close relationship between individual twitches and functional disturbance can be observed in reading where the presence of choreiform movements in the eye muscles produces sudden deviations from the fixation point and from the horizontal saccades following the printed line, thereby hampering reading. Electro-oculographic recordings during reading of a simple text confirmed that the inability in decifering a particular word coincided with the occurrence of a choreiform eye movement. Similarly, the frequent continuation of reading in a wrong line coincided with an involuntary twitch in upward or downward direction (personal observations). However, these observations do not explain dyslexia.

In contrast to this straight forward connection are relationships where the link is considerably less obvious. Comparing choreiform with non-choreiform children at normal elementary schools, Stemmer could not find any association with marks with the exception of marks for writing. The teacher's assessment of intelligence did not differ for the two groups.

Consistent in all studies is the higher incidence of children with moderate and severe choreiform movements in special schools, where the incidence is two to three times higher than in normal schools. The most plausible explanation is the complex association between neurologic dysfunctions and certain traits in behavior and school performance (Wolff & Hurwitz, 1973).

Hertzig (1981) has provided evidence in her 8 year follow-up study of low-birthweight children, that children with minor neurologic dysfunctions are at a higher risk to develop scholastic problems, even if they do not differ on psychometric tests.

CONCLUSION

Choreiform movements are a transient but distinct neurologic sign that can reliably be assessed. They are three to four times more frequently present among boys than girls. The incidence is clearly age-related and was found to be similar in normal school populations in Holland, U.S.A., and Japan. The high incidence of choreiform children in special schools and among juvenile delinquents may be explained by the association of choreiform movements with other minor signs of neural dysfunction and may therefore be an expression of more general neurologic condition.

REFERENCES

Dijkstra J. De prognostische betekenis van neurologische afwijkingen bij pasgeboren kinderen. Thesis, University of Groningen, 1960

Hertzig ME. Neurological “soft” signs in low-birthweight children. Developmental Medicine and Child Neurology, 1981, 23, 778-791

Prechtl HFR, & Stemmer CJ. Ein choreatiformes Syndrom bei Kindern, Wiener Med Wschr, 1959, 109, 461-463

Prechtl HFR, & Stemmer C. The choreiform syndrome in children. Developmental Medicine and Child Neurology, 1962, 4, 119-127

Rutter M, Graham P, & Birch HG. Interrelations between the choreiform syndrome, reading disability and psychiatric disorder in children of 8-11 years. Developmental Medicine and Child Neurology, 1966, 8, 149-159

Rutter M, Graham P, & Yule W. A Neuropsychiatric Study in Childhood. Clinics in Developmental Medicine, Vol 35/36, London, Heinemann, 1970

Stemmer C. Choreiforme bewegingsonrust (een orienterend onderzoek). Thesis, University of Groningen, 1964

Touwen BCL. Examination of the Child with Minor Neurological Dysfunction, 2nd ed. Clinics in Developmental Medicine, Vol 71. London, Heinemann, 1979

Wolff PH, & Hurwitz I. The choreiform syndrome. Developmental Medicine and Child Neurology, 1966, 8, 160-165

Wolff PH, & Hurwitz I. Functional implications of the minimal brain damage syndrome. In Greenblatt M, & Hartmann E (Eds.). Seminars in Psychiatry (Vol. 1). New York: Grune & Stratton, 1973, 105-115

Margaret E. Hertzig

12

Nonfocal Neurological Signs in Low Birthweight Children

Systematic reviews of the literature on the outcome of low birthweight (Abramowitz & Kass, 1966; Benton, 1940; Birch & Gussow, 1970; Davis, 1976; Samaroff & Chandler, 1975) leave little doubt that this condition can have deleterious effects on physical and mental development. The consequences of low birthweight are not uniform, however, and may range from profound physical and mental handicap, through milder degrees of mental retardation, learning disability, emotional and behavioral disturbance; to no discernable disability at all (Davies & Tizard, 1975; Douglas & Gear, 1976; Drillien, 1961; Drillien, Thomson, & Burgoyne, 1980; Fitzhardinge & Ramsay, 1973; Francis-Williams & Davies, 1974; Gunn, Lepore, & Outerbridge, 1983; Janus-Kukulska & Lis; 1966; Kitchen, Ryan, & Richards, et al, 1980). Epidemiologically based investigations have clearly documented an increased frequency of occurrence of nonfocal neurological signs among low birthweight and small for date children (Michelson, Ylinen, & Donner, 1981; Nichols & Chen, 1981). However most investigators tend to view nonspecific deviations in motor, sensory, and integrative functions in low birthweight children at follow-up as incidental findings (Davies & Tizard, 1975; Fitzhardinge, Pope, Arstiakaites, et al, 1976; Fitzhardinge & Steven, 1972). Even Drillien (Drillien et al, 1980), in reporting an association between the minor neurological abnormalities exhibited by some low birthweight children during the first year of life and later suboptimal school performance and adjustment, does not explore relations between concurrently assessed neurologic, cognitive, and behavioral organizations.

This chapter seeks to address this gap in the course of summarizing the finding of a longitudinal study of low birthweight children. Specific con-

SOFT NEUROLOGICAL SIGNS
ISBN 0-8089-1841-9

sideration is directed towards the examination of the relationship between neurological status at 8 years of age and (1) antecedent conditions during pregnancy, birth, and delivery; (2) academic school performance and the presence of psychiatric disturbance, and (3) temperamental organization, in a sample of 66 low birthweight children who had weighed between 1000 and 1750 g at birth and who have been followed through the twelfth year of life. The data deriving from this investigation provide a basis for expanding our understanding of the origin and clinical significance of nonfocal neurological signs as well as of factors that may contribute to variation in outcome among low birthweight children.

DESCRIPTION OF STUDY AND METHODS

The initial sample consisted of a continuous series of 71 socially advantaged infants cared for in 2 premature centers in New York City between 1962 and 1965. Only children who met the following criteria were enrolled in the study: (1) birthweights between 1000 and 1750 g; (2) intact families; (3) social situation of skilled working class or higher; and (4) prenatal registration had occurred during the first trimester and antenatal care had been provided from that time.

Five children were lost to follow-up; of these 2 died, 1 succumbed to "crib death" at 4 weeks of age, and 1 died as a consequence of congenital heart disease at 2 months. An additional 3 families moved to distant areas when their children were 3 months, 5 years, and 6 years old respectively. The remainder of the series, a total of 66 children (31 boys and 35 girls), were followed to at least the eighth year of life. The mean age of the sample at the time of last follow-up was 11 years 8 months.

During the course of the investigations, information has been obtained on (1) the educational and occupational status of the parents; (2) antecedent conditions of the children and their mothers during the perinatal period; (3) clinical neurological status; and (4) behavioral characteristics and temperamental attributes at different age stages of development (Hertzig, 1974; 1981; 1983).

PARENTAL EDUCATION AND OCCUPATIONS

All but 2 of the children's fathers had graduated from high school; 43 (65 percent) had attended college, 28 (42 percent) had graduated from college, and 18 (27 percent) had attended graduate school. All but one of the mothers had graduated from high school; 27 (41 percent) had attended college, 14 (21 percent) had graduated, and 8 (12 percent) had attended graduate school. Thirty (46 percent) of the fathers had occupations at the executive or professional level: these included accountants, engineers, physicians, and professors. Thirteen (20 percent) had clerical, sales, or lower-management jobs, and 23 (35 percent) were skilled workers, artisans, or policemen. Twenty seven (44 percent) of the children had mothers who returned to work before the child's fifth birthday. Of these, 13 were employed full-time and 14 part-time. The occupational distribution of these women was similar to that of their husbands.

At the time of last follow-up, 27 of the children's families were no longer intact; 23 as a consequence of divorce or separation and 4 because of the death of a parent.

ANTECEDENT CONDITIONS

Details of complications of pregnancy, delivery, and neonatal course as well as estimates of gestational age and intra-uterine growth were abstracted from obstetric and neonatal records. The sample included three sets of twins. An additional two children were surviving members of twin pairs, while one child was a twin whose sibling weighed more than 1750 g. Four children (5 percent) were derived from pregnancies that were complicated by first-trimester bleeding, 16 other pregnancies (24 percent) were complicated by third-trimester bleeding, and 5 (7 percent) by preeclampsia. Four children (5 percent) were delivered by cesarean section; 3 of these were repeat sections with the mother in active labor, and 1 was necessitated by the presence of placenta previa.

Gestational age, based on the mother's report of her last menstrual period, ranged from 29 to 39 weeks, with a mean of 32.30 ± 3.19 weeks. Gestational age was estimated to be over 37 weeks in 6 cases. Twenty-eight of the children (42 percent) were small for their gestational dates when the Tanner and Thompson (1970) standards for intrauterine growth were applied. For 20 percent, active resuscitation for the initiation of respiration was required. Postnatal course was complicated by severe respiratory distress, frequent and prolonged periods of apnea, seizures, systemic infections, or jaundice requiring exchange transfusion in 30 percent of cases. In an additional 45 percent, less severe complications including mild respiratory distress, brief and infrequent apneic episodes, or superficial infections of the eyes or umbilicus were noted.

All children were initially nursed in isoletes. Ambient oxygen was monitored frequently and maintained at the lowest concentration possible to prevent cyanosis. Prolonged and severe apnea was treated by manual bag and mask resuscitation. Positive-pressure respirators were not used. Bilirubin levels were determined on all jaundiced infants, and exchange transfusions were performed for an individual bilirubin of 20 mg/100 ml or over. Only one infant received intravenous fluids. Oral feedings were started as soon as possible and consisted of standard formula administered in strengths of 25 calories per ounce of weight for the first 2 or 3 weeks of life and then reduced to 20 calories per ounce. Antibiotics used were penicillin, streptomycin, and chloramphenicol. Length of stay in the nursery ranged from 16 to 86 days with a median of 41 days. Visiting was confined to prescribed hours, and parents were not permitted to handle their infants until they had graduated from the isolettes.

NEUROLOGIC STATUS

First neurological examinations were performed when the infant reached a weight of 2000 g. Subsequent examinations were performed at 6 months, and at 1, 2, 3, 5, and 8 years of age. In all instances the examiner had no knowledge of perinatal events, beyond the fact that the child had been born prematurely. At all ages, localizing signs included standard measures of CNS damage, such as abnormalities in cranial nerves, lateralized dysfunctions, and the presence of pathological reflexes. Between infancy and 5 years, nonfocal signs included disturbances in muscle tone, generalized hyperreflexia, clumsiness of gait, and poor fine motor coordination. The assessment of nonfocal signs at 8 years of age was more complex and was conducted in accordance with procedures initially developed by Lawrence Taft and used in a total population study of mentally retarded children in Aberdeen Scotland (Birch, Richardson, & Baird, 1970). Performance on individual tasks was noted as "within normal limits," "mildly impaired," or "markedly impaired." Tasks were then grouped to permit the development of judgments about the integrity of broader functional areas. As the examination was viewed as a clinical and not a psychometric assessment, no attempt was made to standardize the number of tasks within each of the following functional areas: speech, balance, coordination, gait, sequential finger-thumb opposition, muscle tone, graphesthesia, astereognosis, and choreiform movements. Specific criteria for the assessment of each of these areas of function are fully described in the appendix to this chapter.

All responses were recorded on a specially designed protocol during the course of the examination. Decisions with respect to clinical neurological status were made following review of the entire set of examination protocols by the examiner after an interval of at least 6 months. Between infancy and 5 years of age neurological status was characterized as either "within normal limits" or "abnormal." Abnormalities during this period reflected the presence of any localizing findings and/or any nonfocal signs. More stringent criteria were applied to the examinations conducted at 8 years of age. Children of this age were judged to be neurologically abnormal if (1) any localizing signs of CNS abnormalities were present or (2) if two or more nonlocalizing signs were found. The results of the neurological examinations conducted on 66 children in their eighth year of life are summarized in Table 12-1, where it may be seen that 13 children (7 boys and 6 girls) were found to have localizing findings; 20 children (13 boys and 7 girls) were found to have 2 or more nonlocalizing signs; and 33 children (11 boys and 22 girls) were found to be neurologically normal.

In the analyses to be presented in this chapter, subgroups of low birthweight children are defined in terms of their neurological status at 8 years of age. This decision was based on the following considerations: (1) 93 percent of the original sample of 71 children were examined at this point in time as compared with 75 percent during the first 6 months of life, 70 percent at 1 year, 80 percent at 2 years, 87 percent at 3 years, and 89 percent at 5 years; and (2) the more stringent criteria used to define neurological abnormalities at 8 years permitted a clear distinction to be made between children who displayed localizing and those who displayed nonlocalizing signs. Furthermore, as the data of Table 12-2 indicate, neurological status at 8 years of age did not differ significantly from that determined at earlier points in time.

TEMPERAMENT AND BEHAVIOR

The methods used for the collection of data on temperament and behavior were identical to those utilized in the New York Longitudinal Study (Thomas & Chess, 1977; Thomas et al, 1963; 1968). Parents were the primary source of information with respect to the behavioral characteristics of their children. Interviews were conducted at 6 month intervals during the first 2 years of life and again at 3 years. The interview was designed to elicit detailed descriptions of behavior in everyday life situations. During

Table 12-1
Neurologic Findings at 8 Years of Age

Types of Finding	Male	Female	Total
Localizing signs	7	6	13
Quadriplegia, severe disability	2	2	4
Quadriplegia, moderate disability	0	1	1
Right hemiplegia, moderate disability	0	1	1
Right hemiplegia, mild disability	1	0	1
Left hemiplegia, mild disability	2	0	1
Diplegia, moderate disability	0	1	2
Diplegia, mild disability	1	0	1
Left arm monoplegia	0	1	1
Athetosis. mild disability	0	1	1
Two or more nonlocalizing signs	13	7	20
Balance	7	6	13
Coordination	7	3	10
Choreiform movements	8	0	8
Muscle tone	4	4	8
Gait	3	4	7
Graphesthesia	5	1	6
Finger–thumb opposition	3	2	5
Speech	3	0	3
Astereognosis	2	1	3
Normal	11	22	33
Balance	1	1	2
Finger–thumb opposition	0	2	2
Tone	0	2	2
Gait	1	0	1
Speech	1	0	1
Coordination	0	1	1
Graphesthesia	0	1	1
None	8	15	23

infancy these included routines of feeding, sleeping, dressing, bathing, and diaper changing as well as contact with people. Later interviews also focused on problem-solving behavior, play preferences, and social interactions. The age at which motor and language developmental milestones were achieved was noted. Throughout, emphasis was placed on what and how the children did what they did. Interim reports were obtained annually until 8 years of age and again at 12 years. Changes in familial organization were inquired after and descriptions of the children's behavioral responses

Table 12-2
Stability and Change in Neurologic Status

Age	Status at 8 Years Normal	Abnormal	Total	χ^2	df	p
6 Months						
Abnormal	13	23	36			
Normal	11	6	17	1.8947	1	NS
Total	24	29	53			
1 Year						
Abnormal	5	11	16			
Normal	20	14	34	3.3684	1	NS
Total	25	25	50			
2 Years						
Abnormal	4	15	19			
Normal	25	13	38	3.7647	1	NS
Total	29	28	57			
3 Years						
Abnormal	8	16	24			
Normal	24	14	38	1.1364	1	NS
Total	32	30	62			
5 Years						
Abnormal	7	23	30			
Normal	24	9	33	0.0625	1	NS
Total	31	32	63			

*McNamar Test for significance of changes.

to these and other special events were recorded. In addition, full reports of medical and/or psychiatric consultation and treatment were obtained and school progress was described. Wechsler Intelligence Scale for Children (WISC) IQs, as well as Wide-Range Achievement Test (WRAT) scores in reading and arithmetic, were obtained for each child in the eighth year of life.

Procedures for the analysis of temperament followed those developed in the course of the New York Longitudinal Study. The methods of scoring, together with measures of reliability and validity are fully described in previous publications (Thomas et al, 1963; 1968). In summary, 9 categories of temperament were established by an inductive content analysis of the parent interview protocols covering the first year of life of the first 22 children enrolled in that study. Each child was item-scored to a three point scale established for each category.

To avoid contamination by "halo effects," no successive interviews of a given child were scored contiguously. As the number of scorable items varied from interview protocol to interview protocol, it was necessary to develop a standard method of scaling before quantitative comparisons of temperamental attributes could be undertaken. Standard scores were calculated by converting the raw score in each category to a weighted score, which ranged from 0 to 2. The categories together with their weighted-score points, are summarized in Table 12-3.

The categories are defined as follows:

1. Activity level: The motor component present in the child's functioning.
2. Rhythmicity: The predictability and/or unpredictability in time of such functions as sleep-wake behavior, hunger, feeding patterns, and elimination schedule.
3. Approach-withdrawal: The nature of the initial response to a new stimulus, be it new food, new toy, or new person. Approach responses are positive, whether displayed by mood expression, verbalizations, or motor activity, while withdrawal responses are negative.
4. Adaptability: Responses to new or altered situations over time. In this category, attention is directed towards the ease with which responses can be modified in a desired direction, not on the nature of initial response.
5. Threshold of responsiveness: The intensity level of stimulation that is necessary to evoke a discernible response, irrespective of the specific form the response may take, or the sensory modality affected.
6. Intensity of reaction: The energy level of response, irrespective of its quality or direction.
7. Quality of mood: The amount of pleasant, joyful, and friendly behavior as contrasted with unpleasant, angry, and unfriendly behavior.
8. Distractability: The effectiveness of extraneous environmental stimuli in interfering with or in altering the direction of ongoing behavior.
9. Attention span and persistence: Two categories that are related. "Attention span" concerns the length of time a particular activity is pursued by the child. "Persistence" refers to the continuation of the activity direction.

Table 12-3
Nine Categories of Temperament

Category	Weighted Score
Activity	
High	0
Moderate	1
Low	2
Rhythmicity	
Regular	0
Variable	1
Irregular	2
Adaptability	
Adaptive	0
Variable	1
Nonadaptive	2
Approach–Withdrawal	
Approach	0
Variable	1
Withdrawal	2
Threshold	
High	0
Moderate	1
Low	2
Intensity	
Intense	0
Variable	1
Mild	2
Mood	
Positive	0
Variable	1
Negative	2
Distractibility	
Distractible	0
Variable	1
Nondistractible	2

Validity of the New York Longitudinal Study parents' reports of their children's behavioral characteristics was assessed by subjecting narrative protocols (obtained in the course of 2 direct 4-hour observations conducted at different times within 1 week of the parents' interviews) to the same scoring procedures. Each direct observation was found to agree with the parent's interview at the 1 percent level of confidence. In addition, high levels of both intra- and interscorer reliability at the 90 percent level of confidence were achieved. No separate assessments of validity and reliability were made in the course of the collection and analysis of information obtained from the parents of the low birthweight children, as the two studies were conducted during overlapping time periods by the same personnel.

RESULTS

This chapter will examine three aspects of the data collected in the course of this longitudinal study. Specifically, the relationship of neurological status at 8 years of age to: (1) antecedent conditions of risk; (2) IQ, school performance and psychiatric status; and (3) features of temperamental organization will be explored. The principal focus of consideration will be the comparison of children who exhibited two or more nonfocal neurological signs with those whose neurological examinations were classified as within normal limits.

Neurological Status and Antecedent Conditions of Risk

Despite the fact that the birthweights of these children were confined to a fairly narrow range, there was a wide variation in exposure to additional risk of damage to the central nervous system during the prenatal period. Forty seven (71 percent) of the total sample of 66 children had additional complications. These children were further classified into two groups. Those in which pregnancies had been characterized by bleeding at any time, and/or preeclampsia, as well as those who were small for dates were considered to have sustained additional prenatal complications. Children who had required active resuscitation for the initiation of respiration and/or who experienced severe complications while in the nursery were characterized as having incurred additional postnatal insult. For the purposes of this later classification, nursery complications included one or more of the following conditions: severe respiratory distress, seizures, or frequent and prolonged periods of apnea or jaundice requiring exchange transfusions.

When these criteria were applied, 12 babies (18 percent of the entire sample) were designated as having sustained both prenatal and postnatal complications. Another 27 babies (40 percent) had prenatal complications only, and exclusively postnatal complications occurred in 8 (12 percent). Nineteen of the 66 babies had experienced no complications additional to that of low birthweight.

As may be seen in Table 12-4, 17 of the 33 neurologically normal children (51 percent) were entirely free of additional complications, but this was the case for only 1 child with localizing findings and for only 1 with nonfocal neurological signs. Thus, children with both localizing and non-localizing neurological or clinical examination differed significantly from the normal in this regard ($\chi^2 = 16.6572$, df = 2, $p < 0.001$). Moreover the proportion of children sustaining prenatal complications was virtually identical in the two neurologically impaired groups.

The pattern of association between type of complication and neurological status at 8 years is also of interest. Of the 47 children who sustained perinatal complications additional to that of low birthweight, 31 had abnormal neurological findings at 8 years of age. However, a history of prenatal complications was found significantly more frequently among children who subsequently developed nonfocal neurological signs, while children with localizing findings were more likely to have had postnatal complications (Table 12-5).

IQ, School Performance, and Behavior

The mean IQs and reading and arithmetic quotients (Jastak & Bijou, 1946) of the neurologically normal and NFNS groups are compared in Table 12-6. Although the mean scores of the neurologically normal

Table 12-4
Perinatal Complications in Relation to Neurologic Status at 8 Years of Age

	Hard Signs	NFNS	Normal	Total
Perinatal complications	12	19	16	47
No perinatal complications	1	1	17	19
Total	13	20	33	66

$\chi^2 = .6572$, df = 2, $p < 0.001$

Table 12-5
Type of Perinatal Complications in Relation to Neurologic Abnormalities

	Hard Signs	NFNS	Total
Perinatal complications	4	14	18
Prenatal plus postnatal complications	8	5	13
Total	12	19	31

$\chi^2 = 4.9189$, df = 1, $p < 0.05$

children were consistently higher, no difference between the groups was statistically significant. This examination of group differences suggests that little significance can be attached to the presence of nonfocal neurological signs. However, a more individualized approach to the data does not wholly support this interpretation.

At the time of last follow-up, school performance and adjustment was considered to be entirely adequate in all but 4 of the 33 neurologically normal children (12 percent). One of the four was reported by his parents to be "just getting by"; another was receiving supplementary reading instructions; and the remaining two children were receiving speech therapy.

In contrast, 9 of the 20 children (45 percent) with NFNS were reported to be doing poorly in school or to require special educational intervention. One of these children had been placed in a special class for brain-injured. Although the other eight attended regular classes, four were enrolled in remedial reading and/or mathematics programs; one was receiving special tutoring to maintain barely passing grades; two were reported by their schools to be failing and to be exhibiting emotional problems; and one

Table 12-6
WISC IQ and WRAT Reading and Arithmetic Quotients in the Neurologically Normal and NFNS Groups

	Neurologically Normal			NFNS			
Quotients	No.	Mean	SD	No.	Mean	SD	p
IQ	33	111.55	13.16	20	105.05	15.59	NS
Reading	33	116.85	25.74	20	112.00	29.00	NS
Arithmetic	33	102.52	10.85	20	97.05	12.71	NS

child was receiving speech therapy in school. The difference between the two groups was statistically significant ($\chi^2 = 7.2719$, df = 1, $p < 0.01$).

The frequency into which psychiatric consultation was requested also differed significantly between the two groups. Neurologic status, presenting complaints, and age at which consultation was requested are summarized in Table 12-7. Five children (15 percent) in the neurologically normal group were referred for psychiatric consultation as compared with 10 (50 percent) of those with nonfocal neurological signs ($\chi^2 = 7.4527$, df = 1, $p < 0.01$). Moreover, both severity and chronicity tended to be less pronounced in the neurologically normal children.

In the neurologically normal group, case #333 was seen at the age of 4 ½ years because of parental concern about the child's willfulness and stubborness, but the diagnostic impression was that she was a normal child and follow-up reports indicated no further difficulties. Two other children were seen — one at 6 years (case #111), and one at 8 years (case #321) — because of complaints of frequent temper tantrums and lack of interest in school. Psychiatric opinion was that both children's behavior disorders were reactions to parental separation, and in both instances follow-up reports revealed that all symptoms had subsided with the stabilization of

Table 12-7
Presenting Complaints in LBW Children Who Came to Psychiatric Notice

Case Number	Age at Notice	Neurologic Status	Presenting Complaint*									
			IDL	OA	TT	A/D	IPC	O	OD	PPR	PSP	RB
333	4.5	Negative						+	+			
111	6.0	Negative			+						+	
326	7.5	Negative								+	+	
321	8.0	Negative			+						+	
323	8.0	Negative								+		
334	2.0	NFNS		+	+	+	+					
114	2.5	NFNS	+									+
130	4.0	NFNS	+	+	+							
131	2.5	NFNS	+	+	+							
122	5.0	NFNS		+		+	+				+	
103	6.0	NFNS	+	+			+				+	
331	6.0	NFNS	+	+		+	+			+	+	
116	6.0	NFNS			+		+				+	
108	7.0	NFNS	+				+				+	
324	7.0	NFNS	+		+					+	+	

*IDL = immaturity, developmental lag; OA = overactivity; TT = temper tantrums; A/D = aggressive destructive; IPC = inattentive, poor concentration; O = oppositional; OD = overly demanding; PDR = poor peer relations; PSP = poor school performance; RB = ritualistic behavior; A = anxious.

living arrangements. In another child (case #326), first seen at the age of 7 ½ years, excessive negativism and attention-seeking behavior was also thought to be a reaction to parental separation. However, consultation was requested at the age of 15 because of persistantly poor school performance. The fifth child in the group (case #323), was reported by her mother to be receiving treatment for chronic anxiety and poor peer relationships.

In the group with nonfocal neurological signs, requests for psychiatric consultation were made for five children during the preschool years. One child (case #114) was first seen at the age of 2 ½ years for evaluation of a language lag. Reevaluation at 7 and 13 years revealed that although language had developed relatively normally, he had become isolated, withdrawn, and friendless. He had idiosyncratic preoccupations, and had performed poorly in school. The remaining four children who first came to clinic notice in the preschool period presented with "hyperactivity." For one boy (case #131), this symptom, together with disractability, short attention span, and borderline normal intelligence resulted in special school placement. The others did reasonably well in elementary school, but two have developed additional symptoms in early adolescence: one (case #334) is undergoing treatment for persistent anxiety, and further consultation has been requested for the other child (case #130) because of frequent temper outbursts and increasing social isolation.

Of the five children with nonfocal neurological signs who came to notice after the age of 6 years, 4 were referred because of their school's concerns about immaturity and unreadiness to enter the first grade. Two of these children had moderately impaired hearing and subsequently developed evidence of specific learning disability. One (case #116) has done well and is now successfully attending private school, but the other (case #123) has developed symptoms of school refusal requiring treatment. Two other children also proved to have learning disabilities: one of these children's symptoms of impulsivity worsened after his parent's divorce and he is currently receiving psychotherapy as well as a modified educational program (case #108). The other child's mother reports her as meddlesome, poorly coordinated, and relatively friendless. She receives remedial instruction in school, but no other therapy (case #331). Formal consultation was sought at the age of 7 for the final child in this group (case #324), who was reported to be friendless, unhappy, a management problem at home and doing poorly in school. The diagnostic impression was that she had a reactive behavior disorder and she has been receiving treatment since the age of 11 years.

Temperament in Children with Nonfocal Neurologic Signs

In this chapter, examination of the relationship of temperament to neurological status is confined to a consideration of "difficult" temperament. Thomas and Chess's (1977) clinical description of the "difficult child" has provided the basis for the construction of an "index of difficulty" that is the linear combination of the following five temperamental attributes: rhythmicity, adaptability, approach-withdrawal, intensity, and mood. The higher the numerical value of this index, the more "difficult" the child. The means and standard deviations for the entire sample of LBW children and for each of the neurologically defined subgroups at 1, 2, and 3 years are presented in Table 12-8, and the results of an ANOVA relating "difficulty" to neurological status and age are presented in Table 12-9.

As the data of Table 12-9 indicate, this constellation of developmental attributes is significantly different in children who differ with respect to neurological status. In particular, children with nonlocalizing findings are more difficult than those whose neurological examinations are within normal limits, but less difficult than those with localizing finding. However, the statistical interaction between "degree of difficulty" and age was not significant, indicating that trends over time were similar in all three neurologically defined subgroups. Thus all children, whether they had localizing neurological findings, had two or more nonfocal signs, or were without clinical evidence of neurological abnormality were more "difficult" during the second year of life than at any other time during the preschool period. The increase in degree of "difficulty" is a reflection of the tendency

Table 12-8
"Index of Difficulty" in Neurologically Defined Subgroups of Birthweight Children

	Year 1			Year 2			Year 3		
Findings	n	M	SD	n	M	SD	n	M	SD
Localizing findings	13	2.40	.66	13	2.59	1.05	11	1.79	.82
Nonlocalizing findings	20	2.14	.90	19	2.34	.48	19	2.02	.90
Negative findings	33	1.91	.72	33	1.99	.70	31	1.69	.98
Total	66	2.07	.78	64	2.21	.76	61	1.81	.93

Table 12-9
ANOVA Relating "Index of Difficulty" to Neurologic Status and Age in Low Birthweight Children

Source	Sum of Squares	Mean Square	df	F	p
Neurological status	74186.86	37093.43	2	3.85	<.05
Year	45872.79	22936.40	2	4.59	<.01
Neurological status X year	8681.53	2170.38	4	.43	ns
Subject (neurological)	606493.01	9626.87	63		
Residual error	594480.66	4995.64	119		
Total	1324341.73				

exhibited by children in each of the neurologically defined subgroups to become increasingly intense and nonadaptive in their responses at this point in time (Hertzig, 1983).

The fact that changes in degree of "difficulty" during the first 3 years of life were essentially independent of neurological status makes it possible to consider the entire preschool period as a unit when examining the relations between behavior disturbance, neurological status and "difficulty." The following analyses are based on this strategy, which involved the determination of a composite "index of difficulty" for each child by averaging the "difficulty" scores obtained at 1, 2, and 3 years of age. When this was done it was found that children who came to psychiatric notice were significantly more "difficult" during the first 3 years of life. The mean composite "index of difficulty" among those for whom psychiatric consultation was requested (irrespective or whether they were clinically neurologically normal or had nonfocal neurological signs) was 2.25 ± 0.39 as contrasted with 1.86 ± 0.59 for the remainder (t = 2.81, df = 50, $p < 0.01$). However, within the group of children with 2 or more nonfocal neurological signs, those who came to psychiatric notice were no more difficult than those who did not. The mean composite "index of difficulty" for the 10 children with nonfocal neurological signs for whom psychiatric consultation was requested was 2.26 ± 0.44, as constrasted with 2.02 ± 0.61 for the remaining children with nonfocal neurological signs (t = 1.01, df = 18, NS).

DISCUSSION

It is difficult to make direct comparisons between the findings of this study and the results of other follow-up studies of low birthweight infants (Abramowicz & Kass, 1966; Davies & Tizard 1975; Drillien 1961; 1967;

Drillien et al, 1980; Fitzhardinge & Ramsay 1973; Francis-Williams & Davies, 1974; Janus-Kukulska & Lis, 1966; Kitchen et al, 1980) because of differences in the methods of sample selection, the range of birthweights included, the proportion of infants in the different samples who were small for dates, patterns of neonatal intensive care, age at follow-up, and aspects of function assessed. Nevertheless, the findings described here are consistent with those of previous reports in indicating wide variability in the degree of both neurological impairment and behavioral dysfunction exhibited by low birthweight children. Of the 53 (80 percent of the total sample) children who were without localizing neurological findings, 20 (38 percent) were found to have 2 or more nonfocal neurological signs during clinical assessment conducted at 8 years of age. This finding underscores the association between LBW and NFNS and provides an opportunity for the further exploration of both the origin and functional significance of nonfocal neurological signs.

Shaffer (Shaffer, O'Conner, Shafer, & Prupis, 1983), in reviewing the literature on the origin of nonfocal neurological signs has summarized theories of etiology as including brain damage, nonspecific developmental lag, genetically determined individual differences, or epiphenomena influenced by learning, motivation, attention, or stress. While the data of the present study do not contribute to our understanding of the contribution of either presumed genetic factors or stress to performance on clinical neurological examination, they do confirm the etiologic importance of perinatal risk conditions for both localizing and nonlocalizing neurological abnormality.

However, the pattern of association between type of neurological finding and type of perinatal risk condition suggests that nonfocal and focal neurological signs may well be etiologically distinct.

It appears that whereas nonfocal signs may emerge as a consequence of general developmental disability associated with the complications of pregnancy and failure to grow at expected rates, localizing findings are associated more directly with the effects of such postnatal conditions as respiratory distress, apneic episodes, jaundice, or seizures in a growing and developing nervous system. A high frequency of such conditions among low birthweight babies during the first days and weeks of life is well known and has been attributed to the immaturity of biologic mechanisms underlying these functions. The relative immunity to postnatal complications of the small dates babies in the present study may be a reflection of their relative gestational maturity, and thus their ability to withstand the demands of extrauterine existance in spite of low birthweight.

As for the clinical significance of nonfocal neurological signs, the data from the present study clearly demonstrate that the presence of nonfocal signs is compatible with the normal development of intellectual function, academic school achievement, and behavioral organization in at least half of children so affected. Thus, the findings are consistent with the numerous reports of the occurrence of nonfocal signs in many otherwise normally developing children (Adams, Kocsis, & Estes, 1974; Peters, Romine, & Dykman, 1975; Rutter, Tizard, & Whitmore, 1970; Wolff & Hurwitz, 1966). These findings are also consistent with Shaffer's contention (Shaffer et al, 1983) that the base rate of nonfocal neurological signs in the general population is too high for their detection to be of any clinical value for either screening or prediction.

On the other hand, despite normal intelligence and no significant differences in IQ between the groups, almost half of the children with nonfocal signs required special educational interventions to reach the same overall level of academic school performance achieved by the children who were clinically neurologically intact, 90 percent of whom made satisfactory progress without any modification of school program. This finding, coupled with the high frequency of psychiatric consultation and continuing intervention among the children with nonfocal neurological signs, provides support for the view that these children are indeed at greater risk for the emergence of behavioral and/or school learning problems.

In addition, neurologically defined subgroups of low birthweight children were found to differ systematically in relation to that constellation of temperamental attributes that Thomas and Chess (1977) have labeled the "difficult child." The mean "index of difficulty" reflecting a temperamental pattern of irregularity in biological functioning, occurring in conjunction with an increased tendency to withdraw in new situations, slow adaptability to change, and intense and negative mood, was significantly higher among children with nonfocal neurological signs.

Furthermore, as would be expected in light of the previously reported association between degree of difficulty and behavioral disturbance (Thomas & Chess, 1977), the children of the present sample who came to clinical notice were significantly more "difficult" during the first 3 years of life than were those whose behavior did not lead their parents to request psychiatric consultation. In addition, children with NFNS were significantly more likely to be brought for evaluation than were those who were without clinical evidence of CNS abnormality or dysfunction.

These two sets of findings would appear to suggest that the increased risk of psychiatric disorder among children with nonfocal neurological signs (Shaffer et al, 1983) might well be a consequence of the increased risk of "difficulty" exhibited by these children. Carey (Carey, McDevitt, & Baker, 1979), in a cross-sectional study, has also found that the most "difficult" children among those referred because of behavioral and/or school learning problems were those with clinical neurological findings. Among the children with NFNS in the present sample, however, "difficulty" during the first 3 years of life was not predictive of later behavioral disturbance.

Thus in this sample of LBW children temperament and neurologic status appears to be independently associated with an increased risk of behavioral disturbance. Moreover, the clinical characteristics of the children who came to psychiatric notice are not uniform; they ranged from symptoms characteristic of attention deficit disorder to those more typical of neurotic or reactive behavioral disturbances. This variability suggests that although increased vulnerability may well play a role in the pathogenesis of psychiatric disorder in general, specific symptoms come to be defined in the course of the interaction between a particular child and his familial and broader social environments.

Rutter (1977) too, has suggested that in addition to its effect on temperament and personality, brain damage may lead to psychiatric disturbance through its impact on cognitive capacity as well as on the organization of familial patterns of response. The data of the present study are entirely consistent with the view that the identification of conditions of risk is but one aspect of the multifaceted psychiatric assessment required to provide the data base necessary for the development of appropriate strategies of intervention.

REFERENCES

Abramowicz M, & Kass EM. Pathogenesis and prognosis of prematurity. New England Journal of Medicine, 1966, 275, 878-885, 938-943, 1001-1007, 1053-1059

Adams RM, Kocsis J, & Estes RE. Soft neurologic signs in learning disabled children and controls. American Journal of Diseases of Children, 1974, 128, 614-618

Benton A. Mental development of prematurely born children. American Journal of Orthopsychiatry, 1940, 10, 719-746

Birch HG, & Gussow JD. Disadvantaged Children. Health, Nutrition and School Failure. New York: Harcourt, Brace and World, Inc., 1970

Birch HG, Richardson SA, Baird D, et al. Mental Subnormality in the

Community. A Clinical and Epidemiologic Study. Baltimore: Williams and Wilkins, 1970

Carey WB, McDevitt SC, & Baker D. Differentiating minimal brain dysfunction and temperament. Developmental Medicine and Child Neurology, 1979, 21, 765-772

Davies P. Outlook for the low birthweight baby. Then and now. Archives of Diseases in Children, 1976, 51, 817-819

Davies PA, & Tizard JPM. Very low-birthweight and subsequent neurological deficit. Developmental Medicine and Child Neurology, 1975, 17, 3-17

Douglas JWB, & Gear R. Children of low-birthweight in the 1946 national cohort. Behavior and educational achievement in adolescence. Archives of Diseases in Childhood, 1976, 51, 820-827

Drillien CM. The incidence of mental and physical handicaps in school aged children of very low birthweight. Pediatrics, 1961, 27, 452-464

Drillien CM. The incidence of mental and physical handicaps in school age children of very low birthweight: II. Pediatrics, 1967, 39, 238-247

Drillien CM, Thomson AJM, & Burgoyne K. Low birthweight children at early school age: A longitudinal study. Developmental Medicine and Child Neurology, 1980, 22, 26-47

Fitzhardinge PM, & Steven EM. The small for date infant. II. Neurological and intellectual sequelae. Pediatrics, 1972, 50, 50-57

Fitzhardinge PM, & Ramsay M. The improving outlook for the small prematurely born infant. Developmental Medicine and Child Neurology, 1973, 16, 709-728

Fitzhardinge PM, Pope K, Arstiakaites M, et al. Mechanical ventilation of infants of less than 1,501 gm. birthweight: Health, growth and neurologic sequelae. The Journal of Pediatrics, 1976, 88, 531-541

Francis-Williams J, & Davies PA. Very low-birthweight and later intelligence. Developmental Medicine and Child Neurology, 1974, 16, 709-728

Gunn TR, Lepore E, & Outerbridge EW. Outcome at school-age after neonatal mechanical ventilation. Developmental Medicine and Child Neurology, 1983, 25, 305-314

Hertzig ME. Neurologic findings in prematurely born children at school age. In Rolf M, & Thomas A (Eds.). Proceedings of the Fifth Conference of the Society for Life History Research. Mineapolis: University of Minnesota Press, 1974

Hertzig ME. Neurologic "soft" signs in low birthweight children. Developmental Medicine and Child Neurology, 1981, 21, 778-791

Hertzig ME. Temperament and neurologic status. In Rutter M (Ed.). Developmental Neuropsychiatry, New York: The Guilford Press, 1983

Janus-Kukulska A, & Lis S. Developmental peculiarities of prematurely born children with birthweight below 1250 g. Developmental Medicine and Child Neurology, 1966, 8, 285-295

Jastak J, & Bijou S. Wide Range Achievement Test. Wilmington, DE: C.L. Story, 1946

Kitchen WH, Ryan MM, Rickards A, et al. A longitudinal study of very low-birthweight infants. IV. An overview of performance at eight years of age. Developmental Medicine and Child Neurology, 1980, 17, 63-78

Michelson K, Ylinen A, & Donner M. Neurodevelopmental screening at five years of children who were at risk neonatally. Developmental Medicine and Child Neurology, 1981, 23, 427-433

Nichols PL, & Chen T. Minimal Brain Dysfunction. A Prospective Study. Hillsdale, NJ, Lawrence Erlbaum Associates, 1981

Peters JE, Romine JS, & Dykman RA. A special neurological examination of children with learning disabilities. Developmental Medicine and Child Neurology, 1975, 17, 63-78

Rutter M. Brain damage syndromes in childhood: Concepts and findings. Journal of Child Psychology and Psychiatry, 1977, 18, 1-21

Rutter M, Tizard J, & Whitmore K. Education, Health and Behavior. London: Longmans, 1970

Samaroff A, & Chandler MJ. Reproductive risk and the continuum of caretaking casuality. In Horowitz TD (Ed.). Review of Child Development Research. Chicago: University of Chicago Press, 1975

Shaffer D, O'Connor P, Shafer SQ, & Prupis S. Neurological "soft signs:" Their origins and significance for behavior. In Rutter M (Ed.). Developmental Neuropsychiatry, New York: Guilford Press, 1983

Tanner JM, & Thomson AM. Standards for birthweight at gestation periods from 32 to 42 weeks allowing for maternal height and weight. Archives of Disease in Childhood, 1970, 45, 566-569

Thomas A, & Chess S. Temperament and Development. New York: Brunner/Mazel, 1977

Thomas A, Chess S, Birch HG, et al. Behavioral Individuality in Early Childhood. New York: New York University Press, 1963

Thomas A, Chess S, & Birch HG. Temperament and Behavior Disorders in Children. New York: New York University Press, 1968

Wolff PH, & Hurwitz J. The choreiform syndrome. Developmental Medicine Child Neurology, 1966, 8, 160-165

APPENDIX

The assessment of nonfocal neurological signs was conducted in accordance with the following criteria:

Speech. Each child was engaged in sufficient informal conversation to permit the assessment of clarity and intelligibility. Word-sound production was rated according to the examiner's difficulty in comprehending it. Marked impairment of speech was designated as a "soft" sign.

Balance. Balance was designated as a "soft" sign if performance on at least two of the following three tasks was markedly impaired:

(1) Standing balance. The child was required to stand still for 30 seconds with eyes closed, feet together, arms extended, and fingers spread apart. Marked impairment reflected three or more back and forth movements of the body exceeding one inch of each direction during the observation period.

(2) Hopping. The child was asked to hop ten times consecutively on each foot. Failure to hop at least five times consecutively on both feet was taken as marked impairment.

(3) Walking a line in tandem. The child was asked to take ten steps, placing the heel directly in front of the toe of the other foot (as in walking on a tightrope) with his arms at his side. A failure to approximate heel and toe for at least five consecutive steps reflected marked impairment.

Coordination. Coordination was designated as a "soft" sign if performance on at least two of the following four tasks was markedly impaired:

(1) Finger-to-nose. The child was required to extend each arm laterally and touch his or her index finger to the tip of his or her nose five times with each hand with the eyes open. The sequence was repeated with the eyes closed. Failure to touch the tip of the nose at least three times with both hands with eyes closed indicated impairment.

(2) Alternating pronation/supination. The child stood with one arm relaxed at his or her side and the other elbow flexed at 90° with the hand pointing forward. The child was requested to pronate and supinate the extended hand quickly five times and to repeat the task using the other hand. Impairment was indicated by the movement of both elbows a distance of four or more inches during execution of the alternating hand-movements.

(3) Foot taps. The child was seated in a straight chair and asked to tap the toe of each foot ten times in succession, keeping his or her heel on the floor. The child was then asked to tap both feet together an additional ten times. Failure to sustain simultaneous toe taps indicated impairment.

(4) Heel-shin. The child was again seated in a straight chair with legs extended. The child was required to move one heel down the shin of the opposite leg, from the knee to the big toe, without losing contact. The task was repeated two times with each leg. Impairment was indicated by two or more losses of contact on each of the four trials.

Gait. Gait was observed as the child walked back and forth for a distance of 20 feet. The presence of at least two of the following was designated a "soft" sign: a base wider than ten inches, failure to alternate flexion and extension of the knees smoothly, and absence of a heel-toe gait or immobility of the arms.

Sequential finger-thumb opposition. This task required the child to imitate the examiner in the opposition of thumb to fingers in the sequence: index, fourth, middle, pinky, pinky, middle, fourth, index. The child was requested to repeat each movement before the next was illustrated. The performance of both hands was assessed. Imitative movements were designated a "soft" sign if at least two errors not spontaneously corrected occured with each hand.

Muscle tone. This was assessed in accordance with the procedure described by Rutter et al (1970). Tone in the upper limbs was tested by (1) flapping the hand while holding the lower forearm still; (2) plantar and dorsiflexion of the wrist; (3) flexing and extending the elbow; and (4) dorsiflexing the wrist and bending the fingers back. Tone in the lower limbs was tested by (1) holding the thigh above the knee with the leg hanging and swinging the lower leg, and (2) testing the range of motion of the ankle. In order to ensure that the extremity was limp while these movements were carried out, the child was engaged in conversation about something else to divert his or her attention from the examiner's manipulation. Tone was recorded separately for all four extremities. For tone to be designated a "soft" sign, finding of marked hypotonic or hypertonia in all four extremities was required.

Graphesthesia. Seated with eyes closed, and the hand positioned vertically, with palms facing the examiner, the child was asked to name the letters or numbers he or she felt being written on the palm. A ballpoint pen, with the point retracted, was used to trace the following symbols: right hand 3, a, 2; left hand 8, c, R. If errors were made the child was asked to name the symbols. Graphesthesia was designated as a "soft" sign if at least two failures on each hand occurred in the face of accurate naming.

Astereognosis. By feeling them with each hand in turn, with eyes closed, the child was asked to identify a pocket comb, a key, a quarter, and a penny. Manipulation was permitted but not transfer. After the entire sequence was administered, the objects were shown and the child asked to name them. Stereognosis was classified as a "soft" sign if there were three tactual failures in the face of accurate visual identification.

Choreiform movements. Assessment was made on the basis of the procedure developed by Prechtl and Stemmer (1962). The child was asked to assume the position previously described for the assessment of standing balance, while the examiner watched for small jerky twitches occuring in the fingers, wrist, joints, arms, and shoulders. Choreiform movments were designated a "soft" sign if 10 or more twitches were observed within a 30-second period.

All responses were recorded on a specially designed protocol during the course of the examination. A child was judged to be neurologically abnormal if (1) any localizing signs of central nervous system abnormality were present, or (2) two or more nonlocalizing signs were found. The neurological examination of children without any localizing findings or with fewer than two "soft" signs was considered to be within normal limits.

REFERENCES

Prechtl H, & Stemmer C. The choreiform syndrome in children. Developmental Medicine and Child Neurology, 1962, 4, 119-127

Rutter M, Graham P, & Yule W. A Neuropsychiatric Study in Childhood: Clinics in Developmental Medicine No. 35/36. London: S.I.M.P. with Heinemann: Philadelphia: Lippincott, 1970

Part III

Meaning

Bert C.L. Touwen

13

The Meaning and Value of Soft Signs in Neurology

The term "soft signs" can easily lead to semantic discussions. "Soft" in this connotation is associated with "changeable," "unreliable," and "badly defined" (Concise Oxford Dictionary). If soft signs were as bad as that, they would not be worth talking about. Still quite a few authors use the term, and not always in a derogatory manner. The term is ambiguous, however, and leads to confusion. For instance, Hertzig (1981) after an extensive study, concludes that soft signs may confidently be considered to reflect a primary disturbance in the organization of the central nervous system; but Adams, Kocsis, and Estes (1974) see them only as neurological variations. For Rie, Rie, Stewart, and Rettemnier (1978) the word soft reflects the subjective meaning of the signs, whereas Neligan, Kolvin, Scott, and Garside (1976) define soft signs as having a less evident structural basis than hard signs, which by definition indicate an abnormality of structure. To show some of the confusion of the use of the term, Denckla's (1972) opinion can be forwarded: she states that soft signs are signs that can be consciously feigned by a malingerer, or subconsciously be chosen as a conversion symptom. This sounds rather nonneurological, or referring to more than neurology only; however, she also states that soft signs can be observed as a single manifestation in a certain percentage of so called normal people, but that clusters of soft signs may form hard syndromes, such as Huntington's chorea. In 1978 Denckla appears to single out neurological soft signs as a more or less distinct category consisting of signs of (mild) developmental delay or of light manifestations of traditional neurological abnormalities (Denckla, 1978). In this she follows Rutter, Graham, and Yule (1970).

SOFT NEUROLOGICAL SIGNS
ISBN 0-8089-1841-9

The term "soft" can be replaced by the term "minor," which sounds more neutral. It is doubtful whether this would be very useful as the delineation of minor versus major is probably as complex and difficult as that of soft versus hard (Touwen & Sporrel, 1979). The main problem lies in the significance of the soft (or minor or equivocal) signs: what do they mean and in which way do they contribute to diagnosis. From the point of view of the author of this paper "diagnosis" means "neurological diagnosis." As will be discussed in this chapter, a neurological diagnosis primarily describes a child's neurological condition. It may or may not contribute to a better understanding of a child's behavior at home or at school.

DEFINITION

For the purpose of this chapter soft signs are defined as mild (minor, slight) signs or symptoms that can be observed reliably and consistently during an appropriate neurological assessment carried out by a well-trained examiner. This definition excludes signs or symptoms that involve complex mental operations, such as special concentration or attention, motivation or understanding, or which belong to complex everyday behavior. For example, hyperactivity is not to be considered as a (soft) sign, although neurological soft signs may be involved in awkward or clumsy hyperactivity. Slight coordination difficulties or choreiform dyskinesia are considered soft signs; however, temper tantrums, which may result from continual failures in fine motor activities, can be called behavioral signs (soft or not) but they are not neurological (soft) signs. Also, concentration problems or attention span difficulties are not neurological signs, however important they may be for the child's behavior and for the standardization of the neurological assessment. The search is for the relation between such signs and neurological signs, and, if a statistical relation is found, for an answer to the question whether there is any causality.

The definition also excludes deviant performances in which, besides neurological function per se, nonneurological factors are involved such as intelligence, specific learning capacities, and experience. Examples are poor handwriting, age-inadequate drawing, an inability to dress or to close buttons, to handle scissors, or to put small beads on a cord. These functional abilities imply quite a few neurological functions, which in the case of failure should be examined carefully and specifically.

The question is: what is the meaning of neurological signs of very mild intensity with regard to neurological diagnosis and prediction. Inherent in this question is the notion that the label "soft signs" is not a diagnosis. Identification and particularization of the signs has to precede the question of their interpretation (Carey, McDevitt, & Baker, 1979).

ELICITATION AND RELIABILITY

Many authors have stated that a serious problem with soft signs is the difficulty in elicitation and/or replication (Denckla, 1972; Rie et al, 1978; Rutter, 1977; Rutter et al, 1970; Schain, 1970; 1977). This sounds rather inconsistent. A sign or a symptom that is too vague or diffuse to be clearly and repeatedly observable or elicitable, should not be considered as a proper sign or symptom. It merely reflects soft methods (Page-El & Grossman, 1973). Of course the assessment technique should be appropriate and properly applied. This requirement is of great importance. The developmental neurological maxim that the developing brain's properties, which are age specific, must be respected, so that the examination technique must be accurately adapted to the child's age, is too often neglected (Prechtl, 1972; 1977; Touwen, 1978; 1979). But also with an appropriate assessment technique, a sign is a sign only when it is clearly observable and repeatedly elicitable.

Indications for a Neurological Examination

Three main indications for a neurological examination can be formulated.

1. A child may be referred for neurological assessment because of specific complaints that suggest a neurological origin. Suddenly or insidiously arising problems of posture or motility, diplopia, dizziness, or headaches are examples. In such cases even slight signs of neurological dysfunction may be an indication — an early sign — of an underlying neurological disease, and often repeated examinations are needed to find out whether there is a progressive disorder.
2. Patients may be referred who are known to suffer from a non-neurological disease, and in whom neurological complications are suspected. Leukemia and diabetes mellitus are examples. Again often repeated neurological assessments are required to answer the question of neurological involvement.

3. Nowadays many children referred for a neurological examination belong to a category of patients who have vague or unspecific complaints, which may or may not have anything to do with specific brain function. Behavioral problems and learning difficulties are included in this category of complaints. Remarkably the term "soft signs" is mainly used in connection with such patients. The difference with the two other groups of referrals lies in the empirical fact that in the case of the former two generally time will solve the diagnostic problem, as the neurological disorder will usually be progressive. This will occur hardly ever in the case of children with behavioral and educational problems. Nevertheless, a proper understanding of the significance of possible neurological symptomatology in children with behavioral problems is important, as the presence or absence of such symptomatology may in some instances help to elucidate the behavioral problem. Therefore, in the remainder of this chapter the main focus will be on this category of referrals.

DEVELOPMENTAL DELAY AND NEUROLOGICAL DEVIANCY

The neurological phenomena that are commonly considered as "soft signs" can be divided into two classes: retardation signs and deviant signs in a narrower sense (Rutter, 1977; Rutter et al, 1970; Schain, 1977; Touwen, 1979). A maturational lag as the major origin of the signs was first advanced by Bender (1947), although she also suggested cerebral dysfunction as an origin, and a lag has since been advocated by many authors (e.g., Adams et al, 1974; Barlow, 1974; Kinsbourne, 1973; 1974; Schmitt, 1975; Sommers, 1982). Others have queried this conception (Denckla & Rudel, 1978; Hertzig, 1981; Rie et al, 1978), arguing that a disturbance of the central nervous system may easily lead to a functional retardation, without a retardation being the primary cause of the symptomatology. According to Hertzig (1981) the presence of soft signs may merely reflect an increased vulnerability of the brain during development; at a certain age a combination may be found of signs of developmental delay (neurologically, but also regarding complex behavior) and signs of dysfunction proper. For an adequate evaluation of the child's condition the signs must be differentiated in order to promote proper treatment (Denckla, 1978; Rie et al, 1978).

RETARDATION-SIGNS

Retardation-signs are themselves normal phenomena, which should occur at a younger age than at the actual age when they are found. They may consist of reactions that actually should have disappeared at the age of the examination, such as a persisting plantar grasp reaction, or a (usually phasic) dorsiflexion and spreading of the toes on stimulation of the footsole. A delay in the development of motor functions — in which the performance as such is normal, but incongruous to the child's age — is also a retardation-sign. The delay may be found in gross motor functions, such as walking on tiptoe or on heels, standing on one foot or hopping, and in fine motor functions such as diadochokinesia, fingertip-nose-test, finger-opposition-test etc. (See Touwen, 1979, Table 13-1.)

For a proper evaluation of a developmental delay age-norms are a prerequisite. Age-norms are often either lacking or useless because they are based on various populations, various operationalizations of the functions and reactions and various standardizations of the test-techniques. In some instances developmental-test-scales, e.g., the Denver Developmental Screening Test (Frankenburg & Dodds, 1971; Frankenburg, Goldstein, & Camp, 1971), the Knobloch-Pasamanick Developmental Screening Inventory (Knobloch, Pasamanick, & Sherard, 1966), the Bayley scales (Bayley, 1969), offer norms for a few gross motor functions, but usually up to the age of 6 years only. Fine motor performances are usually described and tested

Table 13-1
Retardation Signs

A. Neurological Items
   1. Age-inadequate mirror and other associated movements, e.g.:
      mouth-opening finger-spreading phenomenon
      a.m. accompanying walking on tiptoe and on heels
      mirror movements accompanying one-sided diadochokinesia
   2. Age-inadequate diadochokinesia
   3. Age-inadequate fingertip–nose, knee–heel, fingertip-touching, finger-opposition, circle tests
   4. Persisting plantar grasp response or (phasic) dorsiflexion of the big toe on the foot sole response.

B. Developmental delay of complex motor functions, such as
   1. Walking on tiptoe or on heels
   2. Standing on one foot
   3. Hopping on one foot
   4. Heel–toe gait

as complex skills in which many neurological mechanisms are involved. Norms for specific neurological tests such as coordination and fine manipulative abilities are virtually absent. Moreover, environmental influences including socioeconomical and cultural and even ethnographical factors may substantially influence normative values. Thus, each examiner should try to get experience in his own population and establish his own norms (cf. Touwen, 1976, 1979).

DEVIANT SIGNS IN SENSU STRICTIORI

In the present connotation deviant signs are signs that do not belong to the normal repertory of a child at any age. They are called signs of an unusual functioning of the brain as they do not occur in the majority of normally and adequately functioning children. Examples are the stereotyped asymmetric tonic neck reflexes or opistotonus in infancy, choreiform dyskinesia or coordination difficulties at (pre)school age, and hypo- or hypertonia or asymmetries at any age (Table 13-2). The signs are called minor or soft if their intensity is mild, in contrast with evident phenomena, which are called hard, or major. The latter designation results from the experience that

Table 13-2
Mild Neurological Deviations*

1. Sensorimotor system:
   - mild hypo- and hypertonia
   - mild asymmetries in posture and motility
   - pathological reflexes (e.g., Babinski)
   - (uni-lateral) loss of muscle power
2. Sensory systems:
   - visual apparatus: eye movements, eye position
   - acoustical apparatus: orientation, localization
   - skin: tactile, discriminatory, stereognostic
   - extinction tests: body scheme(?)
3. Coordination:
   - abnormal fingertip–nose, knee–heel, fingertip-touching tests, dysdiadochokinesia
4. Fine manipulative abilities
   - abnormal finger-opposition, finger following or circle tests
5. Dyskinesia:
   - choreiform dyskinesia, tremors, athetotiform dyskinesia

*Nonhandicapping, often at first glance nonobvious.

they occur in well-known pathological and handicapping conditions, as deteriorating disease or cerebral palsy. This means that a sign such as a Babinski is called hard because it is found in conditions generally recognized as pathological. However, this shows that a reversal is not always justified: a Babinski response may be found in about 4 percent of normal adults (Battine, Fressy, & Coquery, 1965; Maddonick, 1960). Many signs that should not occur in healthy persons at any age, are reported to be present in a small percentage of persons without any complaint. This is not only the case with the Babinski; asymmetric tonic neck reflex activity is another example (Frankstein et al, 1973; Wells, 1944), or an often found slight asymmetry in resistance to passive movements, active power and myotatic reflexes in children between 5 and 8 years, which is probably based on the development of hand- and foot-preference (Touwen, 1979). There are many reports of the prevalence of "soft signs" in children without problems (e.g., Adams et al, 1974; Barlow, 1974; Mangold, 1974; Rutter, Graham, & Birch, 1966; Rutter et al, 1970; Schain, 1977; Sommers, 1982; Werry et al, 1972; Wolff & Hurwitz, 1966). Still it is questionable whether the fact that these signs can be observed in some normal children makes them meaningless if they occur in behaviorally disturbed children. A sound clinical attitude is to consider a sign — whether soft or hard — as meaningful until the opposite is proved. The finding that a sign occurs only in a few persons — meaning that it is normally absent — is a sufficient reason to try and find a possible clinical meaning, which is not always immediately obvious.

It is often difficult to distinguish between deviant signs and retardation signs, e.g., there may be a very slight difference between mild dysdiadochokinesia and a delayed, age inadequate diadochokinesia in which there are too many shoulder movements involved. Also, a delayed performance of the fingertip-nose test can resemble a slightly ataxic fingertip-nose test. The degree in which a clinical condition is caused by a dysfunction in a narrower sense, and in its turn a developmental delay is caused by that same dysfunction, can only be evaluated by an appropriate, that is, a comprehensive and vigorously standardized developmental neurological examination.

SYNDROME AND PROFILES

Before it is feasible to relate the neurological findings to the complaints of the patient, they must be summarized in and interpreted into a neurological diagnosis. Isolated phenomena are rarely of any clinical importance:

their coherence makes the observed signs — major or minor — meaningful as graduators of the neurological integrity. Therefore an effort is made to assemble the findings into syndromes that can be labeled. In Table 13-3 a number of syndromes are listed that can be constructed on the basis of the findings; they consist mainly of very mild forms of traditional neurological syndromes, and furnish a qualitative appraisal of the neurological condition. A further refinement of this qualitative diagnosis is obtained by the construction of a so called neurological profile. For this purpose the neurological test items are grouped into clusters describing discernable categories of neurological display, such as the sensorimotor system, posture, trunk-coordination, coordination of the extremities, fine manipulative abilities, and the presence or absence of dyskinesia (Fig. 13-1, Table 13-4). In the profile of Figure 13-1 a few functional clusters, describing motility, are added, together with an *associated movement* cluster (associated movements are often considered as developmental signs) and a collection of items describing the visual system. Each cluster consists of a number of items, and the number of adequately performed items per cluster, gives a convenient quantification of the neurological condition. The resulting profiles are not diagnostic; they only give a quantification, e.g., a low score on the sensorimotor cluster does not tell us whether a hypotonia, a hypertonia, or a hemisyndrome is present. It implies a quantitative refinement of a qualitative diagnosis, or a presentation of suspect findings that cannot be arranged into a specific and comprehensible syndrome (e.g., the syndrome consisting of the absence of a syndrome, see Table 13-3). Also for therapeutic planning, profiles can be of great use: therapy should be different in patients with clumsiness based on sensorimotor problems, on coordination problems, on fine manipulative disabilities, or on combinations of these.

Table 13-3
Syndromes of Minor Neurological Dysfunction

1. Hemisyndromes
2. Sensorimotor syndromes
3. Dyskinetic syndromes
4. Dyscoordination syndromes
5. Dyspraxia syndromes
6. Sensoric syndromes
7. Retardation syndromes
8. Combinations(!)
9. The syndrome consisting of the absence of a syndrome

Note: The syndromes do not lead to overt handicaps, at most to some clumsiness.

Table 13-4
Groups of Items in the Subsystems of the Neurological Profile

1. *Sensorimotor apparatus*
    - resistance to passive movement
    - muscle power
    - range of movements
    - muscle consistency
    - knee jerk
    - ankle jerk
    - threshold muscle reflexes (legs)
    - biceps reflex
    - triceps reflex
    - threshold muscle reflexes (arms)
    - abdominal skin reflex
    - foot sole reflex
    - other exteroceptic reflexes (big toe)
2. *Posture*
    - sitting, general
    - feet, sitting
    - standing. general
    - legs, standing
    - feet, standing
    - extended arms, standing
    - walking
    - lying in prone and supine position
3. *Balance of trunk*
    - response to push, standing
    - following object with eyes and head
    - Romberg sign
    - rebound phenomenon
    - walking along a straight line
4. *Coordination of the extremities*
    - fingertip–nose test
    - diadochokinesis
    - knee–heel test
    - kicking against examiner's hand
    - fingertip touching test
5. *Fine manipulative ability*
    - finger-opposition test
    - follow-a-finger test
    - circle test
6. *(Dys)kinesia*
    - choreiform movements distal
    - choreiform movements proximal
    - choreiform movements during spontaneous behavior
    - athetotiform movements
7. *Gross motor functions*
    - heel–toe gait during walk
    - walking on tiptoe
    - walking on heels
    - standing on one leg
    - hopping on one leg
    - rising into sitting from lying in supine position
8. *Quality of motility*
    - small motor movements
        - speed
        - smoothness
        - adequacy
    - gross motor movements
        - speed
        - smoothness
        - adequacy
9. *Associated movements*
    - mouth-opening finger-spreading phenomenon
    - a.m. accompanying diadochokinesis in opposite hand
    - a.m. accompanying walking on tiptoe
    - a.m. accompanying walking on heels
    - a.m. accompanying finger-opposition test in other hand
10. *Visual system*
    - position of the eyes
    - directional nystagmus
    - position nystagmus
    - optokinetic nystagmus
    - pursuit movements of the eyes
    - visual fields
    - funduscopy

From Touwen BCL. The Examination of the Child with Minor Neurological Dysfunction. 2nd ed. Clinics in Developmental Medicine, no. 71. London: SIMP with Heinemann, 1979. With permission.

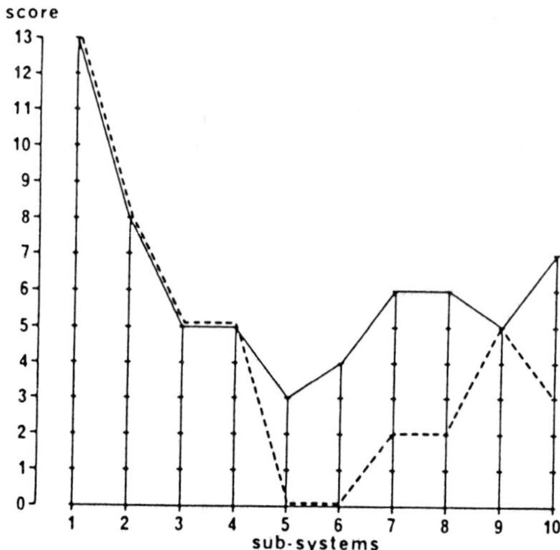

Figure 13-1. The vertical represents the number of test-items scored correctly in each of the ten subsystems (numbered on the horizontal) described in Table 13-4. The solid line represents the highest score possible for each subsystem. The broken line represents the profile of a child with minor neurological dysfunction in fine manipulative ability (score of 0), kinesia (score of 0), and visual system (score of 3). Although gross motor functioning and motility are not optimal, associated movements are not excessive. These findings are too mild to justify a traditional diagnosis. (From Touwen BCL. The Examination of the Child with Minor Neurological Dysfunction. 2nd ed. Clinics in Developmental Medicine, no. 71. London: SIMP with Heinemann, 1979. With permission.)

SIGNIFICANCE

Only now can anything be said about the significance of the neurological signs observed. For the first two categories of referrals for a neurological examination, the answer to the question about the significance is usually sufficiently clear, although follow-up is often required before the answer can be obtained. However, in the third category things are different especially with children in whom neurological findings are present. Generally it must be stated that a direct or causal relationship between the neurological findings and behavioral and/or learning difficulties cannot, or rarely only can, be ascertained. In some instances there may be a plausible relationship between the neurological condition and part of the behavior, e.g., in children with coordination difficulties or dyskinesia and clumsy behavior; to demonstrate this relationship in these children may be of therapeutic importance. The clumsiness may have resulted in (secondary) emotional tension at home or at school, and information about (and treatment of) the neurological basis of the clumsiness may help to lessen the tension. Often, however, such a plausible relationship cannot be shown. In that case an indirect relationship in individual children is a possibility, and should be looked for. One should not forget, however, that comparable behavioral problems may exist with or without neurological symptomatology. This fact emphasizes that neurological (soft) signs need not be causally related to specific behavioural problems. The neurological findings may merely reflect a certain vulnerability of the nervous system, so that the child's ability to cope with his environment in the broadest sense becomes endangered. In that case a child may show neurological signs and behavioral symptomatology that result from the same vulnerability, but which are not causally related. Seen from this point of view a particular environment that is appropriate for a child without neurological dysfunction, may be overtaxing for a child with a neurological dysfunction. This suggests that it is feasible to create environmental conditions in which neurologically dysfunctioning children function adequately or even better than neurologically normal children (Kalverboer, 1975). On the other hand an environment may be so extreme that neurologically normal children decompensate behaviorally. Indeed specific neuro-behavioral relationships, i.e., specific neurological syndromes resulting in specific behavioral and/or learning difficulties are rare, especially in the case of neurological soft signs, and this may be regarded as an argument pro the conception of a diffusely increased vulnerability of the brain (Hertzig, 1981).

Another conception of an indirect relationship between soft signs and behavioral difficulties is the conception that soft signs are one reflection of a "biologically different brain" (Prechtl, 1978) and behavioral problems another, resulting from a rewiring after an early damage, or from a different or unusual wiring during development, even without any evident noxious cause. Finally, a minor neurological dysfunction (the presence of soft signs) can be considered as an indication that the brain's normal variability has decreased, and consequently its adaptability. In this conception the brain is considered as mildly abnormal and the resulting decreased capacity of the brain, reflected neurologically by the presence of the minor signs of dysfunction, leads to a deficient developmental variability of functioning. The resulting lack of adaptive ability is displayed in the often rather stereotyped behavioral and learning problems.

CONCLUSION

Obviously it is often necessary to obtain results of more and other assessments to gain insight into the make-up of a child's individual behavior. Psychometric, psychiatric, behavioral/ethological, socioenvironmental, didactic assessments can be required, and should be carried out blindly. The significance of the neurological assessment and its findings may vary according to the individual child's abilities in other functional areas. As two children are not identical in their environments, it is not surprising that relations between neurological signs or rather — syndromes — and complex behavior are variable, and, if present, statistically only. This does not imply that mild (soft) neurological signs have no significance. They may be significant in some, and may not be so in other children. But they must be identified before anything can be said about them. "Soft signs" is a label without a more than very overall meaning. Identified signs may tell us something about particular functions or mechanisms of the brain. Sets of signs may tell us more, especially if they can be arranged into entities. Asking for a specific meaning of soft signs that can be generalized is asking the wrong question. The proper question states: What is the meaning of this particular neurological set of signs in this particular child? The answer to this question depends on the child.

REFERENCES

Adams RM, Kocsis JJ, & Estes RE. Soft neurological signs in learning disabled children and controls. American Journal of Diseases of Children, 1974, 128, 614-618

Barlow CF. Soft signs in children with learning disorders. American Journal of Diseases of Children, 1974, 128, 605-606

Battini C, Fressy J, & Coquery JM. Critères polygraphiques du sommeil lent et du sommeil rapide. In Sommeil de Nuit, Normal et Pathologique, Etudes Electroencephalographiques et Neurophysiologie Clinique Vol. 2, Paris, Masson 1965, p. 156

Bayley N. Bayley Scales of Infant Development: Birth to Two Years. New York: Psychological Corporation, 1969

Bender L. Clinical study of one hundred schizophrenic children. American

Journal of Orthopsychiatry, 1974, 17, 40-56
Carey WB, & McDevitt SC. Minimal brain dysfunction and hyperkinesis. American Journal of Diseases of Children, 1980, 134, 926-929
Carey WB, McDevitt SC, & Baker D. Differentiating minimal brain dysfunction and temperament. Developmental Medicine and Child Neurology, 1979, 21, 765-772
Denckla MB. Clinical syndromes in learning disabilities. Journal of Learning Disabilities, 1972, 5, 401-406
Denckla MB. Minimal brain dysfunction. In Chall J, & Mirsky A (Eds.). Education and the Brain. Chicago: University of Chicago Press, 1978, pp. 223-268
Denckla MB, & Rudel RG. Anomalies of motor development in hyperactive boys. Annals of Neurology, 1978, 3, 231-233
Frankenburg WK, & Dodds JB. The Denver Developmental Screening Test. Journal of Pediatrics, 1967, 71, 181-191
Frankenburg WK, Goldstein AD, & Camp BW. The revised Denver Developmental Screening Test. Journal of Pediatrics, 1971, 79, 988-995
Frankstein SI, Sergeeva ZN, & Sergeeva LN. Magnus reflexes of the chest musculature in man. Experientia, 1973, 29, 436
Hertzig ME. Neurologic "soft signs" in low birthweight children. Developmental Medicine and Child Neurology, 1981, 23, 778-791
Kalverboer AF. A Neurobehavioural Study in Preschool Children. Clinics in Developmental Medicine No. 54. London: SIMP with Heinemann, 1975
Kinsbourne M. MBD as a neurodevelopmental lag. In De la Cruz FF, Fox BH, & Roberts RH (Eds.). Minimal Brain Dysfunction. New York: New York Academy of Sciences, 1973, pp 267-273
Knobloch H, Pasamanick B, & Sherard ES. A developmental screening inventory for infants. Pediatric Supplement, 1966, 38, 1095-1108
Madonick MJ. Statistical control studies in neurology, X. Journal of Nervous and Mental Diseases, 1960, 131, 547
Mangold B. Psychische Probleme beim Minimal-Brain-Dysfunction-Syndrome. Padiatrie und Padologie, 1974, 9, 95-103
Neligan GA, Kolvin I, Scott DM, & Garside RF. Born Too Soon or Born Too Small. Clinics in Developmental Medicine No. 61. London: SIMP with Heinemann, 1976
Page-El E, & Grossman HJ. Neurological appraisal in learning disorders. Pediatric Clinics of North America, 1973, 20, 599-605
Prechtl HFR. Strategy and validity of early detection of neurological dys-

function. In Douglas CP, & Holt KS (Eds.). Mental Retardation: Prenatal Diagnosis and Infant Assessment. London: Butterworth, 1972, p. 41

Prechtl HFR: The Neurological Examination of the Full-Term Newborn Infant. 2nd ed. Clinics in Developmental Medicine no. 63. London: SIMP with Heinemann, 1977

Prechtl HFR. Minimal brain dysfunction syndrome and the plasticity of the nervous system. Advances in Biological Psychiatry, 1978, 1, 96-105

Rie ED, Rie HE, Stewart S, & Rettemnier SC. An analysis of neurological soft signs in children with learning problems. Brain and Language, 1978, 6, 32-46

Rutter M. Brain damage syndromes in childhood: Concepts and findings. Journal of Child Psychology and Psychiatry, 1977, 18, 1-21

Rutter M, Graham P, & Birch HG. Interrelations between the choreiform syndrome, reading disability and psychiatric disorder in children of 8-11 years. Developmental Medicine and Child Neurology, 1966, 8, 149-159

Rutter M, Graham P, & Yule W. A Neuropsychiatric Study in Childhood. Clinics in Developmental Medicine nos. 35/36. London: SIMP with Heinemann, 1970

Schain RJ. Neurological evaluation of children with learning disorders. Neuropaediatrie, 1970, 1, 307-317

Schain RJ. Neurology of Childhood Learning-Disorders. 2nd ed. Baltimore: Williams and Wilkins, 1977

Schmitt BD. The minimal brain dysfunction myth. American Journal of Diseases of Children, 1975, 129, 1313-1318

Sommers PA. What parents should know about children with learning disabilities. Early Child Development and Care, 1982, 9, 187-192

Touwen BCL. Neurological Development in Infancy. Clinics in Developmental Medicine no. 58. London: SIMP with Heinemann, 1976

Touwen BCL. Minimal brain dysfunction and minor neurological dysfunction. Advances in Biological Psychiatry, 1978, 1, 55-57

Touwen BCL. Examination of the Child with Minor Neurological Dysfunction. 2nd ed. Clinics in Developmental Medicine no. 71. London: SIMP with Heinemann, 1979

Touwen BCL, & Sporrel T. Soft signs and MBD. Developmental Medicine and Child Neurology, 1979, 21, 528-529

Wells HS. The demonstration of tonic neck and labyrinthine reflexes and pontive heliotropic responses in normal human subjects. Science, 1944, 99, 36

Werry JS, Minde K, Guzman A, et al. Studies on the hyperactive child VII: Neurological status compared with neurotic and normal children. American Journal of Orthopsychiatry, 1972, 42, 441-451

Wolff PH, & Hurwitz J. The choreiform syndrome. Developmental Medicine and Child Neurology, 1966, 8, 160-165

H. Gerry Taylor

14

The Meaning and Value of Soft Signs in the Behavioral Sciences

In 1973 Ingram stated that reference to soft neurological signs was "diagnostic of soft thinking" (p. 529). Ingram's conclusion is as true now as it was then. Despite continued study of soft signs in children with learning or behavior problems, the soft sign category is not clearly defined. Investigators do not even agree on the range of behavioral symptoms to include as soft signs. The neurological implications of soft signs and the utility of these signs with respect to diagnosis, prognosis, and treatment are also highly contentious. The fact that the concept of soft signs had its origin in anecdotal observations of children with a wide array of behavior, learning, and neurological disorders probably accounts in part for this state of affairs. Bender (1956) was among the first to bring these symptoms to the attention of the mental health profession. In her studies, soft signs were cited as evidence for the presence of biological antecedents to childhood mental disorders. Following Bender's lead, observations of motor and other complex behaviors have been incorporated into medical examinations, and a good deal of research has been conducted in collaboration with behavioral scientists. Results substantiate soft sign abnormalities in children with a wide range of learning and behavior problems. Soft signs have by now become a common means for documenting *minimal brain dysfunctions* of all sorts.

Like the term "minimal brain dysfunction," the closely related but more specific concept of soft neurological signs has arisen within a historical context that has given increasing acceptance to biological interpretations of behavior and learning disorders (Fletcher & Taylor, 1984; HG Taylor, 1983; Taylor, Fletcher, & Satz, 1984). As a result, researchers and

SOFT NEUROLOGICAL SIGNS
ISBN 0-8089-1841-9

clinicians alike are often uncritical regarding the definition, meaning, and utility of soft signs. As a clinician, I can give personal testimony that soft signs exist. There are multitudes of children with attentional, learning, and language disorders who exhibit sensory-motor difficulties qualifying as soft signs. A large proportion of these children have normal IQs and are free of outright neurological disorder. As a behavioral scientist, however, I am dismayed by the lack of a commonly accepted definition for soft signs. I am also left uneasy by the difficulty one has in distinguishing soft signs from subtle forms of hard neurological signs, or in specifying the relationship of soft signs to neuropathology; and by the frequent failure in discussions of soft signs to come to grips with issues of reliability and validity.

Most of the collection of diverse symptoms in the soft sign category would probably have been dismissed long ago as irrelevant to the neurological examination were it not for two sustained beliefs about these symptoms: (1) soft signs imply a neurological basis for the disorders with which they are associated, even when other more definitive evidence for neuropathology is absent (i.e., soft signs have *neurological* significance); and (2) soft signs are useful in rendering clinical judgments about children with behavior and learning disorders (i.e., soft signs have *psychological* significance).

The first belief amounts to regarding soft signs as *prima facia* evidence for neurophysiological inadequacies. In practice, the process of neurological attribution usually occurs when soft signs are observed in association with a demonstrable clinical disability (e.g., learning problem, attention deficit disorder) and when other more obvious explanations for the disorder, such as outright brain disease, emotional disturbance, or pervasive mental retardation, cannot account for the disability (Satz, 1977). In such cases, reference to soft signs serves to maintain a biological explanation for the disability while relieving the examiner of the need to provide direct evidence for neuropathology. To distinguish the evidence for brain-relatedness provided by soft signs from direct evidence of neuropathology, soft signs are referred to as indices of "neurological immaturity" (Schmitt, 1975; Shapiro, Burkes, Petti, & Ranz, 1978; Wolff, Gunnoe, & Cohen, 1983; Wolff, Gunnoe, & Cohen, 1985), "non-optimal nervous functioning" (Touwen & Prechtl, 1970), or "minor or equivocal degrees of CNS damage or dysfunction" (Denckla, 1973b; Hertzig & Birch, 1968). As I will discuss at greater length later in this chapter, there is no direct neuroanatomical or neurophysiological evidence to support the assumption of clinical-pathological correlates. This first belief rests more on conviction than on fact. Once the belief that soft signs have neurological significance is recognized as a working hypothesis, we can be more objective in examining the evidence. Based on the evidence, we can then decide whether to uphold or reject the belief or to suspend judgment. Existing data furnish some grounds for the belief that soft signs are brain-related, but support is not so clear-cut that we would want to take this belief as established fact. Critical appraisal of this working hypothesis is useful in further clarifying the meaning of soft signs and in highlighting research needs.

The belief that soft signs have clinical utility has been sustained by a variety of evidence linking soft signs to behavior and learning disorders. This evidence includes (1) findings of both concurrent and predictive relationships between soft signs and behavior or learning problems; (2) observations that soft signs may be more associated with some disorders, such as hyperactivity, than with other disorders; and (3) suggestions that soft signs may have implications regarding response to treatment. Unfortunately, empirical support for this second belief is equivocal. Soft signs are found in many children without behavior or learning disturbances, and they are absent in many children with these disturbances.

Furthermore, studies of soft signs that have compared children with behavior-learning disorders to normal children have yielded inconsistent findings. Several studies have failed to find differences. In those studies that have documented a great frequency of soft signs among disordered children, group comparisons have usually been confounded with IQ or other potentially relevant factors. For these several reasons, existing support for the belief that soft signs are clinically useful is less than fully convincing. Further investigation is needed using more reliable measures and more methodologically sound procedures.

The primary purposes of this chapter are to review the soft sign category, the relationship between soft signs and neurological status, and the evidence favoring an association between soft signs and behavior-learning disorders. Methodological shortcomings of existing research will be highlighted, and recommendations made regarding the type of research that is most likely to result in progress. The final section of the chapter summarizes the current status of research on soft signs, outlines research needs, and addresses the implications of this research for the clinician.

THE CONCEPT OF SOFT NEUROLOGICAL SIGNS

Behaviors Included

An enormous variety of clinical findings have been referred to as soft signs. Probably the most extensive single list of soft signs is provided by Peters, Romine, and Dykman (1975). Included in their "special neurological examination" are items ranging from motor and sensory-motor coordination to balance, laterality, right-left orientation, ocular-motor control, oral praxis and speech, somatosensory abilities, writing to dictation, and spelling. Abnormalities on the traditional neurological examination, such as tremors, asymmetries of tone or reflex, ocular-motor problems, and cerebellar findings are also considered soft signs, as long as those abnormalities occur in such a subtle, inconsistent, or isolated fashion so as not to be clearly indicative of neurological disorder (Denckla, 1977; Ingram, 1973). In reports such as that of Peters et al (1975), the soft sign category is so diffusely defined as to include the very behaviors with which these signs were originally said to be associated (i.e., disorders of behavior, learning, or attention), or any of a variety of neuropsychological impairments (see Denckla, 1977).

Among this array of diverse clinical findings is a core of symptoms that fall within the realm of the traditional pediatric neurological examination. This core consists of tests of gross motor coordination and steadiness; motor persistence; facility in performing integrated motor acts (e.g., finger-to-nose pointing, finger-to-thumb apposition, alternating movements); associated movements, or synkinesias; ocular-motor control; and sensory and somatosensory abilities (e.g., graphesthesia, stereognosis, two-point discrimination). Although no soft sign examination has gained wide acceptance, Shaffer et al (1983) have sensibly recommended restricting soft sign evaluations to this category. These researchers do not favor the inclusion of less routinely administered procedures (e.g., the face-hand test, post-rotatory nystagmus, "whirling"), or of standardized psychometric or neuropsychological procedures. Because speech and language assessments are not unique to the neurological examination and because speech pathologists have developed specialized testing procedures in this area, it would also seem reasonable to exclude these assessments from the soft sign category.

There are a number of advantages to restricting the soft sign category in this manner. First, investigators would generally agree that these behaviors are representative of soft signs (Adams, Kocsis, & Estes, 1974; Clements, 1966; Clements & Peters, 1962; Kennard, 1960; Peters et al, 1975; Schmitt,

1975; Touwen & Prechtl, 1970; Werry & Aman, 1976). Second, more restricted designation of soft sign symptomatology prevents overlap with other indices of potential biological significance and thus encourages study of the relationship between these various indices (e.g., the relationship between soft signs and impairments on language or neuropsychological tests). Most importantly, if the existence of soft signs are to be of any value whatever in delineating the nature and origins of learning and behavior problems, they must be defined independently of those disorders. Adopting the more restricted definition of soft signs as proposed by Shaffer et al (1983) satisfies each of these requirements.

Several investigators have suggested that this common core of soft signs be partitioned even further into two or three subsets of signs. Rutter et al (1970) divides soft signs into three distinct subgroups. In the first subgroup are signs that would not be considered abnormal in a younger child. Examples of this subtype are incoordination and motor overflow. Denckla (1977) terms these signs "developmental," and Ingram (1973) refers to them either as a "failure to develop normal behavioral milestones," or as "immature reflex patterns." According to Rutter et al (1970), the second subtype of soft signs is comprised of symptoms such as nystagmus and strabismus. These symptoms may emerge as a result of neurological disease, but they may be also secondary to extra-neurological conditions (e.g., problems in muscle balance, amblyopia, middle ear disease). A third subtype consists of those signs that would not be considered normal for a younger child. Included in this third subgroup are subtle manifestations of more classical neurological signs, such as slight abnormalities in reflexes or tone or minimal athetosis. Rutter et al (1970) warn us that this latter subgroup of signs may be unreliable or difficult to elicit. Denckla (1977) refers to symptoms from the latter two subcategories as "pastel classical neurological signs." Like Rutter et al, she characterizes these latter signs as abnormal for any age, but her descriptions do not suggest that they are particularly unreliable.

One of the virtues of subgrouping soft signs is the selective exclusion of signs that are unreliably present or that may be due to nonneurological factors. Subcategorization of soft signs may also be useful in exploring differential associations with other behavioral or neurological variables. Some soft signs, for example, may prove more valid than others in identifying subtypes of learning and behavior problems, or in discriminating children with and without positive neurological histories. For the time being, however, there is little empirical justification for subgroupings of soft signs and little reason to investigate one type of soft sign over another type. Most signs within the category noted above would be explored in conducting a comprehensive pediatric neurological examination. All of these signs must be evaluated relative to age standards for normalcy, and clinical-pathological correlations are no better established for one sign than for another.

Relationship to Neurological Status

As in the case of "minimal brain dysfunction," referring to a clinical finding as a soft neurological sign is based on a presumption, rather than on proof, of brain-relatedness (HG Taylor, 1983). After all, if the presence of a soft sign allowed us to conclude with any certainty that brain abnormality was present, we could scarcely refer to that sign as soft. In keeping with the definition of soft signs originally proposed by Bender

> "Soft signs" found in an individual should not have a pathognomonic pattern of a kind that would usually indicate one or more clearly localized structural lesions, generalized encephalopathy, or central nervous system (CNS) involvement. (Shaffer et al, 1983, p. 144).

The important question to ask with respect to the neurological significance of soft signs is whether the *presumption* of brain-relatedness is warranted. Specifically, what are the grounds for this presumption, and do these grounds justify retaining the presumption as a working hypothesis?

Before reviewing proper grounds for making this presumption, it is important to expunge common misconceptions concerning the relationship between soft signs and the CNS. Perhaps the most misleading argument in favor of soft signs having neurological significance is the one based on a brain-behavior isomorphism. According to this argument, soft signs may be construed as on a behavioral continuum with, or as minor variants of, those major sensory-motor impairments associated with outright brain disease. Because brain disease exists in degrees, soft signs are assumed to reflect milder and otherwise undetectable forms of neurological disorder. In other words, certain behavioral dysfunctions (i.e., soft signs) are assumed to mirror physiological irregularities of the brain. The problem with this argument is that brain-behavior isomorphisms cannot be supported. There is no straightforward relationship between the extent of brain disease and degree of behavioral impairment (Baumeister & MacLean, 1979; Benton, 1973; Touwen, 1978). Consequently, there is no logical basis for the belief that soft signs, or any other behavior anomalies, constitute direct measures of mild degrees of abnormality. Soft signs are not physiological or anatomical measures. Soft signs are behavioral findings and as such have the same conceptual status as abnormalities in intelligence, memory, or personality.

Two related fallacies about these signs have also fostered misunderstanding regarding their neurological implications. The first fallacy is that there is a sharp distinction between hard signs and soft signs, and the second is that hard signs provide unequivocal evidence for neuropathology. Discussions with many of my neurology colleagues over the last several years make it clear that neurologists do not judge the presence or absence of neuropathology on the basis of a single behavioral sign or group of signs. Even when a child or adult presents with a clear hemiparesis, the history of the symptom, information regarding other events of potential neurological significance (e.g., head injuries, seizure-like behaviors, pre- and perinatal events), and laboratory results (e.g., EEG, CT scan) are all considered in interpreting abnormalities on neurological examination itself (Rutter et al, 1970; Touwen & Prechtl, 1970). Individuals with clear histories of neurological insult may have no residual sensory or motor deficits on examination. Conversely, individuals for whom there is no reason to suspect neurological disease may occasionally exhibit subtle hard signs. Considered in isolation, hard signs do not constitute sufficient grounds for diagnosing brain disease.

The best evidence in this regard is given in the classic Isle of Wight study (Rutter et al, 1970). As part of their investigation of learning and neurological status in this population of children, Rutter et al administered full neurological examinations, including tests of hard and soft signs, to 125 children who showed no evidence of abnormal neurological histories or of cognitive disorders. Neurological examinations were also given to separate groups of children carrying diagnoses of intellectual retardation, specific reading retardation, or neurological abnormality (the latter being determined on the basis of multiple procedures taking into account clinical history as well as examination results). Although "marked" neurological abnormalities discriminated the control and neurologically affected groups quite well, as many as 7 percent of the control children were noted to have one or more prominent abnormalities (e.g., absent right supinator jerk). When severity of neurological deficit was not taken into account, much higher percentages of control children were observed to have abnormalities on "hard signs" portions of the neurological exam. For example, from 3-20 percent of the control children exhibited cranial signs; 4 percent were regarded as having cerebellar dysfunction; 10 percent had tremor; as many as 4 percent exhibited evidence of increased tone; and from 6-33 percent were regarded as having increased or decreased reflexes of one sort or another.

Similar findings emerged in Voeller's (1981) neurological examinations of a group of 90 children with specific learning disabilities. Like Rutter et al, Voeller found a surprisingly high incidence of abnormalities in cerebellar functions, cranial nerves, and deep tendon reflexes. There is no reason to believe that any more than a negligible number of learning disabled children would have a definitive form of neurological disorder (Owen et al, 1971; Taylor, Satz, & Friel, 1979; Thompson, Ross, & Horowitz, 1980). Voeller's findings suggest, therefore, that hard signs do not necessarily imply neurological disease. E. Taylor (1983) also reports a relatively high incidence of isolated hard signs among children for whom neurological problems would not be expected. In his study, Taylor found unequal ankle reflexes in 5 percent of 38 control children, mild facial weakness in 5 percent, and equivocal plantar response in 11 percent. These several observations indicate that diagnosing neurological disorders in children is based on considerations in addition to the presence of abnormalities apparent on the exam itself. Moreover, the degree of abnormality seems to be more critical than its presence or absence.

Questions regarding the distinction between hard and soft signs are additionally raised by the lack of inter-examiner agreement regarding hard signs and by the absence of any criteria on which to base judgments. In the Collaborative Perinatal Project, Nichols and Chen (1981) report substantial differences between research centers in the proportion of children regarded as having neurological disorders. Conventional wisdom regarding neurological diagnosis notwithstanding, even abnormalities in hard signs depend on subjective judgments and may be influenced by expectations created by knowledge of history and other information not given in the standard neurological examination per se. According to Gardner (1979), "One examiner may consider a child to have 2+ deep tendon reflexes (normal) and another may decide that they are 3+ (hyperreflexic)" (p. 119). The fact that both hard and soft signs may occasionally reflect motivational, stress, or practice effects, or may be unreliably elicited, further detracts from their validity as measures of neuropathology (Foster et al, 1978; Rutter, Graham, & Yule, 1970). Whereas more pronounced signs of the classical variety (i.e., prominent hard signs) undoubtedly possess a high degree of validity in relation to neuropathology, there is no clear distinction between hard and soft signs. The relevance of this to the present discussion is that subtle hard signs, even if reliably present, are not necessarily of any greater neurological significance than are soft signs. The fact that certain hard signs are occasionally found in association with soft signs does not justify a neurogenic interpretation of soft signs.

More proper support for the conviction that soft signs have neurological significance is provided by research showing that children with documented histories of brain disease exhibit greater frequencies of these signs than do normal children. Rutter et al (1970) administered tests that fall into the soft sign category. Most of these measures discriminated a group of children with established neurological diagnosis from normal children. Similarly, Bortner et al (1972) examined children from a special school who were diagnosed as brain-damaged and compared this group to age-matched children from regular schools. Bortner et al found that 65 percent of the brain-damaged children displayed two or more soft signs, compared to only 5 percent of the normal children. The results reinforced those of a previous study by the same investigators involving a subset of the brain-injured group tested at a younger age (Hertzig, Bortner, & Birch, 1969). In studies by Cohen et al (1967) and by Woods and Teuber (1978), brain-injured children also showed more motor overflow, or synkinesias, than normal children.

The major problem in citing the preceding evidence is that it is prone to overinterpretation. Lower IQs and increased prevalence of behavioral disturbances are also found in association with brain disease in children (Rutter, 1982). Yet we would hardly claim that neurological limitations explain all cases of limited intelligence or emotional disorder. Although soft signs may be differentially associated with brain disease, like all complex behaviors they are a function of both brain substrate and environmental-historical factors. "Obviously, environmental influences play an important role and there are no two identical brains" (Touwen & Sporrel, 1979, p. 528).

Data suggesting a link between soft signs and earlier medical risk events offer a second body of support for the belief that soft signs have neurological implications. Hertzig (1981) examined the neurological status at 8 years of age of a group of prematurely born children of low birth weight (1000 - 1700 grams). From this total group, 13 had hard signs, 20 had soft signs only, and 33 had normal exams. Hertzig's distinction between hard and soft signs is somewhat questionable. Because the presence of hard signs was apparently judged on the exam alone, it is difficult to know how many of the children with hard signs were suffering from outright neurological disorders. Nevertheless, perinatal complications were much more frequent in children who demonstrated soft signs alone than in children who showed neither soft nor hard signs. In fact, all but one of the 20 children with soft signs had perinatal complications, whereas these complications were present for only 16 of the 33 normal children.

Shaffer et al (1983) compared the early birth histories of children from the Collaborative Perinatal Project who exhibited soft signs at 7 years of age with another group of children from the same project who did not display soft signs. As in the case of Hertzig's study, the usual core group of soft signs was assessed, including involuntary movements, coordination difficulties, and abnormalities in sensory integration. Results showed that the group with soft signs had a lower mean birth weight relative to gestation date than the group without soft signs.

Soft sign sequelae related to early risk events were also discovered in a recent outcome study of *Haemophilus influenzae* meningitis. In this study, conducted by myself and colleagues at the University of Pittsburgh (Taylor et al, 1984), a comprehensive battery of soft signs was administered to each of 24 children who had had meningitis and to 24 school-age siblings. The soft sign battery was comprised of a collection of neuromotor and somatosensory tasks including visual tracking, motor impersistence, choreiform movements, diadochokinesis, motor overflow, finger localization, tactile localization, tactile form perception, double tactile stimulation, and right-left discrimination. Although examination of muscle tone, reflexes, posture, and gait was not carried out, the battery was representative of the core of behaviors most typically included in soft sign assessments. Even when the children with hemiplegias were excluded, comparison of the two groups in terms of age-adjusted soft sign total scores revealed that the post-meningitis group performed more poorly overall than their siblings.

A third general body of support for a relationship between soft signs and neural integrity is provided by associations between these signs and other presumptive indices of brain-relatedness (Taylor & Fletcher, 1983). Presumptive indices include variables that, when found in association with disorders of learning or behavior, might increase one's suspicion that these disorders have a neurological basis. In addition to soft signs, such indices include a family history of disorder, a history of pre- or perinatal complications, minor physical anomalies, a positive response to medications, accompanying neuropsychological deficits or developmental delays, and abnormal electrophysiological findings. Examples of this type of evidence include the association between soft signs and pregnancy-birth risks reported by Hertzig (1981) and the association between soft signs and response to stimulant medications reported by Satterfield (1973). Specifically, Satterfield reports that "minimally brain damaged" children with 4 or more soft signs showed greater response according to teacher ratings to methylphenidate than did children from the same clinical category who manifested no soft signs. In a study having somewhat different implications, Lerer and Lerer (1976) provided additional evidence for an association between soft signs and neurological status. These investigators examined 40 hyperactive children who had 3 or more soft neurological abnormalities. Their results showed a significant reduction in soft signs in response to methylphenidate treatment. Since methylphenidate is known to have neuropharmacological effects, these results can be interpreted as consistent with the notion that soft signs are indeed brain-mediated behaviors.

Evidence for correspondences between soft signs and other presumptive neurological markers include findings of similarities in soft sign status among twins and siblings (Nichols & Chen, 1981; Owen et al, 1971; Rieder & Nichols, 1979), and the association of soft signs with conditions such as hyperactivity, learning disorders, and other specific psychiatric disorders (Quitkin, Rifkin, & Klein, 1976). In a provocative study of 52 dyslexic children, Denckla (1977) explored the relationship of soft sign type to both family history of speech and learning problems and history of neurological risk factors including encephalopathic events. Contrary to expectations, she did not find either of these latter variables to be more closely related to pastel classical soft signs than to developmental soft signs. For the dyslexic group as a whole, however, she reports a high incidence of both positive family history of speech and learning problems and suspect neurological history. Since soft signs were observed in all but three children, these findings raise the possibility that soft signs may co-occur with other indirect indications of neurological involvement.

A final justification for rendering neurological interpretations of soft signs is provided by an absence of association between these signs and social-environmental variables. Although soft signs studies rarely encompass assessment of social variables, existing evidence is supportive. Hertzig (1981) found no relationship between sociometric variables and neurological status in her group of prematurely born children. Likewise, Shaffer et al (1983) report that social and family characteristics failed to distinguish children with and without soft signs. Finally, in our study of post-meningitis children and their siblings, the correlation between the Hollingshead Index of Socioeconomic Status and the aggregate neurological soft sign score was essentially nil. This was despite a significant correlation between the soft sign measure and Full-Scale WISC-R IQ ($r = 0.35, p < 0.05$).

On the other hand, the evidence for an association between soft signs and other presumptive indices of brain-relatedness is not uniformly positive. Many negative findings offset the positive support offered by the above cited investigations. The effect of methylphenidate on the soft neurological status of hyperactive children reported by Lerer and Lerer (1976) was not replicated by McMahon and Greenberg (1977). The latter investigators found soft signs so variable across five separate test occasions as to be useless in measuring response to medications. Other investigators have also challenged the utility of soft signs in predicting response to Ritalin (Barkley, 1976; Werry & Aman, 1976). Similarly, several studies have failed to confirm associations between soft signs and either EEG abnormalities or medical-historical variables (Hart, Rennick, Klinge, & Schwartz, 1974; Kenny & Clemmens, 1971; Paine, Werry, & Quay, 1968; Werry et al,1972; Werry, 1968).

Admittedly, most studies that have failed to demonstrate associations between soft signs and other indirect biological markers have involved children with heterogeneous disorders. In some cases, researchers may have employed unreliable or otherwise inadequate soft sign measures. The results of these studies do not preclude the possibility of finding associations between soft signs and other markers of brain-relatedness, at least with improved methodology. Futher explorations of this issue awaits study of more homogenous groups of children or adults, application of more reliable soft signs tests, and investigation of individual soft signs and behavioral-historical variables as opposed to conglomerate measures (Stevens, Sachdev, & Milstein, 1968; Werry, 1968). More generally, meaningful inquiry into the neurological significance of soft signs requires attention to the three primary *research needs* described in this section:

1. Careful analyses of soft signs in relation to neuropathology in children with definitive forms of brain disease.
2. Investigations of the relationship between soft signs and other presumptive indices including family history, electrophysiological abnormalities, minor physical anomalies, pre- and perinatal complications, neuropsychological and developmental data, and responses to medications.
3. Inclusion of measures of social influences and psychosocial adjustment in order to determine the degree to which soft signs are independent of the latter variables.

UTILITY OF SOFT NEUROLOGICAL SIGNS

Evidence for Criterion-Related Validity

Whether or not one agrees with the direct neurogenic interpretation of soft signs, the relevance of these signs in assessing, predicting, and treating disorders of learning and behavior is an important issue. Evidence in favor of the criterion-related validity of soft signs comes from documented associations between these signs and several independently defined behavioral traits. Concurrent validity has been established by observations that soft signs are more prevalent in groups of children and adults with learning and behavior problems than in groups without these problems. Studies evidencing concurrent validity have involved the following clinical samples:

1. Children and adolescents with diverse forms of behavioral and psychiatric disturbance necessitating referral to mental health centers or institutions (Cohen, Taft, Mahadeviah, & Birch, 1967; Hertzig & Birch, 1968; Kennard, 1960; Wilker, Dixon, & Parker, 1970; Wolff & Hurwitz, 1966).
2. Children diagnosed as hyperactive (Denckla & Rudel, 1978; Mikkelsen et al, 1982; Werry et al, 1972).
3. Children having learning or behavioral problems at school (Adams, Kocsis, & Estes, 1974; Doehring, 1968; Hart et al, 1974; Hertzig, 1981; Lucas et al, 1965; Owen et al, 1971; Peters, Romine, & Dykman, 1975; Stine, Saratsiotis, & Mosser, 1975; Taylor, Satz, & Friel, 1979; Wolff & Hurwitz, 1973; Younes, Rosner, & Webb, 1983).

A greater relative frequency of soft signs is also reported for younger as compared to older children (Connolly & Stratton, 1968; Cohen et al, 1967; Peters et al, 1975; Wolff et al, 1983) and in children with weaknesses in IQ, academic underachievement, general developmental deficits, and personality traits including dependency, withdrawal, and immaturity (Bortner, Hertzig, & Birch, 1972; Carey, McDevitt, & Baker, 1979; Gold, 1979; Hart et al, 1974; Ingram, Mason, & Blackburn, 1970; Mikkelsen et al, 1982; Paulsen & O'Donnell, 1979; Rutter et al, 1970; Rutter & Yule, 1975; Wolff, Gunnoe, & Cohen, 1983, 1985). Kalverboer, Touwen, and Prechtl (1973) have even reported a relationship, albeit weak, between a soft sign-like measure (neurological optimality score) and the quality of play behavior in young boys under nonstimulating play conditions (see also Kalverboer, 1976).

Several additional studies indicate that soft signs may have predictive validity. These studies have shown that children with excessive numbers of soft signs early in life may be at greater risk for academic and learning problems later on. As one example, Peter and Spreen (1979) found that children with soft signs (designated the "minimal brain dysfunction" group) displayed more parent-rated problems of behavior several years after the initial assessment than did either a normal group or a learning disabled group without soft signs. One of the strengths of the Peter-Spreen study is that it explicitly excluded from the soft signs group those children who had definitive forms of neurological disorder. Also, children in both the soft sign and learning disability groups were referred to a clinic for educational handicaps. Both groups, therefore, would have been considered at risk for future problems, making the difference in outcome between these two groups a more impressive one.

Additional confirmation of the predictive validity of soft signs comes from an investigation by Denhoff, Siqueland, Komich, and Hainsworth (1968). In their research, Denhoff et al were able to show a predictive relationship between a collection of soft sign measures (Meeting Street School Screening Test) and success or failure early in school. Bax and Whitmore (1973) likewise found that a short battery of neurodevelopmental tests given at school entrance identified many of the children who later developed reading or behavior problems at school. Finally, Kohen-Raz (1970) discovered that an electronically-generated measure of postural steadiness correlated significantly, in a kindergarten sample, with a teacher rating of school readiness and with performance on an arithmetic readiness test. Although this study examined concurrent relationships between steadiness and academic readiness, a predictive relationship is suggested to whatever extent the readiness ratings and tests themselves predict future educational progress.

Critique of the Evidence and Research Needs

Given that soft signs are associated with age, IQ, and a diverse set of behavior-learning disorders, one of the limitations of these signs may be that they lack clinical specificity. In other words, soft sign measures may tell us nothing new or unique about an individual that we could not learn by means of other psychological test procedures. In support of this possibility, several investigators report that the raised incidence of soft signs is only apparent when comparisons involve groups with more pervasive cognitive-developmental disorders (Ingram, Mason, & Blackburn, 1970; Rutter, Graham, & Birch, 1966). In studies by Rutter et al (1970) and Rutter and Yule (1975), children with specific learning disorders who performed relatively well on IQ tests failed to show any greater prevalence of soft signs than did a control group of nondisabled children. This same trend was apparent in a study conducted under the auspices of Dr. Paul Satz's longitudinal dyslexia project (Taylor, Satz, & Friel, 1979). In this study, 75 children with established problems in reading received neurological examinations. Based largely on soft signs, 4 of the subgroup of 37 children designated as dyslexic (not having other psychosocial or intellectual handicaps) were judged to be abnormal on the neurological exam (11 percent). In contrast, 10 of the subgroup of 38 nondyslexic poor readers were judged to be neurologically abnormal (26 percent). Outright neurological disorder was not responsible for the greater frequency of soft signs in the nondyslexic group.

The implication of this and other findings reviewed here is that soft signs are associated with a host of other problems. If soft signs are considered to have any special utility, they must be shown to have validity independent of their association with other psychological measures. Disabled versus nondisabled comparisons involving groups that are either unmatched or loosely matched on IQ, age, or social variables — as is the case for many of the investigations cited above — provide only a weak form of support for the criterion-related validity of signs. Stronger support for the utility of these signs demands investigation of their *discriminant validity* vis-à-vis other behavioral measures.

Although few studies have dealt with the latter issue in a direct manner, there is some reason to believe that soft signs may indeed possess unique measurement properties. Wolff and Hurwitz (1973), for example, found that children with choreiform movements had more problems in reading, spelling, and behavior than a control group without choreiform movements. Because the two groups did not differ in IQ, the association between soft signs and school problems could be regarded as at least partially independent of IQ. In Hertzig's (1981) study of prematurely born children, children with soft signs were more likely to be referred for psychiatric consultation or to be involved in special educational programs than the children without soft signs, even though there were no significant differences in IQ or in reading and arithmetic achievement test scores.

In what is likely the most well-conceived study of this issue to date, Wolff et al (1985) examined 50 kindergarten and 50 first-grade children. The children were sampled from a normal population and were tested on 3 successive occasions at 6-month intervals. On each occasion, the following neuromotor performances were examined: synkinesias from stress gaits, mirror movements from discrete finger displacements, timed maneuvers, mirror movements from clip pinching, gross motor balance, and fine motor steadiness. In addition to this comprehensive soft sign battery, the investigators administered tests of academic achievement, language and memory abilities, and psychometric intelligence (prorated WISC-R IQ). The relationship of neuromotor status to the criterion tasks of academic achievement and language and memory abilities was analyzed via regression equations into which age and IQ were entered as control variables. Results revealed that neuromotor performance was related both predictively and concurrently to the criterion measures independent of IQ. In fact, neuromotor status accounted for a greater percentage of variance in two specific criterion measures (reading and rapid naming) than did IQ.

Additional although less convincing evidence for discriminant validity comes from studies of hyperactive children. Werry et al (1972) and Hertzig et al (1969) report a greater prevalence of soft signs in hyperactive children than in children with other behavior problems. In the Hertzig et al (1969) investigation there is no information regarding the ages, sexes, IQs, or social classes of the hyperactive and nonhyperactive groups. Consequently, one cannot determine if differences in the latter variables may have contributed to the between-group differences in soft signs. Werry et al (1972) investigated only children with normal IQs and controlled for sex, age, and social class. However, because mean IQs for the hyperactive and nonhyperactive clinic groups are not reported, differences in IQ within the normal range may have at least partially accounted for the differential prevalence of soft signs in their two groups. Mikkelsen et al (1982) also found more soft signs in hyperactive children compared to either control or other clinic-referred groups. The only selection requirement regarding intelligence was that WISC-R IQ be 80 or greater. Again, one cannot rule out the possibility that results reflected between-group differences in normal-range IQ scores. In a study reported by Shaffer et al (1983), in which a group of children having soft signs at age 7 was compared to a similar-aged group without soft signs, differences between the groups in reading and spelling were nonsignificant after adjustments for IQ. Nevertheless, the latter investigators found some evidence for a specific association between hyperactivity and soft signs. Soft signs were associated with hyperactivity, but only for children with IQs less than 80. This result provides one of the rare indications in the literature that it may be best to regard the presence of soft signs as an index of vulnerability, and that the association of soft signs with clinical problems may therefore be relative to the child's status in other respects.

There is also evidence for associations between soft signs and specific forms of psychiatric disturbance. In a follow-up of their children with and without soft signs at ages 16-18 years, Shaffer et al (1983) reported an excess of affective disorders among the children with soft signs. According to these researchers, this differential rate of affective disorder was independent of IQ. Associations between soft signs and psychiatric disturbances are further documented by Hertzig and Birch (1968) and by Quitkin, Rifkin, and Klein (1976). In the Hertzig-Birch study, soft signs were more frequently associated, at least in females, with diagnoses of psychosis than with other mental disorders. However, IQ scores are not reported; and this same differential association was not as apparent for psychiatrically disturbed male adolescents. Quitkin et al found soft signs more prevalent in schizophrenics with premorbid asociality and in persons with emotionally unstable character disorders in comparison to other psychiatric groups. However, the two psychiatric groups with the greatest number of soft signs also had lower mean IQs than the other patient groups. In general, evidence regarding the discriminant validity of soft signs is mixed. Although soft signs have promise in this regard, the issue of discriminant validity has not received the attention it deserves.

Another limitation regarding validation research is the inconsistency of results reported across investigations. Unlike Wolff and Hurwitz (1973), Rutter et al (1966) could not demonstrate an association between choreiform movements and teacher ratings of behavior problems. In their investigation of children on the Isle of Wight, Rutter et al (1970) also failed to find differences between reading retarded and normal children on a more comprehensive neurological examination that included soft signs. Additional negative findings are reported by Erikson (1977) and by Camp, Bialer, Sverd, and Winsberg (1978). The fact that learning disabled and normal children were matched on IQ in Erikson's study makes her findings of particular interest. In other cases, comparisons have revealed greater numbers of soft signs for disabled children than for normal children. However, differences have been so slight and the overlap between disordered and normal groups so extensive that investigators have questioned the clinical utility of soft sign exams (Adams, Kocsis, & Estes,1974; Werry

& Aman, 1976). The predictive validity of soft signs for learning disabled children is also suspect. In an extensive follow-up project by Ackerman, Dykman, and Peters (1977), the results of a special developmental neurological examination administered between 8 and 11 years of age did not predict achievement-level outcomes at age 14.

The lack of close correspondence between soft signs and clinical disorders represents a further limitation to the validity of soft signs. The percentage of learning disabled or hyperactive children without soft signs can range as high as 50 percent (Cantwell, 1975; Dubey, 1976; Taylor, Satz, & Friel, 1979). Even severe forms of reading disability may be found in the absence of any indications of abnormal neurological status (Ingram, Mason, & Blackburn, 1970). Conversely, many normal or even supernormal children exhibit soft signs (Copple & Isom, 1968). Rutter et al (1970) found that 16 percent of a group of children selected on the basis of having good academic skills and no evidence of cognitive dysfunction had between 5 and 10 soft signs each. The existence of soft signs in substantial numbers of normal children has been documented in several investigations (Adams, Kocsis, & Estes, 1974; Hart et al, 1974; Wolff & Hurwitz, 1966).

This lack of one-to-one correspondence between behavior-learning abnormalities and soft sign status suggests that soft signs have limited applicability in the diagnosis or treatment of individual children. However, it would be wrong to conclude that soft signs are of no value whatsoever in clinical practice. I can personally attest to the striking motor and sensory-motor difficulties exhibited by some learning disabled and attentionally deficient children with normal intelligence. Although research findings do not yet permit me to draw any definitive conclusions in these cases, I continue to be intrigued by the possibility that soft sign measures provide useful clinical indices when considered in concert with other findings. The same methodological considerations that make it difficult to interpret soft signs make it equally difficult to dismiss them outright as useless or irrelevant. Fair appraisal of the utility of soft signs demands that further more methodological sound investigations be carried out.

To help resolve some of the outstanding issues regarding soft signs, further investigation must address a number of specific research needs.

Operationalizing measurement. A survey of the research literature reveals that soft neurological signs are typically defined in qualitative rather than in quantitative terms. Exact specifications of even those qualitative aspects of performance that signal the presence-absence of abnormality are lacking. Although there is usually some stipulation regarding the types of behaviors that would indicate abnormality, or the numbers of such behaviors required for the designation of abnormality (e.g., number of choreiform twitches), the features that render a response abnormal and the precise threshold for judging these features to be present are usually unspecified. In some cases, these uncertainties are resolved in a *post hoc* fashion. This procedure assures agreement between observers but does little to communicate procedures to others who might be trying to replicate findings. Trying to remove all subjective factors or create measures that do not rely whatsoever on the experience of the examiner may prove unproductive. Nevertheless, the use of videotapes, the development of refined rating scales, and substantial training in the use of these ratings prior to their formal application may be steps in the right direction.

Neuhauser (1975) describes three fundamental methods for assessing motor skills and movement patterns. The distinctions he draws between these methods suggest avenues along which to refine soft sign measurement. According to Neuhauser, the three methods involve: (1) description of the movement (motoscopy); (2) measurement of performance by means of counting, rating, or timing of movements (motometry); and (3) instrumental recording of movements (motography). Soft sign performances scored in terms of a unit of measurement, as do methods (2) and (3), are likely to show greater inter-observer reliability than measures that are dependent on qualitative observations alone (Werry & Aman, 1976). An additional advantage of quantitative rating scales and instrumentalized recording systems is that they foster the study of the components of soft sign responses (e.g., degree of movement excursion, speed, acceleration). Assessing coordination by counting the number of sequences of movements that can be made within set time limits illustrates sound motometric measurement (Denckla, 1974; Wolff et al, 1983). The motographic approach is exemplified by Bonnevier (1968). Bonnevier measured diadochokinesis in children by taping the child's hand to a rod. When the rod turned, the movement was recorded on a rotating drum. The advantage of his technique over more traditional assessments of diadochokinesis is that his instrument recorded exact rate, timing, and extent of pronation-supination.

An especially good example of how motographic techniques might be applied to the study of soft signs is provided by Schellekens, Scholten, and Kalverboer (1983). These investigators compared children with good and poor neurological optimality scores on a task requiring movement of the child's finger back and forth between lighted buttons. In this study, the exact nature of the child's movement was analyzed by an optical electronic system that allowed for tracing of the hand, arm, and trunk movement and of the positions of the finger, wrist, elbow, and shoulder with respect to one another. Simultaneous with this recording, the investigators videotaped the children in order to render overall ratings of the fluency of their movements and the degree of task orientation. Results confirmed that the group with greater numbers of soft signs (neurological nonoptimality) differed not only in terms of macroscopic variables such as overall ratings of task orientation, movement fluency, and rate of response, but that the groups differed with respect to the more microscopic characteristics of their performance as well. Differences were found, for example, in movement elements, irregularities of movement, time to the "first movement element," and time to "maximal acceleration." Results were interpreted to reflect differences between the groups in the programming of movement components. Further extensions of this type of methodology to the study of soft signs themselves would seem to hold promise as a means of achieving better quantification and of isolating those aspects of performance that may prove to have greatest validity.

Assessments of reliability and stability of measurement. Given the measures of soft neurological status usually applied, poor inter-rater agreement and instability of signs in a given individual across time (McMahon & Greenberg, 1977; Werry & Aman, 1976) should come as no surprise. Personal experience confirms that inter-rater reliability is difficult to achieve without extensive training. An additional hazard is that performance on soft sign tests may be subject to the effects of behavioral epiphenomena such as cooperation, stress, and practice (see Rapoport & Ferguson, 1981; Shafer, Shaffer, O'Connor, & Stokman, 1983). There is no doubt that acceptable levels of inter-observer reliability and test-retest stability can be attained, at least for research purposes (Mikkelsen et al, 1982; Peters et al, 1975; Quitkin, Rifkin, & Klein, 1976; Rutter, Graham, & Yule, 1966; Werry et al, 1972). But the fact that reasonable levels of reliability can be obtained in studies that assess reliability does not assure the reliability of the soft sign measures used in other studies.

Further problems include the fact that reliability is often measured in terms of correlation coefficients or the percentage of ratings in which there is agreement between observers. Considered in isolation, these parameters do not give a true picture of reliability. Correlation coefficients and frequencies of inter-rater agreement are readily inflated by the inclusion of ordinal measures where the occurrence rates are low (and thus agreement regarding the absence of a sign high), or where there is a reasonably high probability of chance agreement. Because soft sign measures often involve ordinal scales with few subcategories, inappropriate assessment of reliability represents a major concern. In such circumstances, the use of the Kappa statistic has been recommended, for it takes both sources of error into account (Cicchetti & Sparrow, 1981; Shafer et al, 1983). Shafer et al review neurological soft signs studies for which Kappa was either calculated or could be derived from available data. Their analyses suggest that acceptable levels of reliability are obtainable (see also Mikkelsen et al, 1982; Quitkin, Rifkin, & Klein, 1976).

Comprehensive assessment of reliability also demands analysis of the consistency of ratings across individual soft sign responses, and even across scale points for a single response. Since inter-rater reliability can vary substantially as a function of the behavior measured (Werry & Aman, 1976), reliability estimates for individual soft sign tests may help to eliminate problematic items and thus shorten the time needed for assessment. In view of the fact that agreement can vary markedly between scale points, it may also be possible to tighten up individual scales by creating more meaningful gradations of judgment. In their case, Rutter et al (1966) found only 34 percent agreement for the "slight movement" subcategory of choreiform movements, compared to 53 percent agreement for "marked movements."

Developing items with good inter-rater reliability will help to assure that measurement methods can be effectively communicated to other investigators and hopefully contribute to the replicability of findings. However, inter-rater reliability does not assure stability of measurement over time. The stability of a given measure is a function of variation within the subject as well as variation within and between raters. To determine to what extent soft sign measures assess constant characteristics of an individual, it is also necessary to employ a test-retest format. In this fashion, the researcher can estimate the amount of intra-subject variability with soft sign responses due either to systematic (e.g., time of testing or practice) or to nonsystematic (error) effects. Variability within clinically disordered groups may be of some interest for its own sake. However, such variability is meaningless unless it can be shown to be independent of systematic environmental influences, and unless reasonable levels of stability exist for normal individuals.

Like inter-rater reliability, test-retest reliability has not received the attention it deserves. Nevertheless, available evidence suggests that soft signs persist across test occasions (Hertzig, 1982; Quitkin, Rifkin, & Klein, 1976; Shapiro, Burkes, Petti, & Ranz, 1978; Rutter, Graham, & Yule, 1970). Quitkin et al (1976) demonstrated a high degree of consistency in the total number of signs observed over two test occasions separated by one or two days (r = .96). In Hertzig's (1982) longitudinal study, 53 children were examined over a four-year test-retest interval. Although the mean number of soft signs diminished across time, the numbers of children who exhibited two or more soft signs did not show a significant decrease. In all of the above-cited studies, the persistence of soft signs across test occasions varied from item to item. In the Hertzig study, consistency ranged from 47-75 percent. Hertzig also found that consistency was related to IQ, with children having lower IQs showing greater numbers of inconsistent findings. The results of these several studies again underscore the importance of evaluating reliability item for item and of not assuming that the findings for one group of individuals will necessarily generalize to all other groups.

Analyses of what is measured by soft signs. Because of the amorphous nature of the soft sign category and because the frequency and reliability of performance varies from item to item, individual soft sign measures require more careful study. Little is known regarding the dimensions of behaviors measured by soft signs or the extent to which individual soft sign items relate to one another or form separable clusters. Information of this sort is essential in designing an efficient soft sign battery and in deciding if soft sign measures add information over and above that provided by other assessments.

There is some reason to believe that aggregate soft sign scores based on a sum of ratings of individual items may prove more reliable and clinically useful than item-by-item comparisons of groups (Gottesman, Croen, & Rotkin, 1982; Rutter, Graham, & Yule, 1970; Touwen & Prechtl, 1970; Werry & Aman , 1976). It has also been suggested that those signs that best discriminate between disordered and normal groups may comprise a more fundamental dimension of motor awkwardness or sensory-motor incoordination (Peters, Romine, & Dykman, 1975; Werry et al, 1972). Several factor analytic studies involving soft signs together with other psychological and neurological variables suggest that a core of soft signs may indeed cluster on a motor incoordination dimension (see Paine et al, 1968; Werry, 1968; 1972).

However, more recent factor analytic work involving other cognitive variables in addition to soft signs fails to provide support for a distinct soft sign dimension. In their study, Rie, Rie, Steward, and Rettemnier (1978) found evidence for several clusters of soft signs. Because various cognitive variables combined with soft signs to form these clusters, the results of Rie et al raise doubts as to whether soft signs should be considered a unified category, or one necessarily distinct from other behavioral measures. One major implication of these latter findings is that it may be profitable to study soft signs in isolation rather than as aggregates. In support of this possibility, Denckla and Rudel (1978) found that motor overflow was more closely related to hyperactivity than were other soft sign measures. Similarly, Wolff et al (1985) discovered that mirror movements, timed fine motor maneuvers, and static balance were more highly related to reading and naming performance than were other soft sign variables. The latter investigators also found that certain measures of associated movement were more age-sensitive than others (Wolff, Gunnoe, & Cohen, 1983). Within the age range of the children studied, overflow from timed sequences of finger movements was, for example, more prominent than overflow from repetitions of a single finger movement.

Review of the neurological soft sign data we collected in our study of post-meningitis children and their siblings lends additional support to the tactic of examining individual soft sign items. As in the case of the Wolff et al (1985) study, our data indicated a high degree of intercorrelation between the three measures of motor overflow we employed. Even after adjusting for age and IQ differences, partial correlations between the three overflow variables (total sample) ranged from .59 to .69. These partial correlations were generally higher than correlations between overflow and other soft sign measures. Analyses of our data further revealed that performances of post-meningitis and sibling groups were significantly different for only a subset of individual soft sign raw scores. Evidently, some of the measures contributed more than others to the overall difference between groups in the age-adjusted total score. Although by no means definitive, these results (unpublished) offer additional confirmation of the need for investigators to inspect the contents of their soft sign batteries. Only in this manner will it be possible to eliminate redundancy and to enhance the overall sensitivity of soft sign measures.

A second implication of the Rie et al (1978) findings is the question they raise about the psychological significance of soft signs — that is, the construct validity of these signs in a psychological rather than a biological sense. Evidence that soft signs tap a primary motor coordination dimension suggests that it may be worthwhile to examine soft sign status in relation to performance on standardized tests of motor ability and praxis. Numerous age-standardized tests of motor skill are available (see Bialer, Doll, & Winsberg, 1974; Gardner, 1979; Graziani, Mason & Cracco, 1981; Gubbay, 1975). Gubbay, Ellis, Walton, and Court (1965) found that children who were severely clumsy had a number of apraxic and agnostic deficits (e.g., difficulties in folding paper and in imitating sequential movements). Compared to their more coordinated peers, the clumsy children were generally fidgety and displayed a more marked lowering of performance relative to verbal IQ on the WISC. Severe difficulties in writing and printing, short attention spans, and articulatory apraxia have also been reported in clumsy children (Walton, Ellis, & Court, 1962). To the extent that soft sign performances overlap with skills assessed by motor batteries, these findings point to potential soft sign correlates. Perusal of the existing literature also confirms correspondences between soft signs and such traits as impulsivity, immaturity, lower performance IQ and perceptual-motor deficits, and hyperactivity (Anderson, 1963; Denckla & Rudel, 1978; Hertzig, Bortner, & Birch, 1969; Paulsen & O'Donnell, 1979; Pretchl & Stemmer, 1962; Werry, 1972; Werry et al, 1972). It may well be that the same common thread of behavior, perhaps something akin to perceptual-motor planning or sequencing, is being tapped in each of these various studies. Wolff et al (1985) suggest that certain neuromotor measures may represent a "manifestation of a genetic mechanism for the serial order control and timing precision of timed distributed functions" (p. 13), and that this mechanism may also predispose the child to problems in other areas, including speech fluency and the temporal organization of expressive speech. In a similar vein, Dykman, Ackerman, Clements, and Peters (1971) argue that basic attention-organizational difficulties account for both motor incoordination and learning disabilities. Although hypotheses of this sort are highly speculative, they do raise the possibility that soft signs tap important behavioral dimensions. Investigation of the psychological correlates of soft signs would help to clarify these traits.

More detailed study of the disorders with which soft signs are associated. Studies of broad groupings of children or adults is unlikely to reveal any relationship between soft signs and clinical disorder. Future research efforts would be well advised to avoid groupings of subjects on the basis of their membership in categories such as learning disability, hyperactivity, minimal brain dysfunction, or psychiatric disturbance. A more promising approach is to examine soft signs in relation to specific features of a given clinical disorder, or to compare highly selected subgroups of disordered individuals with each other and with nondisordered groups. The benefits of more refined analyses of disordered populations is illustrated by Loney, Langhorne, and Paternite (1978). These researchers discovered that soft signs were more frequent in nonaggressive hyperactive children than in hyperactive children who were also aggressive. Previously reviewed studies by Hertzig and Birch (1968) and Quitkin et al (1976) further attest to the differential frequency of soft signs across clinical subgroups. In both of these latter studies, soft signs varied in accordance with specific psychiatric diagnoses. Selection of subjects within relatively restricted age ranges also seems advisable, at least in child studies. Wolff et al (1983) found fairly narrow age-sensitivities for measures of motor overflow. Similarly, Chissom (1971) discovered that motor abilities were related to academic achievement in first grade boys but not in third grade boys.

Use of appropriate multivariate methodology. There are several advantages to studying soft signs in relationship to a multitude of environmental, social, and cognitive variables. One benefit is that multivariate approaches allow the researcher to explore the extent to which group differences in soft signs are a function of differences in these other variables. Only by examining soft signs in association with other measurements will it be possible to discover if these signs tap unique dimensions of behavior and, if so, to begin to cull out from the total soft sign examination those elements that are most unique. If soft signs are to merit continued application in evaluating clinical problems, these signs must tell us something about etiology, behavioral correlates, or treatment alternatives that other measures do not tell us. As noted earlier, confounds between soft signs and other behavioral and environmental measures also shed light on what these signs measure.

A further advantage of multivariate approaches is the opportunity they afford for studying soft signs as indices of vulnerability. Considering the numbers of normal children who manifest soft signs, it may be unreasonable to expect direct relationships between soft signs and clinical problems. Soft signs may only prove worthwhile if studied from an "interactional" perspective. According to this view, soft signs would be regarded as increasing the risk of learning or behavior disorder, but only if certain other risk factors were also present. This concept of vulnerability is best illustrated by Shaffer et al (1983), who as noted earlier found that soft signs were associated with hyperactivity, but only in children with lower IQs. A further example is provided by Waber, Bauermeister, Cohen, Ferber, and Wolff (1981). This research group discovered that the relationship between neuromotor status (based on associated movements) and neuropsychological performance depended on the social status of the groups tested. According to Waber et al, "the particular expression of a psychobiological relationship can differ materially for individuals from different environments" (p. 521).

The importance of studying soft signs within an interactional framework has been emphasized before (Hertzig & Birch, 1968; Prechtl, 1980; Quitkin, Rifkin, & Klein, 1976; Wolff & Hurwitz, 1966; Yule, 1978). In general, however, this sentiment has failed to culminate in research programs that consider soft signs as one variable among others in relation to clinical disorder. If soft signs are conceived of as risk factors, then these signs must be evaluated in conjunction with other problems. A child whose soft signs co-occur with language difficulties, for example, may be more prone to reading disability, whereas a child with a co-existing conduct disorder may be more liable to overactivity. Exploring these and other possibilities demands a multivariate methodology.

A sound multivariate approach involves more than simultaneous measurement of several variables. If this approach is to be productive, methods of data collection and interpretation must be sound. The researcher will need to make sure that soft sign measures meet psychometric standards for reliability and validity and that other dependent measures chosen meet these same standards. Because of the extensive time required for administration of multiple measures, researchers will need to take precautions to avoid any systematic effect of subject fatigue on test results. Due to the subjective nature of some of the ratings of soft signs and possible influences on judgment of such traits as uncooperativeness and fidgetiness (Shafer et al, 1983), investigators may need to be especially careful to avoid examiner biases. One way to minimize potential bias is to simply keep testers blind as to the clinical status of the participant. In addition, administration procedures may need to be closely prescribed, careful instructions and demonstrations provided to assure that the participant understands the task, and videotaping procedures employed as a means of checking for bias.

Finally, it is imperative that appropriate statistical procedures be used to analyze complex multivariate data sets. One potential problem is Type I error. Spurious positive findings are more likely when multiple univariate comparisons are carried out independently. To reduce Type I errors, multivariate analyses of variance or adjustment for the number of comparisons being made via the Bonferroni method are recommended. Other common statistical failings are failure to include enough subjects relative to the number of dependent measures, and the use of covariance procedures to control for the effects of a covariant when that covariant is confounded with the independent variable (Bock, 1975; Evans & Anastasio, 1968; Timm, 1975). The existing soft sign literature is replete with studies in which these basic statistical requirements have been ignored. More sophisticated applications of statistical procedures and rules of inference should enhance the interpretability of future multivariate approaches to the study of soft signs.

SUMMARY AND CONCLUSION

The topic of soft neurological signs is likely to remain a controversial one for some time. In large part, substantive issues regarding the meaning and significance of soft signs will have to be resolved by way of methodologically sound research. Investigators must be fully aware of what we know and do not know about soft signs. They must also be prepared to separate presumptions from facts, develop a familiarity with methodological issues, and work collaboratively with specialists from a variety of fields. The major aim of this chapter has been to discuss areas of contention regarding soft signs; and, in the process, to summarize existing findings, methodological shortcomings, and research needs. Areas of contention involve questions about the boundaries of the soft sign category, neurological implications of soft signs, and their utility in relation to disorders of behavior or learning.

For the time being, the makeup of the soft sign category is determined largely by historical precedent and other a priori considerations. Empirical findings may eventually result in elimination of some items presently included in this category. For example, if certain measures prove to be highly redundant with others or cannot be reliably elicited, these measures would be sensibly excluded from soft sign batteries. Available data, however, fail to provide sufficient grounds for making decisions of this sort. Some investigators may wish to focus more exclusively on one type of soft sign (e.g., associated movements). But inclusion of a broad variety of signs representative of the core group noted earlier in this chapter would also seem well-justified. Due to the lack of established clinical-pathological correlations for signs of the "subtle hard" variety, there is reason to include these measures in soft sign batteries, so long as they can be reliably assessed. Because neurological history is critical to the interpretation of findings on the neurological exam, researchers might also addend collection of this information to the soft sign battery.

At the same time, it is reasonable to impose certain restrictions on the contents of soft sign batteries. Specifically, it is inappropriate to refer to abnormalities on tests of specialized functions assessed by speech pathologists, educators, psychologists, or electrophysiologists as soft signs (Shaffer et al, 1983). Soft signs are most clearly distinguished from other behavioral measures by virtue of their reliance on those aspects of motor and sensory-motor abilities typically assessed in a comprehensive pediatric neurological examination. A more commonly agreed upon and unique referent to the term "soft signs" would be one advantage of imposing such definitional restrictions. Adopting a more restrictive definition would not prohibit the researcher or clinician from administering additional tests of coordination, neuropsychological skill, speech and language, academic achievement, or electrophysiological responsivity. However, these latter measures are less exclusively within the province of the standard neurological examination than are the motor and sensory-motor measures referred to above. Without setting fairly strict boundaries on the soft sign category, and without basing these boundaries on historical precedence, so wide a variety of behavioral abnormalities would qualify as a soft sign as to render the term of little meaning.

The two other areas of contention regarding soft signs cannot be resolved on a priori grounds. The reason is that these issues have to do with *beliefs* about soft signs. Careful evaluation of the data bearing on each belief is required. Suggestions are needed regarding research strategies that are likely to lead to firmer grounds for accepting, rejecting, or modifying these beliefs.

The first belief is that soft signs have special neurological significance. In this regard, it is essential to recognize that there are no established clinical-pathological correlates for soft signs that would constitute proof of their relationship with pathophysiology of the central nervous system. After all, if clinical-pathological correlates were established, these signs could hardly be considered "soft." The term soft is applied, not because these signs represent subtle manifestations of definitive neurological disorders, but because their neurological significance rests on indirect evidence and is therefore uncertain. The brain-relatedness of these signs can only be judged in terms of the extent to which their presence is either correlated with outright neurological disease or, in individuals without clear-cut neurological disorder, is associated with other indirect indications of neurogenecity. Other indirect indices of neuropathology include evidence for genetic influences, associations with developmental delays or with dysfunction in speech and language or neuropsychological skills, minor physical anomalies, pre- and perinatal complications, electrophysiological irregularities, responsivity to medications, and lack of correspondence with psychosocial status (Taylor & Fletcher, 1983).

A review of the relevant literature reveals that soft signs are indeed found in association with a host of developmental, learning, and behavior problems. There is also evidence that these signs may help to predict responsivity to stimulant medications, and that their presence may be relatively independent of socioeconomic factors. In each regard, however, the evidence is sparse and inconsistent. Because soft signs are often accompanied by other abnormalities (e.g. lower IQ), there is reason to question whether soft signs have special neurological significance vis-à-vis other behavioral measures. We cannot reject the possibility that at least some types of soft signs may index "subclinical" neuropathology; or that some signs may be relatively more sensitive to nonpathological variations in structural/physiological brain status than to social-environmental factors, at least compared to other behavioral measures (Shaffer et al, 1983; Wender, 1971; Wolff, Gunnoe, & Cohen, 1983). According to E. Taylor (1983), however, we must also "be prepared to regard such an examination as an index only of motor learning, susceptible to the same influences as other kinds of learning, and like them bearing only a remote relationship to the integrity of the brain" (p. 249).

In summary, the conviction that soft signs carry special neurological implications rests on shaky grounds but cannot be dismissed entirely. Studies of soft signs involving groups of persons with and without outright brain disease, or comparisons between individuals with different forms of brain disease, may help to establish if certain types of soft signs represent subclinical neurological sequelae. Studies of this sort may eventually reveal that certain varieties of soft signs are just as valid as the "harder" residuals of cerebral palsy (e.g., paresis). Whether or not persons with definitive neurological disorders are included for study, assessment of social variables is essential. To the extent that soft signs provide relatively pure measures of neural integrity, researchers should be able to show dissociations with social status or with psychological performance variables known to be relatively dependent on experiential influences. A final tactic for examining the belief that soft signs have special neurological significance is to study associations between these signs and the other presumptive indices of brain-relatedness. The belief that soft signs have neurological implications remains tenable to the extent that soft signs vary in accordance with sex or family history, or are associated with electrophysiological irregularities, minor congenital anomalies, pre- and perinatal complications, specific patterns of developmental delay or neuropsychological impairment, or responsiveness to medications.

A second and separable belief regarding soft signs is that they are useful in making clinical judgments, and thus have criterion-related validity. Soft signs may indeed be useful in specifying diagnosis, prognosis, or preferred treatment, even if these signs have no special neurological significance. Criterion-related validity is evidenced by relationships between soft signs and chronological age, and by the increased prevalence of soft signs in groups of children or adults who are hyperactive or learning disabled or who display other indications of behavioral deviance. A major limitation to the support for the second belief is that there is considerable overlap in soft signs between disordered and normal groups. Other limitations include the fact that some studies have failed to find between-group differences in soft signs. Even where differences have been found, failure to measure or to adequately control for variables such as IQ, sex, age, and social status makes it difficult to interpret these differences. A higher frequency of soft signs in disordered compared to normal groups has been reported in studies that appear to have been free of these confounds (Owen, Adams, & Forrest, 1971; Wolff & Hurwitz, 1973). But other studies fail to substantiate such group differences (Erickson, 1977; Rutter, Graham, & Birch, 1966; Rutter, Graham, & Yule, 1970). For the time being, the belief that soft signs are clinically useful is plausible but not well founded. Further research is required to clarify the criterion-related validity of soft signs.

Improved understanding of the meaning of soft signs is likely to come from attention to several methodological needs. The most obvious of these needs is to develop quantifiable measurement techniques that preserve the content validity of soft signs while simultaneously enhancing both interobserver and test-retest reliability. Improvements in reliability demand a turning away from quantitative rating scales and the provision of examiner training. Videotaping in combination with technologically sophisticated measurement methods may also make it possible to analyze the component movement irregularities that constitute a given soft sign. A second methodological need is to study the measurement characteristics of soft signs in greater detail. This can be accomplished by exploring associations between items within the soft sign category and between soft signs and other psychological measures. Investigating relationships between soft sign items will help to determine whether this category of responses constitutes a single dimension of behavior, or multiple dimensions. Exploring associations between soft signs and other psychological test performances (e.g., tests of sequencing, praxis, motor coordination, attention) will enhance our understanding of what soft signs measure. Of particular interest is the possibility that soft signs measure unique dimensions of behavior — perhaps ones relating to temporal-spatial integration, motor planning, or impulse control. A third prerequisite to more methodologically sound research is to examine soft signs in relation to specific correlates or subtypes of clinical disorders. Soft signs may prove helpful, for example, in subtyping learning disabled or hyperactive children. But it is unlikely that these signs will be of any use whatsoever in distinguishing learning disabled children in general from their nondisabled peers. Finally, a multivariate approach is imperative. Soft signs are not associated in a one-to-one fashion with behavior or learning problems, or even with generalized developmental delays. Moreover, the significance of soft signs varies with age. In light of these facts, it might be best to view deviant performance on soft sign tests as signaling risk more so than actual impairment. The final clinical picture would then be determined by a host of other social-psychological variables.

Taking a multivariate perspective is particularly relevant to clinical interpretation of soft signs in individual children. Considered in isolation, soft signs do not have undisputed neurological significance or clinical value. On the other hand, further study may yet show that particular soft sign measures are quite sensitive to structural-physiological deviations of the central nervous system; or that, independent of their neurological significance, these measures may prove useful as indices of risk or as predictors of the type, course, or preferred treatment of a given clinical disorder. This state of uncertainty need not dissuade the clinician from incorporating soft sign measures into the assessment of individuals with behavior or learning disorders. What is important is that the clinician be aware that soft signs have neurological significance and clinical utility by virtue of conviction more so than fact. When found in association with a behavior-learning disorder, soft signs may raise one's suspicion of constitutional influences (Taylor, 1983). However, soft signs do not prove that there is a constitutional basis for the presenting problem; nor do soft signs help to establish the importance of constitutional considerations, even if we granted these signs etiological significance. In light of what we presently know, soft neurological signs in a given child or adult cannot be said to have any straightforward implications and should only be considered in conjunction with a good deal of other information about the individual.

REFERENCES

Ackerman PT, Dykman RA, & Peters JE. Learning-disabled boys as adolescents: Cognitive factors and achievement. Journal of the American Academy of Child Psychiatry, 1977, 16, 296-313

Adams R, Kocsis J, & Estes RE. Soft neurological signs in learning disabled children and controls. American Journal of Diseases of Children, 1974, 128, 614-618

Anderson WW. The hyperkinetic child: A neurological appraisal. Neurology, 1963, 13, 968-973

Barkley RA. Predicting the response of hyperkinetic children to stimulant drugs: A review. Journal of Abnormal Child Psychology, 1976, 4, 327-348

Baumeister A, & MacLean W. Brain damage and mental retardation. In Ellis NR (Ed.). Handbook of Mental Deficiency: Psychological Theory and Research (2nd ed). Hillsdale, NJ: Lawrence Erlbaum, 1979

Bax M, & Whitmore K. Neurodevelopmental screening in the school-entrant medical examination. Lancet, 1973, 2, 368-370

Bender L. Psychopathology of Children with Organic Brain Disorders. Springfield, Ill: Charles C. Thomas, 1956

Benton AL. Minimal brain dysfunction from the neuropsychological point of view. Annals of the New York Academy of Sciences, 1973, 205, 29-37

Bialer I, Doll L, & Winsberg BD. A modified Lincoln-Oseretsky motor development scale: Provisional standardization. Perceptual and Motor Skills, 1974, 38, 598-614

Bock RD. Multivariate Statistics for the Behavioral Sciences. New York: McGraw-Hill, 1975

Bonnevier J. A study of diadochokinesia in school children. Acta Paedopsychiatrica, 1968, 35, 70-78

Bortner M, Hertzig ME, & Birch HG. Neurological signs and intelligence in brain-damaged children. Journal of Special Education, 1972, 6, 325-333

Camp JA, Bialer I, Sverd J, & Winsberg BD. Clinical usefulness of the NIMH Physical and Neurological Examination for Soft Signs. American Journal of Psychiatry, 1978, 135(3), 362-364

Cantwell DP. Diagnostic evaluation of the hyperactive child. In Cantwell DP (Ed.). The Hyperactive Child: Diagnosis, Management, Current Research. New York: Spectrum, 1975, pp. 17-50

Carey WB, McDevitt SC, & Baker D. Differentiating minimal brain dysfunction and temperament. Developmental Medicine and Child Neurology, 1979, 21, 765-772

Chissom BS. A factor-analytic study of the relationship of motor factors to academic criteria for first-and third-grade boys. Child Development, 1971, 42, 1133-1143

Cicchetti DV, & Sparrow SA. Developing criteria for establishing interrater reliability of specific items: Applications to assessment of adaptive behavior. American Journal of Mental Deficiency, 1981, 86(2), 127-137

Clements SD. Minimal Brain Dysfunction in Children — Terminology and Identification. NINDB Monograph, Washington, DC: U.S. Public Health Service, 1966

Clements S, & Peters J. Minimal brain dysfunction in the school age child. Archives of General Psychiatry, 1962, 6, 185-197

Cohen HJ, Taft LT, Mohadeviah MS, & Birch HG. Developmental changes in overflow in normal and aberrantly functioning children. Pediatrics, 1967, 71(1), 39-47

Connolly K, & Stratton P. Developmental changes in associated movements. Developmental Medicine and Child Neurology, 1968, 10, 49

Copple PJ, & Isom JB. Soft signs and scholastic success. Neurology, 1968, 18, 304

Denckla MB. Development of speed in repetitive and successive finger movements in normal children. Developmental Medicine and Child Neurology, 1973a, 15, 635-645

Denckla MB. Research needs in learning disabilities: A neurologists' point of view. Journal of Learning Disabilities, 1973b, 6, 441-450

Denckla MB. Development of coordination in normal children. Developmental Medicine and Child Neurology, 1974, 16, 729-741

Denckla MB. Minimal brain dysfunction and dyslexia: Beyond diagnosis by exclusion. In Blau ME, Rapin I, & Kinsbourne M (Eds.). Topics in Child Neurology. New York: Spectrum, 1977

Dencka MB, & Rudel RG. Anomalies of motor development in hyperactive boys. Annals of Neurology, 1978, 3, 231-233

Denhoff E, Siqueland, ML, Komich MP, & Hainsworth PK. Developmental and predictive characteristics of items from the Meeting Street School Screening Test. Developmental Medicine and Child Neurology, 1968, 10, 220-232

Dubey DR. Organic factors in hyperkinesis: A critical evaluation. American Journal of Orthopsychiatry, 1976, 46, 353-366

Dykman RA, Ackerman PT, Clements SD, & Peters JE. Specific learning disabilities: An attentional deficit syndrome. In Myklebust HR (Ed.). Progress in Learning Disabilities (Vol 2). New York: Grune & Stratton, 1971 pp. 56-94

Erickson MT. Reading disability in relation to performance on neurological tests for minimal brain dysfunction. Developmental Medicine and Child Neurology, 1977, 19, 768-775

Evans SH, & Anastasio EJ. Misuse of analysis of covariance when treatment effect and covariate are confounded. Psychological Bulletin, 1968, 69, 225-234

Fletcher JM, & Taylor HG. Neuropsychological approaches to children: Towards a developmental neuropsychology. Journal of Clinical Neuropsychology, 1984, 6(1), 39-56

Foster RM, Margolin L, Alexander C, et al. Equivocal neurological signs, child development, and learned behavior. Child Psychiatry and Human Development, 1978, 9, 28-32

Gardner RA. The Objective Diagnosis of Minimal Brain Dysfunction. Cresskill, NJ: Creative Therapeutics, 1979

Gold P. Suspected neurological impairment (SNI) and cognitive abilities: A longitudinal study of selected skills and predictive accuracy. Journal of Clinical Child Psychology, 1979, 8(1), 35-39

Gottesman RL, Croen L, & Rotkin L. Urban second grade children: A profile of good and poor readers. Journal of Learning Disabilities, 1982, 15(5), 268-272

Graziani LM, Mason JC, & Cracco J. Neurological aspects and early recognition of brain dysfunction in children: Diagnostic and prognostic significance of gestational, perinatal, and postnatal factors. In Black P (Ed.). Brain Dysfunction in Children: Etiology, Diagnosis, and Management. New York: Raven, 1981, pp. 131-169

Gubbay SS. The Clumsy Child: A Study of Developmental Apraxic and Agnostic Ataxia. London: WB Saunders, 1975

Gubbay SS, Ellis E, Walton JN, & Court SDM. Clumsy children: A study of apraxic and agnostic defects in 21 children. Brain, 1965, 88, 295-312

Hart R, Rennick PM, Klinge V, & Schwartz ML. A pediatric neurologist's contribution to evaluations of school underachievers. American Journal of Diseases of Children, 1974, 128, 319-323

Hertzig ME. Neurological "soft" signs in low-birthweight children. Developmental Medicine and Child Neurology, 1981, 23, 778-791

Hertzig ME. Stability and change in nonfocal neurological signs. Journal of the American Academy of Child Psychiatry, 1982, 21, 321-236

Hertzig ME, & Birch HG. Neurological organization in psychiatrically disturbed adolescents: A comparative consideration of sex differences. Archives of General Psychiatry, 1968, 19, 528-538

Hertzig ME, Bortner M, & Birch HG. Neurologic findings in children educationally designated as "brain-damaged." American Journal of Orthopsychiatry, 1969, 39(3), 437-447

Ingram TTS, Mason AW, & Blackburn KA. Retrospective study of 82 children with reading disability. Developmental Medicine and Child Neurology, 1970, 12, 271-281

Ingram TTS. Soft signs. Developmental Medicine and Child Neurology, 1973, 15, 527-529

Kalverboer AF. Neurobehavioral relationships in young children: Some concluding remarks on concepts and methods. In Knights RM, & Bakker DJ (Eds.). The Neuropsychology of Learning Disorders: Theoretical Approaches. Baltimore: University Park Press, 1976, pp. 173-183

Kalverboer AF, Touwen BCL, & Prechtl HFR. Follow-up of infants at risk of minor brain dysfunction. Annals of the New York Academy of Sciences, 1973, 205, 173-187

Kennard MA. Value of equivocal signs in neurological diagnosis. Neurology, 1960, 10, 753-764

Kenny TJ, & Clemmens RL. Medical and psychological correlates in children with learning disabilities. Pediatrics, 1971, 78(2), 273-277

Kohen-Raz R. Developmental patterns of static balance ability and their relation to cognitive school readiness. Pediatrics, 1970, 46(2), 276-285

Lerer RJ, & Lerer MP. The effects of methylphenidate on soft neurological signs of hyperactive children. Pediatrics, 1976, 57(4), 521-525

Loney J, Langhorne JE, & Paternite CE. A empirical basis for subgrouping the hyperactive/MBD syndrome. Journal of Abnormal Psychology, 1978, 87(4), 431-441

Lucas AR, Rodin EA, & Simson CB. Neurological assessment of children with early school problems. Developmental Medicine and Child Neurology, 1965, 7, 145-156

McMahon RC. Biological factors in childhood hyperkinesis: A review of genetic and biochemical hypotheses. Journal of Clinical Psychology, 1981, 37(1), 12-21

McMahon SA, & Greenberg LM. Serial neurological examination of hyperactive children. Pediatrics, 1977, 59, 584-587

Mikkelsen EJ, Brown GL, Minichiello MD, et al. Neurologic status in hyperactive, enuretic, encopretic, and normal boys. Journal of the American Academy of Child Psychiatry, 1982, 21, 75-81

Neuhauser G. Methods of assessing and recording motor skills and movement patterns. Developmental Medicine and Child Neurology, 1975, 17, 369-386

Nichols PL, & Chen T-C. Minimal Brain Dysfunction: A Prospective Study. Hillsdale, NJ: Lawrence Erlbaum Associates, 1981

Owen FW, Adams PA, Forrest T, et al. Learning disorders in children: Sibling studies. Monographs of the Society for Research in Child Development (Serial No. 144), 1971, 36(4), 1-77

Paine RS, Werry JS, & Quay HC. A study of minimal cerebral dysfunction.

Developmental Medicine and Child Neurology, 1968, 10, 505-520

Paulsen K, & O'Donnell JP. Construct validation of children's behavior problem dimensions: Relationship to activity level, impulsivity, and soft neurological signs. Journal of Psychology, 1979, 101, 273-278

Peter NM, & Spreen O. Behavioral and personal adjustment of learning disabled children during adolescence and early adulthood: A follow-up study. Journal of Clinical Neuropsychology, 1979, 1, 17-37

Peters JE, Romine JS, & Dykman RA. A special neurological examination of children with learning disabilities. Developmental Medicine and Child Neurology, 1975, 17, 63-78

Prechtl HFR. The optimality concept. Early Human Development, 1980, 4/3, 201-205

Prechtl HFR, & Stemmer CJ. The choreiform syndrome in children. Developmental Medicine and Child Neurology, 1962, 4, 119-127

Quitkin F, Rifkin A, & Klein DF. Neurological soft signs in schizophrenia and character disorders. Archives of General Psychiatry, 1976, 33, 845-853

Rapoport JL, & Ferguson HB. Biological validation of the hyperkinetic syndrome. Developmental Medicine and Child Neurology, 1981, 23, 667-682

Rie ED, Rie HE, Stewart S, & Rettemnier SR. An analysis of neurological soft signs in children with learning problems. Brain and Language, 1978, 6, 32-46

Rieder RO, & Nichols PL. Offspring of schizophrenics, III: Hyperactivity and neurological soft signs. Archives of General Psychiatry, 1979, 36, 665-674

Rutter M. Syndromes attributed to "minimal brain dysfunction" in childhood. American Journal of Psychiatry, 1982, 139(1), 21-33

Rutter M, Graham P, & Birch HG. Interrelations between choreiform syndrome, reading disability, and psychiatric disorder in children of 8-11 years. Developmental Medicine and Child Neurology, 1966, 8, 149-159

Rutter M, Graham P, & Yule W. A Neuropsychiatric Study in Childhood. Clinics in Developmental Medicine (Nos. 35/36). Philadelphia: Lippincott, 1970

Rutter M, & Yule W. The concept of specific reading retardation. Journal of Child Psychology and Psychiatry, 1975, 16, 191-197

Satterfield JH. EEG issues in children with minimal brain dysfunction. Seminars in Psychiatry, 1973, 5, 35-46

Schellekens JMH, Scholten CA, & Kalverboer AF. Visually guided hand movements in children with minor neurological dysfunctions: Response time and movement organization. Journal of Child Psychology and Psychiatry, 1983, 24(1), 89-102

Schmitt BD. The minimal brain dysfunction myth. American Journal of Diseases in Children, 1975, 129, 1313-1318

Shafer SQ, Shaffer D, O'Connor PA, & Stokman CJ. Hard thoughts on neurological "soft signs." In Rutter M (Ed.). Developmental Neuropsychiatry. New York: Guilford, 1983, pp. 133-143

Shaffer D, O'Connor PA, Shafer SQ, & Prupis S. Neurological "soft signs": Their origins and significance for behavior. In Rutter M (Ed.). Developmental Neuropsychiatry. New York: Guilford, 1983, pp. 144-163

Shapiro T, Burkes L, Petti TA, & Ranz J. Consistency of "nonfocal" neurological signs. Journal of the American Academy of Child Psychiatry, 1978, 17, 70-79

Stevens JR, Sachdev K, & Milstein V. Behavior disorders of childhood and the electroencephalogram. Archives of Neurology, 1968, 18, 160-177

Stine OC, Saratsiotis JB, & Mosser RS. Relationship between neurological findings and classroom behavior. American Journal of Diseases of Children, 1975, 129, 1036-1040

Taylor E. Measurement issues and approaches. In Rutter M (Ed.). Developmental Neuropsychiatry. New York: Guilford, 1983, pp. 239-255

Taylor HG. MBD: Meanings and misconceptions. Journal of Clinical Neuropsychology, 1983, 5(3), 271-287

Taylor HG. Minimal brain dysfunction in perspective. In Tarter RE, & Goldstein G (Eds.). Advances in Clinical Neuropsychology (Vol. 2). New York: Plenum, 1984, pp. 207-229

Taylor HG, & Fletcher JM. Biological foundations of "specific developmental disorders": Methods, findings, and future directions. Journal of Child Clinical Psychology, 1983, 12(1), 46-65

Taylor HG, Fletcher JM, & Satz P. Neuropsychological assessment of children. In Goldstein G, & Hersen M (Eds.). Handbook of Psychological Assessment. New York: Pergamon Press, 1984, pp. 211-234

Taylor HG, Michaels RH, Mazur PM, et al. Intellectual, neuropsychological, and achievement outcomes six to eight years after recovery from *Haemophilus influenzae* meningitis. Pediatrics, 1984, 74(2), 198-205

Taylor HG, Satz P, & Friel J. Developmental dyslexia in relation to other childhood reading disorders: Significance and clinical utility. Reading

Research Quarterly, 1979, 15(1), 84-101

Thompson JS, Ross RJ, & Horwitz SJ. The role of computed axial tomography in the study of the child with minimal brain dysfunction. Journal of Learning Disabilities, 1980, 13(6), 48-51

Timm N. Multivariate Analysis. Monterey: Brooks-Cole, 1975

Touwen BCL. Minimal brain dysfunction and minor neurological dysfunction. In Kalverboer AF, van Praag HM, & Mendelwicz J (Eds.). Advances in Biological Psychiatry, Minimal Brain Dysfunction: Fact or Fiction? (Vol. 1). Basel: S. Karger, 1978, pp. 55-67

Touwen BCL, & Prechtl HFR. The Neurological Examination of the Child with Minor Nervous Dysfunction. Clinics in Developmental Medicine (No. 38). Philadelphia: Lippincott, 1970

Touwen BCL, & Sporrel T. Soft signs and MBD. Developmental Medicine and Child Neurology, 1979, 21, 528-529

Voeller K. A proposed extended behavioral, cognitive, and sensorimotor pediatric neurological examination. In Ochroch R (Ed.). The Diagnosis and Treatment of Minimal Brain Dysfunction in Children: A Clinical Approach. New York: Human Sciences, 1981, pp. 65-90

Waber DP, Bauermeister M, Cohen C, et al. Behavioral correlates of physical and neuromotor maturity in adolescents from different environments. Developmental Psychobiology, 1981, 14(6), 513-522

Walton JN, Ellis E, & Court SDM. Clumsy children: Developmental apraxia and agnosia. Brain, 1962, 85, 603-612

Wender P. Minimal Brain Dysfunction in Children. New York: Wiley-Interscience, 1971

Werry J. Studies of the hyperactive child. IV. An empirical analysis of the minimal brain dysfunction syndrome. Archives of General Psychiatry, 1968, 19, 9-16

Werry JS. Organic factors in childhood psychopathology. In Quay HG & Werry TS (Eds.). Psychopathological Disorders of Childhood. New York: Wiley, 1972, pp. 83-121

Werry JS & Aman MG. The reliability and diagnostic validity of the Physical and Neurological Examination for Soft Signs (PANESS). Journal of Autism and Childhood Schizophrenia, 1976, 6(3), 253-262

Werry JS, Minde K, Guzman D, et al. Studies in the hyperactive child. VII. Neurological status compared with neurotic and normal children. American Journal of Orthopsychiatry, 1972, 42, 441-450

Wilker A, Dixon JF, & Parker JB. Brain function in problem children and controls: Psychometric, neurological, and electroencephalographic comparisons. American Journal of Psychiatry, 1970, 127(5), 634-645

Wolff PH, Gunnoe CE, & Cohen C. Associated movements as a measure of developmental age. Developmental Medicine and Child Neurology, 1983, 25, 417-429

Wolff PH, Gunnoe CE, & Cohen C. Neuromotor maturation and psychological performance: a developmental study. Developmental Medicine and Child Neurology, 1985, 27, 344-345

Wolff PH, & Hurwitz J. The choreiform syndrome. Developmental Medicine and Child Neurology, 1966, 8, 160-165

Wolff PH, & Hurwitz I. Functional implications of the minimal brain damage syndrome. In Walzer S, & Wolff PH (Eds.). Minimal Cerebral Dysfunction in Children. New York: Grune & Stratton, 1973, pp. 105-115

Woods BI, & Teuber HL. Mirror movements after childhood hemiparesis. Neurology, 1978, 28, 1152-1158

Younes RP, Rosner B, & Webb G. Neuroimmaturity of learning-disabled children: A controlled study. Developmental Medicine and Child Neurology, 1983, 25, 574-579

Yule W. Diagnosis: Developmental psychological assessment. In Kalverboer AF, van Praag HM, & Mendelwicz J (Eds.). Advances in Biological Psychiatry, Vol. 1. Minimal Brain Dysfunction: Fact or Fiction? Basel: S. Karger, 1978, pp 35-54

Part IV

Appendices: Contemporary Soft Sign Examinations

National Institute of Mental Health

*Appendix A**

Physical and Neurological Examination for Soft Signs

*Source: Guy W (Ed.). ECDEU Assessment Manual for Psychopharmacology. Rockville, MD: N.I.M.H., 1976, pp 383-406. In the public domain. Appreciation to reprint the PANESS is gratefully acknowledged to the Department of Health and Human Services and to the authors.

The Physical and Neurological Examination for Soft Signs (PANESS) consists of two parts; the first part is a physical examination while the second part is a scored neurological examination for soft signs. Investigators may employ one or both sections of the PANESS in their studies. The content of the physical examination — though new to the Early Clinical Drug Evaluation Unit (ECDEU) battery — should be very familiar to physicians. The neurological section, on the other hand, attempts to "quantify" a number of standard clinical procedures and may require additional training. The physical examination has been developed within the ECDEU program; while the neurological section has been developed by Abbott Laboratories and Dr. Close. Applicability for the battery is with children to age 15.

THE PANESS PHYSICAL STATUS EXAMINATION

This 15-item section of the PANESS will not be described here in detail; the reader is referred to the ECDEU Manual for further details. Items include:

1. Age (in months)
2. Height (in inches or centimeters)
3. Weight (in lbs. or kgs.)

4. Head Circumference (in inches or centimeters)
5. Pulse (per minute)
6. Blood Pressure (systolic and diastolic)
7. Visual Acuity (right and left)
8. Opthalmoscopic (normal/abnormal)
9. Audiogram (normal/abnormal)
10. Handedness (right/left/mixed)
11. Physical Examination (normal/abnormal) in the following areas: 1. HEENT, 2. Neck, 3. Cardiovascular, 4. Pulmonary, 5. Liver, 6. Kidney, 7. Spleen, 8. Other abdominal, 9. Musculoskeletal, 10. Gross neurologic, 11. Skin, 12. Lymphatics, 13. Genito-urinary.
12. Scored Neurologic Exam conducted? (yes/no)
13. Past Medical History (specify)
14. Abnormal Physical Findings (specify)
15. Diagnosis (specify per ICD classification)

MANUAL FOR THE NEUROLOGICAL EXAMINATION FOR SOFT SIGNS

(Abbott Laboratories and John H. Close, M.D.)

I. Introduction

This scored neurological examination is designed to assist the observer in determining whether neurological soft signs are present in a child. Because this is not a test of learning, it is important that the patient fully understand what is expected of him. The examiner (who need not necessarily be a physician) should demonstrate every task to be performed while giving the verbal instructions in the test description. Prefacing instructions should be used in an identical manner from one child to the next, utilizing a set routine of presentation. The time usually required to perform this test is 15 to 20 minutes.

At the beginning of testing, the child's attention should be obtained by making the statement, "Pay attention and watch what I do because you will have to do it after me." Since many items require stopwatch timing, the caution must be given, "Don't start until I say NOW, Okay?" immediately after the description and demonstration of each task. Proper instruction and clear demonstration are important contributors to the effectiveness of this scored examination.

A positive atmosphere should be maintained throughout the examination, accompanied by verbal praise and reinforcement. Incentive, such as the promise of a choice of a toy upon completion of testing from a box of inexpensive toys, may also be used.

II. Materials and Equipment

The room used for the test should be adequately lit, have a minimum noise level and be as free as possible from extraneous materials. One wall should be darkened by a black felt cloth or blackboard to provide a black background for the test of opticokinesia. Other needed items include the examiner's chair (facing away from the dark wall), a chair for the patient which faces a table or desk, and a convenient drawer for examining materials. Adhesive tape, 1½ inches in width sould be used to make a six-foot long, straight line on the floor, away from any nearby obstructions.

The following materials are needed:

1. A standard-lined 8 ½ x 11 inch writing tablet. On the cardboard back, clearly inked geometrically attractive figures of a square, a six, a circle, a three, and an X, approximately one inch high.
2. Three or four sharp, soft lead pencils.
3. A ball point pen.
4. A toy cricket or other hand-held device for making clicking noises.
5. A stop watch (expensive models are unnecessary).
6. A two-point discriminator with one-centimeter separation.
7. A ring (simple wedding band type).
8. A car key.
9. A coin (nickel).
10. A standard two-inch safety pin.
11. Box of small, cheap toys.

III. Administration and Scoring

Rapport should be established by a few minutes of conversation. Acclimatization to test circumstances may then be phased in by one or two simple unscored tasks, such as, "Can you show me your right foot? Good! Now point to your left ear." (Gentle correction is used with an incorrect gesture, and the gesture repeated). Above all, a completely encouraging, nonpunitive atmosphere is required. In all the directions that follow, quotation marks indicate verbal instructions; parentheses enclose a physical description of the demonstration. Right or left handedness should be recorded before the test begins. (Item 10).

A. Tests 1–20

1. Finger to Nose

"I want you to touch a finger to your nose. Begin with your arm out here." (Extend the arm laterally with the hand in a loose fist, index finger extended as pointer.)

"Now do like this." (Make a wide sweep medially to touch the nose.)

Score: **1**–Smoothly and accurately performed.

2–Slowly, jerkily, and missing the target, then correcting. (If 10 seconds pass with no attempt, instruct and demonstrate again.)

3–Same as 2; but done only after encouragement or a repeat instruction and demonstration.

4–Same as 3; but without correcting target error.

2. Contralateral Finger to Nose

"Now do the other hand." (Demonstrate again.)

Score as in Test No. 1

3. Finger to Nose, Eyes Closed

"Now close your eyes and do that again." (No demonstration necessary.)

Score as in Test No. 1

4. Contralateral Finger to Nose, with Eyes Closed

"Close your eyes again and do it with the other hand." (No demonstration necessary.)

Score as in Test No. 1

5. Heel to Shin

"Touch your heel against the front of the other leg, up high like this." (Demonstrate the heel touching just beneath the patella.)

Score as in Test No. 1. Either foot may be used acceptably.

6. Contralateral Heel to Shin

"Now do it with the other heel." (Demonstrate again.)

Score as in Test No. 1

7. Heel to Shin, Eyes Closed

"Now close your eyes and do that last one again." (No demonstration necessary.)

Score as in Test No. 1

8. Contralateral Heel to Shin, Eyes Closed
"Now close your eyes and try it with the other heel." (No demonstration necessary.)
Score as in Test No. 1

For questions 9–16, the child is told to turn to the table; a sheet of paper is taken from the pad and placed in front of the child and the date written in the upper right-hand margin. Tape or thumbtacks may be used to securely fix the page in front of the child. The child is then given a pencil and told to write or print his name at the upper left. No matter how poorly this is performed, the child should be told that it is well done.

For drawing on the child's hand, one should try to imagine a frame that consists of a line bordering one-half inch within the proximal, distal, and lateral margins of the hand. All numerals and figures should be drawn in the palm in the same aspect that the child would look at it when reading. All figures should be drawn with the nonwriting end of the ball point pen. On all graphesthesia and stereognostic samples, the child should be told, "Now turn your face up toward the ceiling and close your eyes." One must be certain that the demonstration cannot be visualized. Having been told this, take the palm of the child's hand in your hand and slowly (about 3 seconds) and smoothly draw a numeral or figure, the base of which should be at the thenar and hypothenar portions of the palm. The child should then be told "Open your eyes and draw the figure on the paper." Practice one or more times with each hand until the child understands the procedure. The actual examinations are then initiated.

The child is told "Draw on the paper each of the things I draw in your hands while your eyes are closed. I may draw another number, or I may draw figures, like a circle or a square."

9.–16. Graphesthesia

"Now turn your face up and close your eyes while I draw. There. Now open your eyes and see if you can draw it."

These verbal instructions are used prior to each of the tasks listed to the right.

9. Draw a square—right hand.
10. Draw an x—left hand.
11. Draw a circle—right hand.
12. Draw a square—left hand.
13. Draw an x—right hand.
14. Draw a 3—left hand.
15. Draw a circle—right hand.
16. Draw a 3—left hand.

If the child is unsuccessful after the first tracing, make the remark "That's fine; close your eyes and let me do it again." If after the second time the child is still unable to draw the figure, raise the pad off the table so that the figures drawn on the back are visible. "Can you pick out the one I drew? Fine; draw it." The child is allowed to draw the figure while still visualizing the example on the back of the pad.

Score: 1–If the child does the figure correctly after the first trial.
2–If the child does the figure successfully after the second example.
3–If the child picks the figure from those drawn on the pad.
4–If the child is still unsuccessful after two examples and the visualization of the figure on the pad.

Questions 17–20 involve stereognosis. Different objects are placed in the hands without bilateral repetition of the same object (17. Coin: right hand; 18. Ring : left hand; 19. Safety pin: right hand; 20. Key: left hand). The method of testing and of scoring here is similar to that in the preceding description. The child's face should be directed toward the ceiling with eyes closed at all times when the objects might be in sight. The box of objects is kept beneath the table out of sight. Each object is placed in the child's hand for a period of approximately 5 seconds, and then the child is told, "Now give it back. Without looking, tell me what it is." If at that point the child is unable to identify the object, it is replaced in the hand with the remark, "Feel it and think what it could be." After 5 seconds, it is removed and replaced in the box with the other objects. If the child is still unable to identify it, the box is brought into sight with the question "Can you pick it out of here?"

Score: 1–If the child names the object successfully on the first trial.
2–If the child names the object after the second placement in the hand.
3–If the child is successful only after seeing the object.
4–If the child is unable to pick the object out of the box.

B. Questions 21–29

Here, the straight line taped on the floor is used for testing. As long as the patient's foot is touching the tape in any way, it is not considered a miss.

21. Walking Tiptoe

"Walk this line to the end up on your toes." (Demonstrate while up on the balls of the feet; arms hanging naturally, carefully walk the line.)

"Be sure you stay on the line."

The examiner should wait at the end of the line. This serves two purposes; first, the examiner remains close to the child to protect against falling; and secondly, he or she will be positioned for the next demonstration, the return trip. An error count is made for each time the child misses the line or puts a foot down flatfooted. This actual count, 0, 1, 2, or 3, is scored. If a greater number of misses occurs, score as "3".

22. Heel Walking

    "Now go back on your heels like this." (Arms at side, walk on heels on the line.)

    Score: The same method as in Test No. 21 is used.

23. Hopping on One Foot

    "Can you hop all the way without missing the line? Be sure not to put the other foot down." (Demonstrate a hop on the line.)

    The examiner should again remain at the end of the line.

    Score: An error occurs if the child misses the line or if the elevated foot is allowed to touch the floor.

24. Hopping on the Other Foot

    "Now hop back on the other foot." (Demonstrate accordingly.)

    Score as in Test No. 23

25. Tandem Walking Forward

    "Now be sure you put your heel against your toe and walk to the end staying on the line." (Demonstrate heel–toe walking on line and remain at the end.)

    Score: An error consists of not placing the heel to toe or missing the line completely.

26. Tandem Walking Backward

    "Now do the same thing backwards." (Demonstrate accordingly.)

    Score as in Test No. 25

In Test Nos. 27, 28, and 29 the child is seated at the side of the table with hands on knees. Three (3) clear examples are given in each case before actual counting begins. The examples should always be given exactly the same way. The test should be performed on the dominant side; in a right-handed child the right cheek and right hand should be employed. Again, the child's face is directed upward with the eyes tightly closed.

27. Face–Hand Test

"I am going to brush your hand and face at the same time."	(With a light fluff of cotton in each hand, the dorsum of the hand and the cheek beneath the malar eminence should be brushed simultaneously and softly with as nearly equal pressure as is possible.)
"Did you feel it?"	
"Now I'm going to brush only your face."	(This is then performed.)
"Did you feel it?"	

On the third example, the hand only is brushed, and again with the forewarning:

"Now I'm going to brush only your hand."	(This is then performed.)
Begin actual test—	
"Now I'm going to do this some more and I want you to tell me what I do each time."	(First, hand only; second, face only; third, face–hand combination; each time asking the child *"There, what did I do?"*)

Score: If the child misses none of these, "**0**" is marked; if he misses one, "**1**" is marked; and so on, up to a total of missing all three.

28. Face–Noise Test

This test is similar, except that the face is brushed at the same time a cricket toy is clicked in the ipsilateral ear. Again, three variations are performed as examples. First, the cricket only is clicked; second, the cricket is clicked and the face is brushed; third, the cricket is clicked without brushing the face. Note that the cricket is clicked in every example.

Begin actual test— (First the cricket is clicked and face simultaneously brushed.)	*"Can you tell me what I did?"*
(Second, the cricket is clicked without brushing.)	*"Can you tell me what I did?"*
(Third, the cricket is clicked and face brushed again.)	*"Can you tell me what I did?"*

Score: As in the case of Test No. 27, the number of errors is counted; if the child misses none of the trials, "**0**" is marked; if one of the examples is missed, "**1**" is marked; if two are missed, "**2**" is marked; and if all three are missed, "**3**" is marked.

29. Two-Point Discrimination

Again, three examples are given utilizing the one-centimeter separation, two-point discriminator on the dorsum of the digiti minimi.

"You see, I have only touched you with one point."	(Only one point is touched.)
"I used two points on you that time. Could you tell it?"	(Both points are used.)
"Now only one point again."	(One point only is again used.)

Begin actual test—

"What did I do that time?"	(Using two points.)
"What did I do that time?"	(Using one point.)
"What did I do that time?"	(Using two points.)

Score: Same as in Tests 27 and 28, appropriate number is marked for 0 through 3 errors.

C. Questions 30–36

These tests require the use of a stopwatch and accurate timing of the child's performance. It is necessary that the child know clearly when the test starts, and that he is told to keep doing the task until the examiner tells him to stop. For scoring purposes, if the child persists in the task for 20 seconds or more "**1**" is marked; 15 to 19 seconds, "**2**" is marked; 10 to 14 seconds, "**3**" is marked; and 0 to 9 seconds, "**4**" is marked. At the outset of these tests the child is told *"Now I am going to tell you some things to do; be sure that you don't start doing each one of them until I say to begin. Do you understand? Also, be sure you continue doing them until I tell you to stop."*

30. Tongue Extrusion

    "Watch me now." (The examiner should stick out his tongue for a period of 3–4 seconds.)

    "Did you see what I did? All right, now when I tell you to start do it a long time until I tell you to stop. Ready—begin!"

31. Arms Extended

    "Hold your arms in front of you like this until I tell you to stop." (The arms should be extended directly in front of the examiner, palms down.)

    "Could you see how I did that? Are you ready to start? All right—begin!"

    Presence of drift does not alter the timed nature of scoring in this task.

32. Eyes Closed

    "Watch how tightly I can close my eyes." (Close the eyes very tightly.)

    "Now you do it when I tell you to. Ready—begin!"

33. Stand on One Foot

    "Now I'm going to stand on one foot without moving it." (Stand up on either foot with the arms hanging naturally down at the sides.)

    "It doesn't matter which foot you stand on. Did you see how I did that? Are you ready? Begin!"

34. Stand on the Other Foot

    "Now do the same thing when I tell you to start, standing on the other foot. Are you ready? Begin!" (No demonstration necessary.)

35. Romberg

"Now stand up like this on both feet but keep your eyes closed."

(The examiner stands in front of the child on both feet, erectly, with his hands at his sides and his eyes tightly closed.)

"Are you ready to do that? All right, begin!"

36. Tandem Romberg

"Now put one heel against the other toe and stand with your eyes closed until I tell you to stop. Either foot may be in front."

(Demonstrate eyes closed, tandem stance, arms at sides.)

D. Questions 37–43

In these tests, the examiner should assure himself of exactly what constitutes a four-per-second beat. A general tendency is to make this beat faster than it should be. The examiner should appraise his or her own sense of rhythm by listening to a four-per-second example; either with a clock or, if available, a metronome. A typical alarm clock or wrist watch (but not a stopwatch) ticks at a four-per-second rate.

Each test is of five seconds duration. The child is seated at the table facing the dark background wall, and the examiner's demonstrations should be clear and perhaps exaggerated. The child should be allowed 3 or 4 seconds practice at Nos. 37, 39, 41, and 43. If a mistake is seen for which the child would be downgraded, such as a lack of smooth delivery, the child should be informed. He should also be told at the outset not to move the rest of his body, but rather just the part that is supposed to be moving.

Adventitious movement will be considered any movement unnnecessary to the task at hand, whether it be a jerk, twitch, grimace, body contortion, sticking out of the tongue, etc. Contralateral rigidity is not considered adventitious. The starting point of each of these tasks for the purpose of timing should be a clear-cut signal.

37. Finger Tapping

"Now watch how I tap only my finger just this fast. Notice that I leave my other arm down at my side."

(Demonstrate sitting erectly with the tapping motion mainly comprised of finger action not hand motion.)

"You see that I am just moving my finger and not my hand and arm? Would you like to practice that quickly before we start?"

At this point, if the child is going too slowly he should be told *"Go a little faster"* and allowed to practice again.

"That looks good. Are you ready now? All right, begin!"

Score: The examiner is actually grading three things at once. A brief familiarization and practice is needed to accomplish this. The first type of scoring is the actual count of the number of taps performed in the five-second period. The child must be shown the proper rate of tapping at the beginning. The number of taps is scored in the proper position. Simultaneously, one is making mental note of adventitious movements. Their number represents a separate score and is indicated by a mark in the proper position.

"Quality" is also scored 1 through 4; the examiner marks the appropriate number based on his or her best judgment of performance. This evaluation is not meant to reflect absolutely correct rhythmicity, but rather the smoothness of delivery overall. Points should not be taken away if the child ends the task at a more rapid or more slow tapping rate than that with which he began, as long as he phases in and out of such changes smoothly. We downgrade the child for sporadicism, or for the appearance of "bursts" in his sequencing. If the child only makes one such change in rhythm, he will receive a score of **1** in the quality position; if he makes this error twice, he will receive a score of **2**; three times, a score of **3**; and a score of **4** could represent a completely arrhythmic performance.

38. Finger Tapping—Other Hand

"Now we are going to do it with the other hand; why don't you practice that for a moment?"

(No repeat demonstration necessary.)

"That's fine. Are you ready now? Begin!"
Scoring as in Test No. 37

39. Foot Tapping

"Now watch how I sit and tap only my foot just this fast. Would you like to practice that for a moment?" (Demonstrate accordingly. The heel remains on the floor. Assure that there is moderate extension at the knee or the resultant angle on the foot makes the task difficult.)

"That's fine. Are you ready now? Begin!"
Scoring as in Test No. 37

40. Foot Tapping—Other Foot

"Now let's do it with the other foot; you may practice for a moment." (No repeat demonstration necessary.)
Scoring as in Test No. 37

41. Finger and Foot Synchronization

"Now we are going to try the finger and the foot at the same time. You must tap them together at the same rate you have been tapping them separately. Watch how I do it." (Examiner must be careful to synchronize finger and foot tapping through several repetitions at an adequately fast rate. Like sides are always paired; right hand with right foot, left hand with left foot.)

"Do you want to practice that now?"

"That's fine. Do you think you are ready to start? All right. Begin!"

Score: The scoring of tap count and adventitious movement count is the same here as in previous examples. However, the "quality" score now reflects the actual number of times the child deviates from synchronized tapping. A complication of this scoring immediately becomes obvious; that is, if the child is unsynchronized from the start. In such a circumstance one must grade quality according to the amount of time during the test asynchrony is apparent. A quality score of **1** is well synchronized, hand and foot, throughout the entire study. If the child is not well synchronized for some portion of the test, divide total test time into thirds. If the child's tapping is not synchronized for one-third of the time, a quality score of **2** is recorded; if two-thirds of the time asynchrony is demonstrated, a score of **3** is received; and a quality score of **4** is recorded for gross asynchrony throughout.

42. Synchronous Finger and Foot Tapping—The Opposite Side

"Now I want you to tap your foot and finger on the other side together. Do you want to practice that? All right, begin."

(No repeat demonstration necessary.)

Scoring as in Test No. 41

43. String Test

This is an opticokinetic test performed with a rapid and a slow component. An object on the examiner's hand should serve as a target on which the child may fix his gaze; a ring on a finger or a piece of chalk between fingers is adequate. The motion is made against the dark background, and through a distance of about two feet. The test hand is moved away from the body rather quickly, then brought back to the examiner's side more slowly. It is performed approximately two feet from the child with first the right and then the left hand. The examiner should step to the right or left far enough so that the demonstrating hand will be directly in front of the child's face. The child's head must remain still, following only with the eyes.

"Now I'm going to pretend that I am pulling on a piece of string several times that is hooked to my belt. I want you to follow my hand with your eyes everywhere it moves. But you can't move your head. It may help you if you watch this ring on my finger."

(The hand is moved away from the body in a quick motion and then more slowly brought back medially. This is done five consecutive times rhythmically.)

"Now I'm going to do it on the other side."

It is permissible for the examiner to place a hand on the child's head, if it would help to stabilize him. The number of times the patient successfully follows the target movement out of the possible five is scored. If nystagmus is present, the direction of the fast component should be noted.

Margaret E. Hertzig

Appendix B

Neurologic Evaluation Schedule

The Neurologic Evaluation Schedule was initially developed by Dr. Lawrence Taft for the purpose of assessing the neurologic status of 8-10-year-old children as part of a study of the epidemiology of mental retardation in the community of Aberdeen, Scotland (Birch, Richardson, Baird, et al, 1970). Subsequently the schedule has been utilized in studies of low birthweight children (Hertzig, 1974; 1981; 1983); children educationally designated as brain-injured (Hertzig, Bortner, & Birch, 1969) and children who were malnourished during the first 2 years of life (Richardson, 1976). Studies of normal controls have indicated that fewer than 5 percent of children attending regular school in both Scotland (Birch et al, 1970) and the United States (Hertzig et al, 1969) exhibit 2 or more nonfocal signs.

The examination can be easily performed by an individual with general medical training. The reliability of two examiners independently rating the responses of the same patient at the same time is high (Quitkin, Rifkin and Klein, 1976), however both short-term (Quitkin, Rifkin, & Klein, 1976) and long-term (Hertzig, 1982) stability of response to particular items is more variable. Nevertheless children who exhibited two or more nonfocal signs when between 8 and 12 years of age continue to do so when examined 5 years later (Hertzig, 1982).

The schedule provides for an assessment of both localizing and nonfocal signs. Localizing signs include such standard findings of central nervous system damage as cranial nerve abnormalities, lateralized dysfunctions and the presence of pathologic reflexes. Assessment of the presence or absence of nonfocal signs is more complex. Performance on individual tasks is rated as being within normal limits, mildly impaired, or markedly impaired. Tasks are grouped to permit the development of

SOFT NEUROLOGICAL SIGNS
ISBN 0-8089-1841-9

judgments about the integrity of broader functional areas. As the examination is viewed as a clinical and not a psychometric assessment no attempt has been made to standardize the number of tasks within each area. The following methods and criteria are employed:

1. Speech: Each is engaged in sufficient informal conversation to permit the assessment of clarity and intelligibility. Word sound production is rated in accordance with the examiners difficulty in comprehension. Marked impairments are required for the designation of speech as a nonfocal sign.
2. Balance: Balance is designated as a nonfocal sign if performance on at least two of the following three tasks is markedly impaired.
   a. Standing balance. The child is required to stand still with eyes closed, feet together, arms extended, and fingers spread apart for 30 seconds. Marked impairment is reflected in three or more back and forth movements of the body exceeding 1 inch in both directions during the observation period.
   b. Hopping. The child is asked to hop 10 consecutive times on each foot. Marked impairment reflects a failure to hop at least 5 consecutive times on both feet.
   c. Walking a line in tandem; the child is asked to take 10 steps placing the heel directly in front of the toe of the other foot (as in walking on a tightrope) with his arms at his side. Marked impairment reflects a failure to approximate heel and toe for at least five consecutive steps.
3. Coordination: Coordination is designated as a nonfocal sign if performance on at least two of the following four tasks is markedly impaired:
   a. Finger-to-nose. The child is required to laterally extend each arm and touch his index finger to the tip of his nose 5 times with each hand with his eyes open. The sequence is repeated with the eyes closed. Marked impairment reflects a failure to touch the tip of the nose at least three times with both hands with eyes closed.
   b. Alternating pronation supination. This test is performed with the child standing one arm relaxed at his side. The other elbow is flexed 90 degrees with the hand pointing forward. The child is requested to quickly pronate and supinate the extended hand five times and to repeat the task using the other hand. Marked impairment is reflected by the movement of both elbows a distance of 4 or more inches during execution of the alternating hand movements.
   c. Foot taps. The child is seated in a straight chair and asked to tap

the toe of each foot in succession a total of 10 times while maintaining his heel on the floor. He is then asked to tap both feet together an additional 10 times. Marked impairment reflects a failure to sustain at least 5 simultaneous toe taps.

d. Heel-shin. This task is performed with the child seated in a straight chair with his legs extended. He is required to move one heel down the shin of the opposite leg from the knee to the big toe without losing contact. The task is repeated two times with each leg. Marked impairment reflects two or more losses of contact on each of the four trials.

4. Double simultaneous stimulation: The child is seated with his hands resting on his thighs and his eyes closed. He is told "I am going to touch you, I want you to show me where." He is touched lightly on the right cheek and left hand. If the child indicated he had been touched only once he is asked "anywhere else?" No further questions are asked as the left cheek-right hand, cheek, and both hands are stimulated. The entire sequence is repeated once. In order to eliminate the possibility that errors in reporting were a consequence of right-left confusion the child is asked to point to the part of the body touched rather than to name it. Any error on the second trial results in the designation of DSS as a nonfocal sign.
5. Gait: Gait is observed as the child walks back and forth a distance of 20 feet. Designation as a nonfocal sign requires the presence of at least two of the following: a base of more than 10 inches, a failure to smoothly alternate flexion and extension of the knees, absence of a heel-toe gait or immobility of the arms.
6. Sequential finger-thumb opposition: This task requires the child to imitate the examiner in the opposition of thumb to fingers in the following sequence; index, fourth, middle, pinky, pinky, middle, fourth, index. The child is requested to repeat each movement before the next is illustrated. The performance of both hands is assessed. Imitative movements are designated as a nonfocal sign if at least two errors (not spontaneously corrected) occur on each hand.
7. Muscle tone: Muscle tone is assessed in accordance with the procedure described by Rutter, Graham, and Yule (1970). All four extremities were examined as follows; tone of the upper limbs was tested by (a) flapping the hand while holding the lower forearm, (b) planter and dorsiflexing the wrist, (c) flexing and extending the elbow, and (d) dorsiflexing the wrist and bending the fingers back. Tone of the lower limb is tested by (a) holding the thigh above the knee with the leg hanging down and flapping the knee, and (b) testing the range of mo-

tion of the ankle. In order to insure that these movements are carried out while the extremity was limp the child is engaged in conversation about something else to divert his attention from the examiner's manipulation. Tone is recorded separately for all extremities. A finding of marked hypo or hypertonia in all four extremities is required for tone to be designated as a nonfocal sign.

8. Graphesthesia: The child is seated with his eyes closed, his hand positioned vertically facing the examiner, and asked to name the letters or numbers he feels being written. A ball point pen with the point retracted is used to trace the following symbols; right hand ... 3, a, 2; left hand ... 8, c, R. If errors were made he is asked to identify the symbols visually. Graphesthesia was designated as a nonfocal sign if at least 2 failures on each hand occur in the face of accurate visual identification.
9. Astereognosis: The child is requested to identify the following objects by feeling them with each hand in turn with his eyes closed: a pocket comb, key, quarter, and penny. Manipulation is permitted but not transfer. After the entire sequence is administered visual identification is requested.
10. Choreiform movements are assessed by asking the child to assume the position previously described for the assessment of standing balance while the examiner watches for small jerky twitches ocurring in the fingers, wrists joints, arms, and shoulders. Choreiform movements are designated as a nonfocal sign if 10 or more twitches are observed within a 30 second period.

Neurologic Examination

Protocol.

General Behavior

Cooperative_______________ Uncooperative_______________

Comments:____

____

____

Speech

Absent___________ Stutters__________ Stammers__________

Lisps_________ Echolalia_________ Incomprehensible_______

Expressive Aphasia__________ Receptive Aphasia__________

Comments: ____

____

____

Knowledge of Left and Right

R hand____________ L ear____________ R eye____________

Hand Dominance

a) Throw a ball______________________________

b) Turn a door knob______________________________

c) Use scissors______________________________

d) Write______________________________

Eye Dominance

a) Kaleidoscope______________________________

b) Sight rifle______________________________

c) Paper______________________________

Eye_________________ Shoulder_________________

Foot Dominance

a) Kick

Pref.__________ Other__________ Better__________

Right–Left Awareness Items (Piaget)

1. Show me your right hand. __________
   Now show me your left hand. __________
   Show me your right leg. __________
   Now show me your left leg. __________
2. (E sits opposite S) Show me my right hand. __________
   Now my left. __________
   Show me my right leg. __________
   Now my left leg. __________
3. (Place coin on table left of a pencil in relation to S).
   Is the pencil to the right or to the left? __________
   And the penny—is it to the right or to the left? __________
   (Have S move around to the opposite side of the table and repeat questions.)
   Is the pencil to the right or to the left? __________
   And the penny—is it to the right or to the left? __________
4. (S is opposite E; E has a coin in right hand and a bracelet or watch on left arm).
   You see this penny. Have I got it in my right hand or in my left? __________
   And the bracelet—is it on my right arm or my left? __________
5. (S is opposite three objects in a row: a pencil to the left, a key in the middle, and a coin to the right.)
   Is the pencil to the left or to the right of the key? __________
   Is the pencil to the left or to the right of the penny? __________
   Is the key to the left or to the right of the penny? __________
   Is the key to the left or to the right of the pencil? __________
   Is the penny to the left or to the right of the key? __________
   Is the penny to the left or the right of the pencil? __________

Comments:____

____

____

Cranial Nerves

Eyes (2nd, 3rd, 4th, & 6th nerves)

Gross vision (Snellen chart)

R_____ L_____ Both_____

Pupils

R_____mm L_____mm

Reaction to Light R_____ L_____

Accommodation R_____ L_____

Nystagmus________________________________
Comments: ________________________________
____

E.O.M.

Intact_________________________________
Abnormality____________________________

Visual field by confrontation

Single stimulation

Intact____________________
Abnormality_______________

Double simultaneous stimulation

Intact____________________
Abnormality_______________

Fundi

Disc	N1_____	Abnormality______
Retina	N1_____	Abnormality______

Corneal sensation

Right	Intact_____	Absent_________
Left	Intact_____	Absent_________

7th Nerve

Facial asymmetry Absent______________
Absent______________

8th Nerve-Audition

Gross hearing	Intact_____	Abnormal______
Double simultaneous stimulation	Intact_____	Abnormal______

10th Nerve

Gag reflex Present_____ Absent_____

12th Nerve

Tongue

Midline_____
Deviated to the right_____
Deviated to the left_____

Standing Balance (30 seconds)

Normal________ Mildly impaired_________

Markedly impaired_________

Comments: ____

____

____

Hopping (10 times each foot)

Normal________ Mildly impaired_________

Markedly impaired_________

Comments: ____

____

____

Choreiform movements	**None**	**Slight**	**Marked**
Shoulder	________	________	________
Arm	________	________	________
Fingers	________	________	________

Comments: ____

____

____

Arm drifts: ______________________________________

____

Subject to hold hands and arms extended with eyes closed for 30 seconds

Muscle tone

	Right			**Left**		
Upper extremities	**Hyper**	**NL**	**Hypo**	**Hyper**	**NL**	**Hypo**
Hand flap						
Wrist flex/ext.						
Elbow flex/ext.						
Hyperext. fingers						
Lower extremities						
Knee flap						
Ankle						

Comments: ____

____

____

Muscle strength

Upper extremities________________________________

Lower extremities________________________________

Reflexes

	B.J.	T.J.	Radial	Abd.	K.J.	A.J.
right						
left						

Clonus

	Absent	Sustained	Unsustained
right	________	________	________
left	________	________	________

Plantar response

	Flexion	Extension	Equivocal
right	________	________	________
left	________	________	________

Comments: ________________________________

____

Finger to nose

	R Impairment			L Impairment		
	Normal	Mild	Marked	Normal	Mild	Marked
eyes open						
eyes closed						

Comments: ________________________________

____

Finger–Thumb Opposition:

	R	L
1		
3		
2		
4		
4		
2		
3		
1		
Consec. Movts.		
Overflow Mvts.		

Comments: ________________________________

____

Pronation–Supernation

	R Impairment			L Impairment		
	Normal	Mild	Marked	Normal	Mild	Marked

Overflow mvts.____________________
Comments: ____________________

Foot taps

	R Impairment			L Impairment		
	Normal	Mild	Marked	Normal	Mild	Marked
one foot						
two feet						

Overflow movt.____________________
Comments: ____________________

Heel–Shin

	Right	Left
Normal		
Mildly Impaired		
Markedly Impaired		

Comments: ____________________

Sensory

Face Hand Test (eyes closed)

	F	H
RF–LF		
LF–RH		
RF–RH		
LF–LH		
F–F		
H–H		
RF–LF		
LF–RH		
RF–RH		
LF–LH		
F–F		
H–H		

Comments: ____________________

Sensation

Pinprick______________________________

____

Light touch____________________________

____

Position______________________________

____

Graphesthesia

Right hand	3________	a________	2________
Left hand	8________	c________	R________

Comments: ______________________________

____

____

Astereognosis

	R	L
Key	__________	__________
Quarter	__________	__________
Penny	__________	__________
Comb	__________	__________
Pencil	__________	__________

Comments: ______________________________

____

____

Gait

		Impairment	
	Normal	**Mild**	**Marked**
base			
knee flex/ext.			
heel–toe–gait			
arm movement			

Comments: ______________________________

____

____

____

Walk a Line in Tandem

Normal_________Mildly Impaired_________

Markedly impaired_________

Comments: ____

____

____

Neurologic Examination—
Summary of Findings

Code: 0=normal ?=mild impairment +=marked impairment

Behavior

Speech

Cranial Nerves
(eyes)

2, 3, 4, 5, 6
7

8
10

12

Muscle Strength

Upper R
L
Lower R
L

Muscle Tone

Upper R
L
Lower R
L

Reflexes

Biceps R
L

Triceps R
L

Radial R
L

Knee R
L

Ankle R
L

Ankle Clonus R
L

Plantar
Responses R
L

Balance
Standing
Hopping
Line in tandem

Coordination

Finger to Nose
Pronation–
Supernation

Foot taps
Heel–Shin

DSS

Finger–Thumb
Opposition R
L

Graphesthia R
L

Astereognosis R
L

Choreatiform
Movements

Gait

Neurologic Diagnosis:

_______ Localizing findings_______________________________

____

_______ Non-localizing findings # Signs_______________

_______ Normal

Non-Localizing Findings

	Sp.	Bal.	Cood.	DSS	FTO	Tone	Graph	Aster.	Choreif.
+									
-									

REFERENCES

Birch HG, Richardson SA, Baird D, et al: Mental Subnormality in the Community. A Clinical and Epidemiologic Study. Baltimore: Williams and Wilkins, 1970

Hertzig ME: Neurologic findings in prematurely born children at school age. In Rolf M, & Thomas A (Eds.). Proceedings of the Fifth Conference of the Society for Life History Research. Minneapolis: University of Minnesota Press, 1974

Hertzig ME: Neurologic soft signs in low birthweight children. Developmental Medicine and Child Neurology, 1981, 21, 778-791

Hertzig MD: Stability and change in nonfocal neurological signs. Journal of the American Academy of Child Psychiatry, 1982, 21, 231-236

Hertzig ME: Temperament and neurologic status. In Rutter M (Ed.). Developmental Neuropsychiatry. New York: The Guilford Press, 1983

Hertzig ME, Bortner M, & Birch HG: Neurologic findings in children educationally designated as "brain-damaged." American Journal of Orthopsychiatry 39:437-446, 1969

Quitkin F, Rifkin A, & Klein D: Neurologic 'soft' signs in schizophrenia and character disorders. Archives of General Psychiatry, 1976, 36, 665-674

Richardson SA: The influence of severe malnutrition in infancy on the intelligence of children at school age: An ecological perspective. In Walsh RN & Greenough WT (Eds.). Environments as Therapy for Brain Dysfunction. New York: Plenum Press, 1976, pp. 256-271

Rutter M, Graham P, & Yule W: A Neuropsychiatric Study in Childhood. (Clinics in Developmental Medicine nos. 35/36). London: Hienemann, 1970

John E. Peters

Appendix C

A Special or Soft Neurological Examination for School Age Children

In 1960 when I first made a selection of items for use in testing for "soft" or integrative neurological signs in children with learning and behavioral problems, there were very few persons who had done research or clinical work in this field. Among the early names were Strauss (Strauss & Lehtinen, 1947; Strauss & Kephart, 1955), Teicher (1941), Gesell (Gesell & Amatruda, 1947), Bender (1956), Passamanick (Passamanick, Rogers, & Lillienfied, 1956), Eisenberg (1957), Laufer (Laufer, Denhoff, & Solomons, 1957), Kennard (1960), and Denhoff (1961). Our basic assumption then, as now, was that due to prenatal, perinatal, or early childhood brain damage, or due to genetic deviations, or combinations of these, there were deficits in the integrative aspects of the nervous system controlling movement that were not usually detected in the routine neurological examination; that the presence of such motor signs often co-existed with and suggested a relationship to dysfunctions in still more complex areas such as writing, drawing, reading, and various intellectual functions; and that these soft signs might assist in diagnosing and understanding the limitations of "these children" who at that time had no unifying designation and were rarely recognized. They were often dismissed as merely stupid, unmotivated, bad, or emotionally blocked. In the 1940s, 1950s, and 1960s, the prevailing theories in psychiatry and psychology posited that dyslexia and hyperactivity and the symptoms frequently associated with them, such as impulsiveness and inattentiveness were entirely due to psychodynamic or experiental factors and not at all due to central nervous system (CNS) deviations. At that time such children were often mishandled by schools and some were subjected to extended psychotherapy in the expectation of

SOFT NEUROLOGICAL SIGNS
ISBN 0-8089-1841-9

curing the reading problem and/or the hyperactivity by that means.

Clements and the present author in 1962 (Clements & Peters, 1962) took the strong position that the symptoms in question were largely due to CNS deviations whatever other contributory factors may exist, and that these children needed specific educational and behavioral remediation directed to their deficits; i.e., beginning instruction at whatever the current level of skills happened to be. As a result of the frustration in the child resulting from his deficits, his behavior often became disturbed to a lesser or greater extent, depending of course on how well he was accepted and handled by his family and his teachers. Our position did not exclude the fact that some of these children who also had significant emotional problems benefitted from various forms of psychotherapy including behavior modification (Gardner, 1974). Because the symptoms were highly variable from child to child, we opted for a broad inclusive term that pointed to brain deviations as the primary source of the symptoms and not to the attitudes and behavior of parents and teachers. We selected the term minimal brain dysfunction (MBD), which still had advantages in facilitating communication and understanding among professionals, but not much value as a specific diagnostic term indicating what the treatment or remediation should be. A similar defense for an inclusive concept can be made for the term cerebral palsy — which signifies a more obvious affliction than MBD. We theorized that there could exist numerous discrete dysfunctions based on deficits or deviations in specific cell systems of the brain; that some children would have singular deficits and others would have multiple deficits; that by trying to delineate distinct clusters of symptoms (Clements & Peters, 1972; 1981) we might achieve a better understanding of both etiology and treatment. As it turns out the clusters have had some value for our conceptual understanding, but at the practical level we still have to delineate the specific areas of deficit in skills such as language, arithmetic, motor performance, and behavior and then design correspondingly specific remedial programs for those areas.

What purpose does a soft-sign examination serve? Even though there is great theoretical and research interest in these signs and symptoms, practically speaking a school diagnosis of learning disability can be made on a child of average intelligence on the basis of poor reading, spelling, and writing whether or not hyperactivity or other special neurological signs are present (Peters, Davis, Goolsby, et al, 1973; Peters Dykman, Ackerman, & Romine, 1974; Peters, Romine, & Dykman, 1975). Even so the examination is useful in a number of ways. For a trainee in psychiatry or psychology the examination provides a way of *learning to perceive* the subtle but important abberations in movement, stance, directionality, associative movements, and visuo-motor coordination that so often exist in these children. In testing for these and especially in watching the child in the act of writing and spelling, the trainee becomes aware of the frustration the child experiences in trying to keep up with his classmates. The soft sign findings add certainty to the diagnosis in cases that are not immediately obvious. In more severe cases the test items are helpful in monitoring the child's development and improvement over time. The test results provide a quite tangible evidence of CNS deviation that is helpful for all the members of the diagnostic team; particularly so for the physician who may be involved in prescribing and monitoring medication. It becomes for the physician the principal and personal contact with the pathology.

In our clinic, however, we do not perform the special neurological examination on every child. With a very experienced team of clinicians the case for learning disability and/or attentional deficit is fairly apparent. If trainees are present or if additional corroboration is needed, the examination is done. If the diagnosis is at all unclear, the examination may be helpful in resolving the uncertainty.

I must add that the coincidence of various soft signs and learning disability/attention deficit disorder is far from 100 percent; i.e., there are a good many children with attention deficit disorder and/or learning disabilities whose signs are either faint or outgrown (Peters et al, 1975) or simply absent. No one sign is pathognomonic, and some normal children have lesser degrees of the signs.

For a short practical examination I selected certain high yield items based upon both research and clinical experience (Peters et al, 1974; 1975).

More involved children such as autistic, pervasive developmental, schizophrenic, and mild cerebral palsy usually show more signs, and some of these show a greater degree of abnormality of certain signs than do MBD children.

Here is the battery of tests and descriptive explanations that I have used for over 20 years:

SPECIAL NEUROLOGICAL EXAMINATION FOR CHILDREN

1. *Head rotation (passive)* — The child is told, "Stand up, put feet together, and close your eyes. Now, put your arms straight out in front of you — spread your fingers a little — don't touch your thumbs together." Some immature children do not understand "out in front." If the child fails

to comprehend the instructions, he is reinstructed; if he fails again, examiner places the arms and hands in proper position. After observing for arm fatigue, the examiner asks child to lower his arms and relax. After allowing a momentary rest of arms, examiner says, "This time I'm going to put my hands on your head and turn it; don't help, let me do it, and keep your arms straight out in front." He was then asked to place arms out in front again and to close eyes. Examiner then slowly rotated the child's head 90 degrees in the horizontal plane in one direction, held the position a few seconds, and then rotated the head 180 degrees in opposite direction. The rotation was repeated several times. *Very light* finger pressure was used to turn the head unless child resisted.

Examiner looks for signs of motor stance fatigue — "drooping" of one or both arms, arm divergence or overlap, flexion of elbows, and irregular or "spooning" positions of wrists, hands and fingers. With passive rotation of the head, the examiner looked for exaggeration of these same signs, and for exaggerated "corrective movements" of hands; but in addition he looked for the "whirling" phenomenon (Bender, 1956),a tendency for body to follow head as it is gently turned by examiner. Examiner scored degree of torso twisting with the feet stationary. If the entire body, including the feet, turned as the head rotated, the subject received a score of 4+. We have observed that by age 6-7 there is usually good separation of head movements from the body as a stationary base, as "background," so to speak. Torso or body turning is an associative movement.

Many MBD's show choreoathetoid movements of fingers, hands, arms, neck, and torso. One can sense these little jerks in neck and torso through the hands as the child's head is turned.

2. *Imitate finger movement* — This item obtains an estimate of the child's ability to observe and copy movements of particular fingers. Child sits facing examiner and is asked to copy finger movements that examiner makes with the fingers of either his right or left hand. Examiner extends both arms with fingers a little up and palms toward the child, saying, "Do exactly as I do." Child then imitates finger-thumb touching as done slowly by examiner, e.g., if examiner touched left thumb to left index finger, then child executed the same maneuver with thumb and index finger of his right hand. Child duplicates the examiner's movements as the latter switches about from hand to hand. In the event a child copies left to left, he was asked to copy on the same side as examiner. This is a complex item dealing with power of discriminative observation and motor coordination. It yields additional information on finger agnosia in that some children need to glance at their fingers in order to decide which one to move; this is espe-

cially so with the ring and middle fingers.

Many MBD's show moderate to severe fatigue of the extended arms. The nonhyperactive dyslexic child usually does not show this sign. Atypical children with multiple developmental deviations may show a severe degree of it. In MR's and autistic children the concept of a requested stance may be lacking; in many MBD's there is actual tonic muscle fatigue.

3. *Hop on one foot* — Child is asked to hop across the room on one foot and then back on the other foot. (This is a place to begin observing for knowledge of right and left, but no comment is made to child). Note quality of execution.

4. *Skip* — Child is asked to skip across the room and back. The examiner looks for poor sequencing; also, excessive arm flinging (associated movement). At age 7 the average child, female or male, can skip.

5. *Fingers-thumb* — Examiner sits close to and facing the child with hands on knees, palms up. He says, "watch me first; look, I touch my thumb to each finger, one, two, three, four, slowly, one, two, three, four; now you do it. Now a little faster. Now the other hand." Examiner looks for inability to curl fingers, missed contacts, poor sequence, slowness, stickiness of release, reckless speed with inaccuracy, and associative movements.

6. *Alternating movements of hands* — Examiner places his hands on his knees, palms down, and demonstrates *very slowly* slapping the knees alternately with palms and backs of hands. Child asked to do same, first with both hands, then with each hand separately; at first he is told to "go slow" and then "faster" and then "very fast;" scored for disorganization, and slow sticky turns, either hand or both. If child uses edge of hand as a pivot, he is asked to lift hands off leg between each turn. Observe also for excessive vigor of slaps on knees — often seen in hyperactives.

7. *Thumb and Index finger tapping* — Child is shown how to tap his curled index finger at the distal joint of the thumb and told, "Do it as fast as you can." Younger children are naturally slower. Look for slow, clumsy execution. Associated movements of thumb, wrist, arm, jaw, or foot are noted under item 8. Speed of foot-tapping may be tested — MBD's often can't establish a rhythm; often one foot is slower than the other.

8. *Associated movements, items 2 thru 7* — Symmetrical associated movements in items 2, 5, and 6 are more pronounced in younger and less pronounced in older children. They have usually disappeared in normal children by age 10. In MBD-LD children this "soft" sign is often prominent and still present at age 10-14. The greater mirroring is from the dominant hand to the nondominant.

Nonsymmetrical associated movements may appear in the upper extremities in items 3 and 4. In item 7, in order of severity of the spill-over of excitation, the thumb, other fingers, arm, jaw, and foot may move in rhythm with the index finger. A firm open-mouthed setting of the jaw suggests a resisting of this extraneous movement.

9. *Right-left confusion*

a. Examiner and child sit facing each other and examiner says, "Put your right hand on your left ear; put your left hand on your right knee; put your left on your left ear," etc. Degree of hesitancy and inaccuracy determine the score: 1+ for slight hesitation; 2+ for initially wrong then corrects, or for a long hesitation; 4+ for reversal or random accuracy. If results are unclear examiner returns to this item later, being careful to give the child no further clues as the correctness of right-left.

b. Child was asked to point to the examiner's left hand, right foot, right hand, left ear, etc. Because of chance "correct" response, this may need to be repeated at end of the examination.

c. Examiner asks child to stand with feet together and says slowly, with appropriate pauses, "Turn to the right, turn to the left, turn to the left again, turn to the right, and turn to the right again," etc. This item was scored for confusion concerning left-right.

d. (Peters' sign) Some children return to starting position in item c before turning again, but others may smile or shrug their shoulders, implying "That's silly; I have already turned right." Still others stand silent and do nothing. This response is often shown by children 8 years old and younger. The normal response appears between ages 8 and 9. It is often found in MBD's beyond this age.

10. *Eye-tracking (quality of, and associated head movements)*

a. This item tests the ability of the child to hold his head fixed while examiner checks extra-ocular movements. Examiner says, "follow my finger with your eyes, but keep your head still." If the child's head turns as his eyes tracked the finger, examiner says, "Keep your head still and move just your eyes." If the child persists in head following, his head is held by examiner. This is another example of differentiation of movements. In most children age 5, eyes and head are more bound. Some MBD clinic cases show this at age 6, 7, and 8. If the head moves after the initial instructions, the score is 1+ or 2+, depending on degree; if the head returned to following after the child was reminded to hold it still, the score was 3+; and if it was necessary for examiner to hold the child's head, the score was 4+.

b. The quality of tracking is scored according to whether the eyes follow only approximately, in jerks, preceed the finger, or grossly overshoot. Nystagmus can also be tested for at this time.

c. Distracted to examiner's face.

d. Esophoria or exophoria is noted.

11. *Speech dysfluences* — the child was asked to repeat sounds, words, and sentences; th, r, thr, z, pl, and l; "The thin man threw the ball," "Please run quickly," and "Three zebras boarded a plane. The child was also asked to say "la, la, la, la, la, as fast as you can." Slowness is noted. Stuttering during the examination observed and noted. Dysarthric speech (clumsy, thick, separated sounds) also noted.

12. *Writing to dictation* — the child is given unlined paper and pencil without an eraser and asked to write the following dictated sentences: (1) A boy had a dog. (2) The dog saw a bird. (3) My name is ___________. (4) Please come quickly. For children 10 years or older add: (5) The question was about the constitution, or (6) It was a question of constitutionality.

Examiner looked for letter reversals such as "d" and "b." One reversal was scored 2+ at age 8, 3+ at age 9, 4+ at age 10. Spelling score is estimated according to age and grade, and especially degree of departure from "logicalness" or "phoneticness."

The finished product is insufficient for judging; examiner must observe the *act of writing*. Look for labored or slow "drawing" of letters. Eraser is not permitted — if child is dissatisfied, he can write it again below. Thus a permanent record of his efforts is obtained. Rate the writing re escalation in size, which is often seen in hyperactives. Look for hesitation and false starts in direction of starting letters.

SPECIAL NEUROLOGICAL EXAMINATION FOR CHILDREN

Name:_______________ Age:____ Grade:_____ School:__________

	Mild	Moderate	Severe
1. Head rotation (passive; knows "arms in front"?)			
A. Arms drop or spread__________	+	++/+++	++++
B. Irregular position, wrist, hand, or fingers	+	++/+++	++++
C. Whirling of torso or body	+	++/+++	++++
D. Choreoathetoid movements	+	++/+++	++++
2. Imitate finger movement:			
A. Slow, sticky, or clumsy	+	++/+++	++++
B. Wrong copying; has to glance at fingers	+	++/+++	++++
C. Fatigue of extended arms (in 1 and 2)___	+	++/+++	++++
3. Hop on one foot, then the other:__________	+	++/+++	++++
4. Skip (note both quality and sequencing):	+	++/+++	++++
5. Fingers–thumb: sequence; slow; clumsy; reckless	+	++/+++	++++
6. Alternating movements of hands: disorganized; too vigorous_______________	+	++/+++	++++
7. Thumb and index finger tapping:	+	++/+++	++++
8. Associated movements, items 2 thru 7:			
A. Symmetrical____________________	+	++/+++	++++
B. Nonsymmetrical__________________	+	++/+++	++++
9. Right–left confusion:			
A. Hand on opposite ear or knee (by age 7)_____	+	++/+++	++++
B. Point to examiner's knee, etc. (by age 8)_____	+	++/+++	++++
C. Stand, turn right, left, etc. (by age 8)_____	+	++/+++	++++
D. Returns to fixed base or immobile and puzzled (relative R&L by age 9)_____	+	++/+++	++++
10. Eye-tracking:			
A. Doesn't hold head fixed (assoc. movement)	+	++/+++	++++
B. Quality of tracking________________	+	++/+++	++++
C. Distracted to examiner's face__________	+	++/+++	++++
D. Esophoria or exophoria_____________	+	++/+++	++++
11. Speech dysfluences and tongue:__________	+	++/+++	++++
12. Written to dictation: A boy had a dog; a dog saw a bird; my name is __________; please come quickly; the question was about the constitution.			
A. Reversals____________________	+	++/+++	++++
B. Labored, slow, confused letter attack___	+	++/+++	++++
C. Spelling; departure from "phonetic logic"	+	++/+++	++++
D. Reckless speed—escalates size, poor spacing	+	++/+++	++++

13. Observations (circle appropriate words): Hyperactive, restless, hypoactive, distractable, overtalkative, impulsive, meddlesome, aggressive, absent-minded, bizarre, thought or behavior disorganized, slow of speech or movement.
14. Temperament; emotional state (circle appropriate words): Cold, shy, sullen, suspicious, hostile, fearful, gentle, quiet, respectful, friendly, forward, tense, anxious, acutely upset.

    Comments:

BIBLIOGRAPHY

Bender L: Psychopathology of Children with Organic Brain Disorder. Springfield, Ill: C.C. Thomas, 1956

Clements SD, & Peters JE: Minimal brain dysfunction in the school age child. Archives of General Psychiatry, 1962, 6, 185-197

Clements SD, & Peters JE: Minimal brain dysfunctions in children: Concepts and categories. World Medical Journal, 1972, 19, 54

Clements SD, & Peters JE: Syndromes of minimal brain dysfunction. In Black B (Ed.). Brain Dysfunction in Children. New York: Raven Press, 1981

Denhoff E: Emotional and psychological background of the neurologically handicapped child. Exceptional Child, 1961, 27, 347-349

Dykman RA, Ackerman PT, Clements SD, & Peters JE: Specific learning disabilities: An attentional deficit syndrome. In Myklebust HR (Ed.). Progress in Learning Disabilities, Vol. II. New York: Grune & Stratton, 1971

Eisenberg L: Psychiatric implications of brain damage in children. Psychiatric Quarterly, 1957, 31, 72

Gardner RA: Psychotherapy of minimal brain dysfunction. In Masserman J (Ed.). Current Psychiatric Therapies, Vol XIV. New York: Grune & Stratton, 1974

Gesell A, & Amatruda CS: Developmental Diagnosis. New York: Paul B. Hoebner, Inc., 1947

Kennard MA: Value of equivocal signs in neurological diagnosis. Neurology, 1960, 10, 753

Laufer MW, Denhoff E, & Solomons G: Hyperkinetic impulse disorder in childrens' behavior problems. Psychosomatic Medicine, 1957, 19, 38

Passamanick B, Rogers ME, & Lillienfield AM: Pregnancy experiences and the development of behavior disorders in children. American Journal of Psychiatry, 1956, 112, 613

Peters JE, Davis JR, Goolsby CM, et al: Physician's Handbook: Screening for MBD. Amsterdam: Ciba Foundation, 1973

Peters JE, Dykman RA, Ackerman PT, & Romine JS: The special neurological examination. In Conners CK (Ed.). Clinical Use of Stimulant Drugs in Children. Amsterdam: Excerpta Medica, 1974

Peters JE, Romine JS, & Dykman RA: A special neurological examination of children with learning disabilities. Developmental Medicine and Child Neurology, 1975, 17, 63

Silver AA: Psychological aspects of pediatrics, postural and righting responses in children. Journal of Pediatrics, 1952, 41, 493

Strauss AA, & Kephart NC: Psychopathology and Education of the Brain-Injured Child, Vol II. New York: Grune & Stratton, 1955

Strauss AA, & Lehtinen L: Psychopathology and Education of the Brain-Injured Child. New York: Grune & Stratton, 1947

Teicher JD: Preliminary survey of motility in children. Journal of Nervous and Mental Disease, 1941, 94, 277

Compiled by David E. Tupper

Appendix D

Composition of Other Published Soft Sign Examinations

1. *Examination for Soft Neurological Signs*
   Richard A. Gardner
2. *Neurological Dysfunctions of Children*
   James W. Kuhns
3. *Quick Neurological Screening Test (Revised edition)*
   Margaret Mutti, Harold M. Sterling, and Norma V. Spalding
4. *Examination of the Child with Minor Neurological Dysfunction (2nd edition)*
   Bert C.L. Touwen
5. *Extended Neurological Examination*
   Kytja Voeller

1. EXAMINATION FOR SOFT NEUROLOGICAL SIGNS

In his excellent book on the objective diagnosis of minimal brain dysfunction, Dr. Richard Gardner devotes a chapter to the assessment of soft neurological signs. He classifies them as two types: (1) the soft developmental type of soft neurological sign and (2) the soft neurological type of soft neurological sign. Gardner emphasizes strongly the use of objective, standardized, well-designed measurement instruments in the evaluation of soft neurological signs and he recommends a selective choice of test procedures to be added to the routine neurological examination. Thus, he does not have a soft sign battery per se, but does recommend a variety of useful test procedures to be used, which he describes well in his book and for which he includes normative data. His procedures are generally used for children ages 5 to 15 years.

Organization and Recommended Procedures:

A. The Soft Developmental Type of Soft Neurological Sign
 1. Primitive Reflexes — those that disappear with age
 — those that appear with age
 2. The Developmental Milestones
 3. Speech — articulation (the Articulation Screening test)
 4. Pencil Grasp — the simian grasp
 — intermediate grasp (with extended distal interphalangeal joints)
 — the pincer (tripod) grasp

B. The Soft Neurological Type of Soft Neurological Sign
 1. Tremors and Choreiform Movements
 2. Motor Impersistence
 Denckla's test of balancing on one foot
 Lincoln-Oseretsky Scale (test 32)
 Denver Developmental Screening Test (foot balancing)
 McCarron Asssessment of Neuromuscular Development (foot balancing)
 Southern California Perceptual-Motor Tests (standing balance)
 Garfield's Impersistence tests
 Gardner Steadiness Tester
 3. Motor Overflow
 Touwen and Prechtl Mouth-Opening Finger-Spreading Phenomenon
 Kinsbourne's Finger Stick Test
 Abercrombie, Lindon, and Tyson's Finger Movement Test
 Cohen et al. Tests of Motor Overflow

Source: Adapted from Gardner RA: The Objective Diagnosis of Minimal Brain Dysfunction (Chapter 6). Cresskill, NJ: Creative Therapeutics, 1979. With permission.

2. NEUROLOGICAL DYSFUNCTIONS OF CHILDREN (NDOC)

The NDOC is an 18-item screening evaluation for soft neurological signs that, unlike a strict neurological examination, is designed to be used by psychologists, physicians, school psychologists, nurses, or other professionals. Its goal is to assist the examiner in identifying neurologically based learning disorders in school age children so they may be referred for further neurological evaluation. The NDOC manual provides not only a complete description of the administration of each item but also a theoretical interpretation of each item and common clusters. Thus, it has much to offer the inexperienced clinician in the interpretation of soft signs in the individual case. The exam consists of 16 tasks that the child is asked to perform as well as 2 items covering measurement of head circumference and developmental history using a structured parental interview. Each item is scored either *yes* (impaired) or *no* (normal) and all items are considered in terms of developmental age. The age range covered for the NDOC is 3-10 years of age.

Items

1. Hand Kicking — left and right foot
2. Walking Along a Straight Line
3. Walking on Tiptoe
4. Walking on Heels
5. Standing on One Leg — preferred and nonpreferred leg
6. Hopping on One Foot — preferred and nonpreferred leg
7. Foot Stimulation Reflex — left and right foot
8. Posture with Arms Extended — left and right arm
9. Finger to Nose — left and right hand
10. Fingertip Touching — left and right hand and arm
11. Finger Opposition — left and right hand
12. Visual Positioning — left and right eye
13. Visual Fixation
14. Visual Pursuit
15. Involuntary Eye Movements
16. Tongue Movements
17. Head Circumference
18. Developmental History

Source: Adapted from Kuhns JW: Neurological Dysfunctions of Children. Monterey, CA: Publisher's Test Service, 1979. With permission.

3. QUICK NEUROLOGICAL SCREENING TEST (Revised edition)

The Quick Neurological Screening Test (QNST) is designed to be used by nonneurologists and functions, as does the NDOC, as a soft sign screening evaluation. It consists of 15 face valid items (listed below) testing hand skill, figure recognition and production, eye tracking, double simultaneous stimulation, repetitive hand movements, and other soft signs. Each item is given a numerical score but the most informative aspect of the test for the individual child is the qualitative information gained on each item. The QNST manual provides ranges of classification for the total test score of high, suspicious, and normal, and it suggests that suspicious and high scores represent the children at risk for learning disabilities (based on correlational research described in the manual). The manual also includes several interpretive and medical considerations for the items, and there is a section on educational implications of the results. It is appropriate for a wide age range of children from preschool through later school age.

Items

1. Hand Skill
2. Figure Recognition and Production
3. Palm Form Recognition
4. Eye Tracking
5. Sound Patterns
6. Finger to Nose
7. Thumb and Finger Circle
8. Double Simultaneous Stimulation of Hand and Cheek
9. Rapidly Reversing Repetitive Hand Movements
10. Arm and Leg Extension
11. Tandem Walk (10 feet)
12. Stand on One Leg
13. Skip
14. Left-Right Discrimination
15. Behavioral Irregularities

Source: Adapted from Mutti M, Sterling HM, & Spalding NV: QNST: Quick Neurological Screening Test (Revised edition). Novato, CA: Academic Therapy Publications, 1978. With permission.

4. EXAMINATION OF THE CHILD WITH MINOR NEUROLOGICAL DYSFUNCTION (2nd edition)

Dr. Touwen's minor neurological sign examination is more of a traditional neurological examination than some of the others presented. It is, however, a rather comprehensive, standardized examination including

(1) assessment of sitting, standing, walking, lying; (2) examination of the motor system and reflexes and the functioning of various parts of the body including the trunk and the head; and (3) specific tests for coordination, involuntary and associated movements, as well as a consideration of general data about the child. The exam is appropriate for children from ages 3 to 12 years. Each item in the examination is defined in terms of an optimal response, rather than a normal response. They are then scored numerically in relation to the optimal response (0 = absent response, 2 = weak response, 3 = strong optimal response). No data are reported regarding either reliability or validity of the examination, although Touwen describes the interpretation of various clusters of items (see also his chapter in this book) so that it is meant to be primarily a clinically useful examination. It does, however, require some experience to administer.

OUTLINE — PROFORMA

- Assessment of Sitting
  - Spontaneous motility
  - Involuntary movements
  - Posture
  - Reaction to push against shoulder
  - Following an object
- Examination of the Motor System
  - Muscle power
  - Resistance to passive movements
  - Range of movements
  - Kicking
- Examination of Reflexes
  - Tendon reflexes
  - Plantar response
  - Other reflexes
- Assessment of Standing
  - Posture
  - Spontaneous motility
  - Involuntary movements
  - Pronation of arms (20 seconds)
  - Supination of arms (20 seconds)
- Test for Involuntary Movements (20 seconds)

Tests for Co-ordination and Associated Movements
- Finger-nose test
- Fingertip-touching test
- Finger opposition test
- Follow-a-finger test
- Circle test
- Standing with eyes closed
- Reaction to push against shoulder

Assessment of Walking
- Posture
- Gait
- Placing of feet
- Walking along a straight line
- Other gross motor functions

Assessment of the Trunk (Standing)
- Inspection of the back and spine
- Skin reflexes

Assessment of Lying
- Prone
- Posture of legs and feet in prone position
- Posture of legs and feet in supine position
- Knee-heel test
- Sitting up without help of hands

Assessment of the Head
- Facial musculature
- Position of eyes
- Fixation
- Pursuit movements
- Convergence
- Nystagmus
- Optokinetic nystagmus
- Pupillary reactions
- Visual acuity
- Visual field
- Choreiform movements of the face
- Ears
- Tongue
- Pharyngeal arches
- Spontaneous motility

Funduscopy
General Data

Source: Adapted from Touwen BCL: Examination of the Child with Minor Neurological Dysfunction, Second edition (C.D.M. No. 71). London: Hienemann, 1979. With permission.

5. EXTENDED NEUROLOGICAL EXAMINATION

Much like Gardner's examination, Voeller's proposed Extended Neurological Examination is more of a flexible incorporation of neuropsychological assessment techniques into a standard neurological examination than a well-defined soft sign examination. Nevertheless, in a chapter from a book on MBD outlining his suggestions, Voeller provides an extensive list of follow-up procedures for the routine neurological examination, including measures of hand preference, fine motor functioning, language processing, body image, visuospatial processing, and others. The chosen tests are generally well-standardized and reliable and can be used to follow up more closely minor difficulties noted during the standard neurological exam. The age range for use of his suggested procedures is not noted but most likely they cover preschool through school age. Hence, Voeller also suggests careful, systematic following up of individual children with suspected neurological dysfunction.

Components

Physical Examination
Behavioral Responses
Standard Neurological Examination
  Level of consciousness
  Cranial nerves
  Gross motor
  Sensation
Extended Neurological Examination
  Hand preference
  Foot and eye preference
  Fine motor battery
    Purdue pegboard

- Use of pencil
- Body image
  - Human figure drawing
  - Right-left orientation
  - Finger naming
- Language processing
  - Fluency, articulation, grammar, running speech
  - Picture description
  - Color naming
- Graphomotor-constructional
  - Bender-Gestalt
  - Beery
- Visual-spatial processing
  - Raven's Progressive Matrices
  - Block design
  - Object assembly
- Receptive language
  - Illinois Test of Psycholinguistic Ability
  - Peabody Picture Vocabulary Test
  - Token test
  - Digit span
- Academic
  - Woodcock Reading Mastery Test
  - Wide Range Acheivement Test

Source: Adapted from Voeller K: A proposed extended behavioral, cognitive, and sensorimotor pediatric neurological examination. In Ochroch R (Ed.). The Diagnosis and Treatment of Minimal Brain Dysfunction in Children. New York: Human Sciences Press, 1981, pp 65-90. With permission.

Index